Understanding and Treating
Tardive Dyskinesia

FOUNDATIONS OF MODERN PSYCHIATRY
David J. Kupfer and Richard Jed Wyatt, Editors

UNDERSTANDING AND TREATING TARDIVE DYSKINESIA
Dilip V. Jeste and Richard Jed Wyatt

UNDERSTANDING AND TREATING
Tardive Dyskinesia

DILIP V. JESTE AND RICHARD JED WYATT

Foreword by Ross J. Baldessarini

THE GUILFORD PRESS
New York and London

This book was written by Dilip V. Jeste and Richard Jed Wyatt in their private capacity. The views expressed herein do not necessarily reflect those of the National Institute of Mental Health.

© 1982 The Guilford Press
A Division of Guilford Publications, Inc.
200 Park Avenue South, New York, N.Y. 10003

Printed in the United States of America

LIBRARY OF CONGRESS CATALOGING IN PUBLICATION DATA
Jeste, Dilip V.
  Understanding and treating tardive dyskinesia.

  (Foundations in modern psychiatry)
  Bibliography: p.
  Includes index.
    1. Tardive dyskinesia.   2. Psychotropic drugs—Side
effects.   I. Wyatt, Richard Jed.   II. Title.
III. Series.
[DNLM: 1. Dyskinesia, Drug-induced. WL 390 J58u]
RC394.T37J47   616.8′3   81-7059
ISBN 0-89862-175-5   AACR2

To my parents, my uncle, Sonali, and Shafali
—D.V.J.

Acknowledgments

We are grateful to Ross J. Baldessarini, MD, for reviewing this book thoroughly and carefully, for making many valuable suggestions, and for writing a foreword. We wish to thank Daniel Tarsy, MD, who also reviewed the manuscript in its entirety and made numerous useful suggestions. We also thank Steven Matthysse, PhD, Janice R. Stevens, MD, and Jacob Brody, MD, who reviewed certain chapters. Seymour Weingarten, Editor-in-Chief, and Judith Grauman, Managing Editor, of The Guilford Press, were very helpful, encouraging, and tolerant.

We wish to express our gratitude to the editors and publishers of the following journals for permitting us to reprint some portions of articles published therein: *American Journal of Psychiatry* (1981, *138*, 297–309), *Psychiatric Annals* (1980, *10,* 39–51), *Schizophrenia Bulletin* (1979, *5,* 251–293), and *Archives of General Psychiatry* (in press).

Last, but not least, we are indebted to our colleagues and our patients who actively participated in the research.

Foreword

Modern clinical psychopharmacology began in 1949–1952 with the introduction of lithium salts, reserpine, and chlorpromazine (Thorazine) into the treatment of severely disturbed patients. Chlorpromazine led to the development of other similar antipsychotic ("neuroleptic") agents. Many of these have proven to be effective and relatively safe antipsychotic medications useful in schizophrenia, paranoid disorders, mania, and some severe forms of depression, as well as other neuropsychiatric disorders. The study of these and other psychotropic agents gave rise to the new scientific discipline of psychopharmacology — all since the early 1950s. The antipsychotic psychopharmaceuticals rapidly diminish psychotic symptoms and behavior and have important preventive effects, both of a direct pharmacologic type and by reduction of untoward complications of prolonged illness or institutionalization. The use and evaluation of such drugs have been accompanied by revolutionary changes in the practice and theory of psychiatry.

These and other new forms of medical treatment of psychiatric patients as well as changing policies and social attitudes, strongly encouraged by the availability of effective new treatments, led to important changes in current patterns of clinical care of the severely psychiatrically ill. Notable changes include a much-reduced prevalence of psychiatric hospitalization, the phasing out of many public mental institutions, the early return of hospitalized patients to home and work, the development of open psychiatric units in general hospitals, and an increased reliance on local community and outpatient treatment facilities. Many patients with even severe psychiatric illnesses are treated effectively by physicians without specialized training in psychiatry, as well as by psychiatrists.

In addition, the use and study of such agents have helped to draw psychiatry even closer to the rest of medicine, have encouraged more critical differential diagnosis and rational therapeutics, and have gained support for biomedical approaches to psychiatry that complement psychosocial theories and therapies.

The available antipsychotic agents, while highly effective and reasonably safe, are not perfect drugs. Virtually all of those available in current American practice are "neuroleptic," or capable of inducing undesirable neurologic effects. Current research is aimed at trying to develop effective antipsychotic agents that are less neurotoxic. In the meantime, we must use the available agents as wisely as possible. With the increased application of neuroleptic agents to long-term management of patients with chronic or severe psychiatric disorders, late neurologic complications associated with such long-term treatment are becoming evident.

Although this monograph deals only with tardive dyskinesias, an important neurological problem associated with prolonged use of the neuroleptic agents, it is important to place the problem in an appropriate perspective. The use of neuroleptic drugs has had highly beneficial effects on patient care and they are generally as safe as many other drugs essential to the treatment of other serious illnesses. With careful clinical use, the risk of late dyskinesias can be minimized.

In this monograph on tardive dyskinesia, Drs. Jeste and Wyatt have taken on a large and complex task. They have carried out a masterful job of scholarship in compiling, analyzing, and synthesizing the clinical and preclinical scientific literature on this important and timely topic, which presents many clinical, scientific, industrial, and medicolegal challenges. Their highly unified and balanced work presents a consistent and reasoned point of view that complements and is an advance beyond other multi-authored monographs on the subject that have appeared recently (*Tardive Dyskinesia: Research and Treatment,* W. E. Fann, R. C. Smith, J. M. Davis, and E. F. Domino, Eds., Spectrum Publications, New York, 1980; and *Tardive Dyskinesia,* Task Force Report 18, Task Force on Tardive Dyskinesia, American Psychiatric Association, Washington, D.C., 1980). This monograph represents not only the most up-to-date, but also the most extensive and thorough, review of the subject now available.

Ross J. Baldessarini, MD

Preface

"Doctors give drugs of which they know little, to patients of whom they know even less," wrote Voltaire. Although there is obviously some truth in this statement when applied to psychopharmacology, continuing clinical and basic research is trying to reduce the areas of ignorance regarding psychotropic drugs as well as psychiatric disorders. As new discoveries seek to improve the management and understanding of illnesses, they also create problems of their own. The introduction of neuroleptics, which opened one of the two important eras (the other being that of psychological awareness through psychoanalytic theory) in the recent history of psychiatry, also brought with it the problem of tardive dyskinesia.

This book has been written with the aim of providing an overview of the rapidly expanding literature on tardive dyskinesia, not only for clinicians, but also for others who may have to deal with neuroleptics directly or indirectly. Our hope is that this book will stimulate further research on tardive dyskinesia. The history of psychopharmacology shows that a number of clinically undesirable side effects of drugs have proved to be "valuable" for improving insights into and management of psychiatric disorders. Thus the observation of sedation associated with the use of antihistamine drugs was one of the antecedents that eventually led to the discovery of antipsychotic phenothiazines. Cade, an Australian investigator, noticed lethargy in guinea pigs who had been injected with lithium salts and decided to try lithium in the treatment of mania. Reserpine-induced depression, along with other data, suggested a likelihood of monoamine depletion in endogenous depression, and offered a rationale for the use of monoamine oxidase inhibitors in that disorder.

Could tardive dyskinesia, too, in the long run prove to be a blessing in disguise?

Dilip V. Jeste, MD
Richard Jed Wyatt, MD

Contents

*Understanding and Treating
Tardive Dyskinesia*

CHAPTER I

Introduction

NEUROLEPTICS

The entry of neuroleptics into psychiatry in the early 1950s revolutionized the treatment of psychotic disorders, especially schizophrenia. Jean Delay and Pierre Deniker of Paris were the first to report successful use of chlorpromazine in the treatment of psychiatric patients (Delay & Deniker, 1952). Since then a large number of similar drugs have been added to the therapeutic armamentarium of clinicians to help in the battle against schizophrenia. These drugs were initially called "major tranquilizers." It soon became apparent, however, that these chemical agents did not produce merely tranquility or sedation, but also a relief of psychotic symptoms in large numbers of patients. They also induced neurologic reactions. Today these drugs are usually called "neuroleptics" or "antipsychotic drugs." Although neither term is totally satisfactory, we and many others prefer the label "neuroleptic" to "antipsychotic drugs." The term "psychosis" includes not only schizophrenia, but also other conditions such as affective disorders. (Although neuroleptics may relieve symptoms in patients with certain affective disorders, most clinicians treat such patients with other drugs instead of or in addition to neuroleptics.)

Neuroleptics have improved the overall management of schizophrenic patients to a greater extent than has any other psychiatric treatment. However, neuroleptics do not cure schizophrenia. They relieve or reduce acute psychotic manifestations and lower the chances of relapse in chronic schizophrenic patients. Neuroleptics are at least partially responsible for the dramatic decline in the number of public mental hospital inpatients since the late 1950s (Davis, 1980). Numerous studies have shown that

1

maintenance neuroleptic medication significantly reduces relapse rates in chronic schizophrenic patients when compared with placebo treatment. Lehmann (1975) contends that the most significant achievement of long-term neuroleptic therapy has been its impact on the high relapse rate in chronic schizophrenic patients in remission. Indeed, much of the medical profession believes that the community mental health movement would not have been possible without the benefit of neuroleptics (Crane, 1973a). As evidence of the widespread use of neuroleptics, Ayd (1970) estimated that about 250 million people had received neuroleptic treatment until 1970.

Neuroleptics have been useful from another perspective: They have led to a surge of investigations into the biochemistry of schizophrenia and other related disorders. The mechanism of action of neuroleptics is still not precisely understood, but it is generally thought that their anticatecholaminergic activity (chiefly by blockade of postsynaptic dopamine receptors) is primarily responsible for many of their actions. Indeed, the hypothesis of dopaminergic hyperactivity in schizophrenia is based partly on the assumption (which is supported by a number of experiments) that neuroleptics exert their antipsychotic effects by blocking dopamine receptors. Various aspects of neuroleptic actions are considered later in appropriate chapters.

Table 1-1 summarizes the relative clinical potencies (on a milligram basis) of different neuroleptics. The drugs are classified according to their chemical structures.

Like most potent drugs in medicine, neuroleptics also produce serious side effects in some patients. The one side effect that has caused most concern in recent years has been tardive dyskinesia. There are two main reasons for this concern: a progressively increasing prevalence and a tendency to become irreversible in some patients. Crane (1973a, 1973b) asserts that tardive dyskinesia is likely to be a major limiting factor in long-term prescription of neuroleptics. Tardive dyskinesia has raised some disconcerting ethical and legal dilemmas. A number of patients have sued clinicians and hospitals for a failure to prevent or reverse persistent dyskinesia. A debate is now going on over the need to obtain a written informed consent from patients before starting neuroleptic treatment.

In spite of the growing literature on tardive dyskinesia, controversies abound regarding its pathogenesis, pathophysiology, course, prognosis, and management. It would be useful to start by defining the term.

Table 1-1. Relative Potencies of Neuroleptics

Generic name	Brand name	Relative potency (mg)[a]
Phenothiazine derivatives		
Aliphatic		
Chlorpromazine	Thorazine	100
Triflupromazine	Vesprin	26
Piperidine		
Thioridazine	Mellaril	108
Mesoridazine	Serentil	45
Piperacetazine	Quide	19
Piperazine		
Trifluoperazine	Stelazine	3.7
Prochlorperazine	Compazine	14
Perphenazine	Trilafon	8.8
Acetophenazine	Tindal	22
Thiopropazate	Dartal	24
Butaperazine	Repoise	10
Fluphenazine	Prolixin, Permitil	1.2
Thioxanthene derivatives		
Aliphatic		
Chlorprothixene	Taractan	35
Piperazine		
Thiothixene	Navane	3.2
Butyrophenones		
Haloperidol	Haldol	2.4
Benzoquinolizines		
Tetrabenazine[b]		40
Diphenylbutylpiperidines		
Pimozide	Orap	1.2
Penfluperidol[b]		2 (weekly)
Indolic derivatives		
Molindone	Moban	6.8
Dibenzazepines		
Loxapine	Loxitane, Daxolin	9.2
Dibenzodiazepines		
Clozapine[b]		79
Rauwolfia alkaloids		
Reserpine	Serpasil, etc.	1.1

Note. Adapted from Wyatt (1976).

[a]Standard: chlorpromazine = 100 mg.

[b]Considered experimental in the United States.

DEFINITION OF TARDIVE DYSKINESIA

Tardive dyskinesia may be defined as a syndrome consisting of abnormal, stereotyped involuntary movements, usually of choreoathetoid type, principally affecting the mouth, face, limbs, and trunk, which occurs relatively late in the course of drug treatment and in the etiology of which the drug treatment is a necessary factor. Each clause in this definition is discussed below:

1. "Tardive dyskinesia is a syndrome": It is not a unitary illness with identical symptomatology, etiopathology, course, and prognosis. A "syndrome" (Greek, meaning a running together) refers to a conglomeration of signs and symptoms indicating an abnormal condition, which may have different subtypes. Several identifiable subtypes of tardive dyskinesia have been described (see Chapter 3).
2. "Consisting of abnormal, stereotyped involuntary movements": "Stereotypy" refers to a constant and apparently meaningless repetition of certain movements.
3. "Usually of choreoathetoid type": The definitions of chorea, athetosis, and other types of abnormal movements are given in Chapter 3.
4. "Principally affecting the mouth, face, limbs, and trunk": These are the common localizations of dyskinesia, although other areas, such as the pharynx, larynx, and respiratory and diaphragmatic muscles, may also be involved in unusual cases.
5. "Which occurs relatively late in the course of drug treatment": "Tardive" is a French word referring to late onset of the characteristic manifestations of this condition (*Taber's Dictionary,* 1973). Abnormal movements that occur within a few hours or days of instituting drug treatment have different courses, prognoses, and management approaches and should not be confused with late-occurring dyskinesias. Although the distinction between "early" and "late" occurrence is vague, a cutoff point of 3 months' drug treatment may be justified on clinical grounds (see Chapter 3).

We have specifically used the term "drug treatment" in the definition of tardive dyskinesia to indicate that certain drugs other than neuroleptics can also produce late dyskinesia. L-Dopa and amphetamine are the major examples of such nonneuroleptic drugs. It should be pointed out, however, that L-dopa induces dyskinesias primarily in patients with Parkinson's disease and that amphetamine-induced dyskinesias are not common enough to pose a serious problem. Hence, in this book, we have generally restricted the discussion of tardive dyskinesias to neuroleptic-induced tardive dyskinesias. For the purposes of a broad definition of tardive dyskinesia, however, the term "drug treatment" is preferred.

6. "In the etiology of which the drug treatment is a necessary factor": Dyskinesias can occur in the absence of any drug treatment—for example, as a result of ill-fitting dentures or Huntington's disease. By the same token, the presence of dyskinesias in a patient who has a history of drug treatment does not necessarily mean that his or her abnormal movements were produced by the drugs. It is useful to attempt to rule out nonpharmacologic causes of dyskinesia before attributing the patient's movement disorder to drugs. The differential diagnosis of tardive dyskinesia is discussed in Chapter 3.

It is worth stressing that permanence or irreversibility is not a necessary part of the definition of tardive dyskinesia. Neuroleptic-induced tardive dyskinesia is reversible in a little over one-third of the patients, and tardive dyskinesias caused by nonneuroleptic drugs are almost invariably reversible when the offending drugs are discontinued.

OTHER EXTRAPYRAMIDAL SIDE EFFECTS OF NEUROLEPTICS

Tardive dyskinesia is thought to be an extrapyramidal side effect of neuroleptics. There are three other extrapyramidal side effects, which differ from tardive dyskinesia in that they occur much earlier in the course of neuroleptic treatment and are, as a rule, reversible. These include acute dystonias, akathisia, and parkinsonism. Rabbit syndrome is a parkinsonism-like extrapyramidal reaction; it is also reversible. These other extrapyramidal side effects are discussed in Chapter 3.

"DISCOVERY" OF TARDIVE DYSKINESIA

Other extrapyramidal reactions of neuroleptics, such as acute dystonias, akathisia, and parkinsonism, were identified soon after the introduction of neuroleptics into clinical psychiatry. It took half a decade after the in-

itial use of chlorpromazine as a neuroleptic, however, before tardive dyskinesia was first described in the literature. Schönecker (1957) is usually given
the credit for first reporting neuroleptic-induced tardive dyskinesia. His
brief case descriptions suggest a diagnosis of reversible tardive dyskinesia
in three of his four patients. In a German article, the title of which may be
translated as "A Peculiar Syndrome in Oral Region as a Result of Administration of Megaphen," Schönecker reported on four patients with oral
dyskinesias induced by Megaphen (chlorpromazine). The first patient, an
18-year-old student, had acute oral dyskinesias along with dystonias, both
of which responded quickly to parenteral administration of anticholinergic
medication. In the other three patients, women with cerebral arteriosclerosis, lip smacking was seen after 2 to 8 weeks of Megaphen treatment and
did not improve with the antiparkinsonian drug Akineton (biperiden hydrochloride). The symptoms persisted for weeks or months until neuroleptic use was reduced or discontinued.

It was J. Sigwald and his associates (1959) in Paris who provided the
first detailed descriptions of the syndrome of tardive dyskinesia. The title
of their French article may be translated as "Four Cases of Faciobuccolin-
gual Masticatory Dyskinesia with a Prolonged Course, Secondary to
Treatment with Neuroleptics." With remarkable precision, the authors
divided neuroleptic-induced dyskinesias into three subtypes: (1) acute dyskinesias, which occur early in the course of treatment with piperazine
phenothiazines and which show rapid improvement; (2) subacute dyskinesias, which become manifest later in the course of neuroleptic use and
which are unrelated to the type of neuroleptic, disappearing within 1
or 2 weeks of stopping the drugs; and (3) chronic dyskinesias, which are
much less common but which pose a serious problem because of their tendency to continue for several weeks or longer after withdrawal of medication.

Sigwald, Bouttier, Raymondeaud, *et al.* (1959) then went on to describe four patients with chronic dyskinesia, which persisted for months
after neuroleptics were discontinued. All four patients were nonschizophrenic women between 54 and 69 years of age. The primary diagnoses included anxiety state, obsessive–compulsive neurosis, trigeminal neuralgia,
and herpatic neuralgia. The following case provides a vivid description of
tardive dyskinesia.

A 54-year-old woman had continuous facial pain despite bilateral alcohol injections into Gasserian ganglia. She had received alternating treatment with prochlorperazine and levomepromazine for 8 months when she

was noticed to have involuntary chewing movements and pharyngeal paresthesia. Stopping the neuroleptics resulted in an increase in the facial pain, necessitating reinstatement of the drugs. A few months later, she developed other abnormal involuntary movements, such as protrusion of the tongue, opening of the mouth, dyskinesia of the lips, and rocking movements of the trunk. Her speech also became unintelligible. The oral dyskinesia was temporarily reduced by swallowing or speaking and increased by voluntary movements of the hands. The patient could not be taken off neuroleptics for long periods because of aggravation of facial pain. The dyskinesia was still present 2 years after it first made its appearance.

Sigwald *et al.* (1959) described three other cases of tardive dyskinesia. The authors believed that, although neuroleptics induced the dyskinesias, the type and the dose of neuroleptics were not important in the etiology of tardive dyskinesias. After stating that the treatment of tardive dyskinesias was unsatisfactory, Sigwald *et al.* raised the question of whether these movements were permanent. The investigators believed that the dyskinesias would probably disappear slowly over a period of time.

Uhrbrand and Faurbye (1960) from Roskilde, Denmark, published the first epidemiologic survey of "Reversible and Irreversible Dyskinesias after Treatment with Perphenazine, Chlorpromazine, Reserpine and Electroconvulsive Therapy." The authors concluded that prolonged use of neuroleptics was likely to induce dyskinesias in some patients, especially the elderly and those with brain damage, and that these dyskinesias tended to be irreversible in certain cases.

Walter Kruse (1960) of Danver State Hospital, Hathorne, Mass., was probably the first American psychiatrist to report tardive dyskinesia. In an article entitled "Persistent Muscular Restlessness after Phenothiazine Treatment," Kruse described three patients with phenothiazine-induced abnormal involuntary movements that did not respond to antiparkinsonian medication and that were still present long after the neuroleptics were stopped. Legs were most affected in his cases, although involuntary movements of lips and tongue were also seen in one patient, and those of arms in another. All three patients were schizophrenic women in their 50s.

Since the mid-1960s there has been a progressive increase in case reports as well as epidemiologic studies of tardive dyskinesia. Crane (1968b, 1973b) computed the number of articles on tardive dyskinesia in the medical literature and found that it had risen from the 21 published before 1966 to 60 from 1966 through 1971. Despite this growing interest in the subject, there was little understanding of the pathophysiology of tardive dyskinesia during the 1960s. From a therapeutic viewpoint, the only principal treatments tried during this period included either administration or withdrawal of neuroleptics.

It was the increase in the reports of L-dopa-induced dyskinesias in patients with Parkinson's disease since the late 1960s that aroused speculation about the mechanisms underlying neuroleptic-induced tardive dyskinesias. The hypothesis of striatal postsynaptic dopamine receptor supersensitivity proved to be of heuristic value since it led to a number of animal studies on a possible model of tardive dyskinesia. Experiments with longterm administration of neuroleptics to monkeys during the 1970s provided the most valid available model of tardive dyskinesia.

Drugs that were found to be useful in the treatment of L-dopa-induced dyskinesias or Huntington's chorea received clinical trials in patients with tardive dyskinesia during the 1970s. Although most of these drugs were found to have only limited value in the management of tardive dyskinesia, such drug studies reduced the therapeutic nihilism that had earlier surrounded the notion of "irreversible" tardive dyskinesia.

The last few years have seen a number of well-conducted clinical, biochemical, neuropathological, and therapeutic studies in patients with tardive dyskinesia. Although the solution is not in sight, at least steps are now being taken to seek answers to a number of questions. An important step in this direction was the formation of the Task Force on Tardive Dyskinesia by the American Psychiatric Association (Baldessarini, Cole, Davis, *et al.*, 1980).

"ACCEPTANCE" OF TARDIVE DYSKINESIA

It has been almost a quarter of a century since Schönecker (1957) first described neuroleptic-induced tardive dyskinesia. Yet there is still some controversy about the existence of this syndrome.

The main contention of the critics of the concept of tardive dyskinesia is that a causal association between neuroleptics and this syndrome has not been satisfactorily demonstrated. Turek (1975), in an article entitled "Drug Induced Dyskinesia: Reality or Myth?," suggested that the dyskinesia may be related to the primary psychiatric disorder for which neuroleptics are prescribed rather than to the drugs themselves. Arguing along somewhat similar lines, Garber (1979) noted that dyskinesia-like disorders were described by Kraepelin long before neuroleptics were introduced.

The epidemiologic data (see Chapter 2) show rather convincingly that neuroleptic-induced tardive dyskinesia is indeed a real clinical entity and that its prevalence has been steadily increasing over the past two decades. It may therefore appear curious that there is still some doubt about its existence.

The principal reason for the controversy is the considerable time lag between the initiation of neuroleptic treatment and the appearance of dyskinesia. This makes it difficult to establish a cause-and-effect association between the drugs and the untoward reaction. Other characteristics of the syndrome, such as the tendency to become worse on neuroleptic withdrawal and to be suppressed on increasing the neuroleptic dosage, add to the problem. According to Paulson (1975), there may be another factor responsible for the delayed recognition of tardive dyskinesia—namely, a resistance to accept iatrogenic disorders. This may be particularly true when the drugs have proved to be the single most effective treatment for such a chronic disabling illness as schizophrenia.

From a broader perspective, neuroleptics are following the so-called "Law of the New Drug" (Figure 1-1). Soon after they were discovered, they were hailed as a panacea for numerous psychiatric disorders; they were thought to have few serious side effects. Now the pendulum could swing to the other extreme, leading to the impression that these drugs are toxic substances with limited clinical use. The truth lies somewhere between these two extremes. There is a need for a rational acceptance of two facts: Neuroleptics are very helpful when used properly, and tardive dyskinesia is a genuine problem with long-term neuroleptic treatment.

Figure 1-1. Law of the new drug.

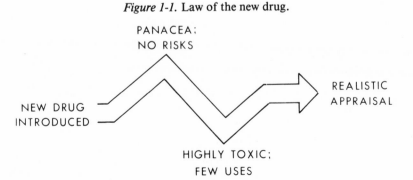

CHAPTER II

Epidemiology

SOME CONCEPTS IN EPIDEMIOLOGY

The *Living Webster Encyclopedic Dictionary* (1975, p. 330) defines "epidemiology" as "the science concerned with the study and control of epidemic diseases." It goes on to define an "epidemic" (Greek *epi* upon + *demos* people) as a widely prevalent condition "common to or affecting a whole people, or a great number in a community at the same time," such as a contagious disease. In psychiatry, epidemiology refers to the study of the occurrence of psychiatric disorders within a specified population, often expressed in terms of incidence and prevalence (Hinsie & Campbell, 1974, p. 270).

EPIDEMIOLOGIC TERMS

To maintain some uniformity in reporting epidemiologic data, the results of epidemiologic surveys should, whenever possible, be mentioned in terms of incidence and prevalence. Incidence is the number of new cases that appear during a specified period in a unit population, whereas prevalence is the number of all cases (new and old) of a disease that exist currently within a unit population. Prevalence may be expressed in three ways: (1) "Point prevalence" refers to the number of cases that exist at a specific time, for example, on July 1, 1980; (2) "period prevalence" is the number of cases that exist within a defined period of time, for example, from January 1 through December 31, 1980; and (3) "lifetime prevalence" refers to the number of people who may have a disease anytime during their lifetimes (Hinsie & Campbell, 1974, p. 270). Incidence and prevalence are usually expressed in percentages or as ratios (per 1000 or 100,000 population).

METHODS FOR COLLECTING EPIDEMIOLOGIC DATA

Epidemiologic data on conditions such as tardive dyskinesia can be collected by direct and indirect methods, the former being more desirable, but also more difficult (Morris, 1975). Direct methods include:

1. Prospective longitudinal studies of patients and controls.
2. Quasi-longitudinal studies, which are really cross-sectional studies on populations from different age groups, for example, 31 to 50 years and 51 to 70 years. Here it is assumed that, when the younger group gets older, it will have the same characteristics that the older group now has.
3. Cross-sectional studies of point prevalence.

Indirect methods for accumulating epidemiologic data include:

1. Retrospective studies, such as reviewing patient charts.
2. Questionnaires that are sent to clinicians to get an impression of the approximate prevalence of a condition.
3. Review of the literature. The number of articles on a particular disease and the number and types of cases reported in those articles may give clues to historical trends, syndrome identification, possible causes, and so forth.

PROBLEMS IN EPIDEMIOLOGIC STUDIES
OF TARDIVE DYSKINESIA

GENERAL PROBLEMS IN PSYCHIATRIC EPIDEMIOLOGY

Psychiatric epidemiologic studies should, but often do not, satisfy three basic requirements. The first requirement is development of an acceptable and clinically useful definition of the syndrome to be studied. Second, there is a need for specifying rather objective criteria for diagnosis. Third, some measure of quantitative assessment of the severity of the condition is usually warranted. Since it is difficult to exclude subjective bias totally in psychiatric evaluation, having two or more examiners and assessing the subject on several different occasions is recommended. Unfortunately, the number of studies on the epidemiology of tardive dyskinesia that satisfy these criteria is quite small.

PROBLEMS IN EPIDEMIOLOGIC STUDIES OF DRUG-INDUCED ILLNESS

Jick (1977) has outlined problems and research needs for studying drug-induced illnesses. He considers the magnitude of two risks—the added risk of illness experienced by the users of a drug and the baseline risk in the absence of that drug use. Somewhat arbitrarily, Jick defines each risk as being "high" if the rate of newly occurring illness exceeds 1 per 200 persons (at risk) per year, as "low" if the rate is less than 1 per 10,000 persons (at risk) per year, and as "intermediate" if the rate falls anywhere in between. Identification of a drug-induced syndrome may be considerably delayed if the time necessary to induce the illness is long. It is apparent that epidemiologic studies of drug-induced tardive dyskinesias should be complemented by similar work on spontaneously occurring dyskinesias in order to define the risk of drug-induced illness as well as the baseline risk of developing dyskinesias. Only then can we have some notion about the relative risk and the attributable risk of drug-induced tardive dyskinesia. "Relative risk" may be defined as the ratio of the incidence of the disorder in those exposed to the drugs to the incidence in those not exposed (*A Psychiatric Glossary,* 1980, p. 81). "Attributable risk" is the incidence of the disorder in exposed individuals that can be attributed to the exposure. It is derived by subtracting the incidence of the disorder in the nonexposed population from that in the exposed population (*A Psychiatric Glossary,* 1980, p. 76).

SPECIFIC PROBLEMS IN EPIDEMIOLOGIC STUDIES OF TARDIVE DYSKINESIA

Neuroleptic-induced tardive dyskinesia has not yet been universally accepted as a distinct syndrome. Following are a number of reasons for the controversy surrounding the causal relationship of neuroleptics to tardive dyskinesia:

1. Dyskinesia occurs spontaneously in a certain proportion of patients who have never received neuroleptics. Thus neuroleptics are not a necessary cause for the production of dyskinesia.
2. Only a minority of patients treated with neuroleptics develop tardive dyskinesia. Neuroleptics are therefore not a sufficient cause for inducing dyskinesia. Predisposing constitutional factors also seem to play a role in the etiology of tardive dyskinesia.
3. Tardive dyskinesia, as the name indicates, develops late in the course of neuroleptic therapy, usually after years of treatment. Hence a temporal cause-and-effect relationship is difficult to prove.
4. In a variable percentage of patients, the dyskinesia does not disappear on discontinuing the presumably responsible neuroleptics. It may persist for years and may even be irreversible in some cases.
5. Paradoxically, the dyskinesia may first appear on reducing the dose of a neuroleptic or on stopping the medication. To complicate the matter further, neuroleptics are probably the most effective suppressing agents for dyskinetic symptoms (Chapter 10).

It is therefore necessary to specify criteria for judging evidence to be used in establishing neuroleptic-induced tardive dyskinesia as a real entity. Similar criteria might also be useful for other late-onset side effects, such as the controversial lithium-induced nephrotoxicity.

CRITERIA FOR ESTABLISHING TARDIVE DYSKINESIA AS A DISTINCT SYNDROME

Criteria are presented here for both direct and indirect evidence.

CRITERIA FOR DIRECT EVIDENCE

Prospective, controlled, long-term, double-blind studies of groups of patients matched at baseline should show that the incidence of dyskinesia is significantly greater among the drug-treated patients than among non-drug-treated, matched patients. Such studies would, however, be not only impractical, but also unethical, in part because they would deliberately seek to induce a neurological disorder in some patients; on the other hand, they would deny neuroleptics to other patients who would otherwise be treated with those drugs. We therefore need to consider criteria for indirect evidence to be used in establishing tardive dyskinesia as a syndrome.

CRITERIA FOR INDIRECT EVIDENCE

Possible criteria for indirect evidence are:

1. Prevalence of dyskinesia should be significantly higher in neuroleptic-treated patients than in non-neuroleptic-treated patients matched for age, sex, race, and primary diagnosis.
2. A significantly greater proportion of patients given long-term neuroleptic therapy should have dyskinesia than patients who have had short-term neuroleptic therapy.
3. Prospective studies of neuroleptic-treated patients should show an increasing prevalence of tardive dyskinesia with increasing length of treatment.
4. Factors related to neuroleptic therapy should be important primary discriminating variables in multifactorial analyses comparing dyskinetic patients with nondyskinetic patients.
5. Tardive dyskinesia should be shown to occur in patients from diverse diagnostic categories and from different parts of the world, who have shared the common factor of neuroleptic treatment.
6. Biochemical, neuropathological, or other presumably relevant differences should be sought between patients with persistent tardive dyskinesia and those without dyskinesia so as to suggest possible neural mechanisms underlying persistent tardive dyskinesia.
7. A tardive-dyskinesia-like syndrome should be induced with prolonged neuroleptic administration in animals.

It is apparent that none of these seven criteria alone is sufficient to establish the entity of tardive dyskinesia. Taken together, however, they provide strong indirect evidence for the existence of the syndrome. Experimentally testable hypotheses to explain the paradoxical aspects of tardive dyskinesia (e.g., the appearance or the worsening of the symptoms on withdrawal of neuroleptics, or suppression of the dyskinesia by increasing neuroleptic dosage) will be of further help. It is probable that, with rapid advances in neurochemistry and neuropathology, the task of understanding the relationship between neuroleptics and tardive dyskinesia may become somewhat easier in the years to come. Work on animal models may also establish a more direct cause-and-effect relationship between neuroleptics and tardive dyskinesia than is possible in clinical studies.

Evidence for the seven criteria will be considered later in this chapter, as well as in Chapters 4, 5, 6, and 10. Although there is a need for more research, the available evidence strongly suggests that tardive dyskinesia *is* a distinct, recognizable syndrome which is attributable to long-term neuroleptic treatment.

IS TARDIVE DYSKINESIA MORE COMMON THAN SPONTANEOUS DYSKINESIA?

One criticism of the concept of tardive dyskinesia is that dyskinesia frequently occurs spontaneously among chronic psychiatric patients, especially the elderly—the group that is also most prone to develop tardive dyskinesia. It has also been asserted that similar movement disorders were described in mental hospital patients long before neuroleptics were introduced into psychiatry (Garber, 1979). We should therefore look at studies conducted both before and after neuroleptic use.

PRENEUROLEPTIC STUDIES

There were few formal studies of abnormal involuntary movements of dyskinetic or choreoathetoid type prior to 1955. In his classical book, *Dementia Praecox and Paraphrenia,* Kraepelin (1919/1971) referred to a number of bodily symptoms of schizophrenia. In the subcategory "spasmodic phenomena," Kraepelin (p. 83) describes movements of the musculature of the face and of speech as follows: "Some of them resemble movements of expression, wrinkling of the forehead, distortion of the corners of the mouth, irregular movements of the tongue and lips, twisting of the eyes, opening them wide and shutting them tight, in short, those movements which we bring together under the name of making faces or *grimacing,* they remind one of the corresponding disorders of choreic patients. Nystagmus may also belong to his group" (italics in original). He goes on to include smacking and clicking with the tongue, sudden sighing, sniffing, laughing, clearing the throat, fine twitchings of lips, tremor of outstretched fingers, and sprawling, irregular movements called "athetoid ataxia." He completes the list of spasmodic phenomena with tremor of the muscles of the mouth, which "may completely resemble that of paralytics," and twitchings of the muscles of the mouth on tapping lower branches of the facial nerves. Later in the book, under the caption "Prognostic Indicators," Kraepelin (pp. 206–207) states that the appearance of abnormal involuntary movements is a sign of poor prognosis, indicating loss of volitional control, and may herald the onset of "incurable terminal states."

It is instructive to note the differences between Kraepelin's description given here and the characteristics of tardive dyskinesia. Kraepelin labeled the disorders as "spasmodic phenomena," a term that would be closer to dystonias (disturbances of muscle tone) rather than dyskinesias (disturbances of movement), although such a distinction is not always made. Some of the movements described by Kraepelin—for example, smacking of the lips, choreoathetoid movements of extremities—resemble those of tardive dyskinesia, whereas others, such as nystagmus, laughing, or tremors of outstretched hands, are not a part of the tardive dyskinesia syndrome. Had the rather characteristic symptom complex of tardive dyskinesia been as prevalent among mental hospital patients in Kraepelin's day as it is today, an astute phenomenologist like Kraepelin would have given more specific descriptions of this syndrome. (Kraepelin has given longer descriptions of "seizures" than of "spasmodic phenomena" as symptoms of schizophrenia.) Furthermore, the abnormal involuntary movements in Kraepelin's patients occurred in poor-prognosis, late-stage schizophrenics. There is no evidence that tardive dyskinesia patients have schizophrenia with a worse prognosis than nondyskinetic patients chronically treated with neuroleptics. Indeed, tardive dyskinesia has also been reported in schizophrenic outpatients and in patients with neurotic and affective disorders who have received neuroleptics (see Chapter 4).

Mettler and Crandell (1959) conducted a study of neurologic disorders at a state hospital in 1955—before neuroleptics had been introduced into general use there. They found that only about .5% of the total hospital population had chorea or athetosis.

The main issue here is not whether dyskinesia existed in the preneuroleptic period, but whether a tardive-dyskinesia-like syndrome was as prevalent then as it is today. There are probably few clinical entities that man-made drugs can produce and that Nature cannot. Usually the drugs produce syndromes similar to the naturally occurring ones, although the frequency may be different. The available evidence suggests that a tardive-dyskinesia-like syndrome was uncommon in the preneuroleptic years.

POSTNEUROLEPTIC STUDIES

We found 12 studies[1] comparing the prevalence of dyskinesia among neuroleptic-treated and non-neuroleptic-treated patients. These are summarized in Table 2-1.

Of these 12 studies, 10 found a significantly higher prevalence of dyskinesia among neuroleptic-treated than among non-neuroleptic-treated patients. Although they might not have used identical criteria for the diagnosis of dyskinesia, they all looked for abnormal involuntary movements in the orofacial region, with or without choreiform movements of extremities. All the studies were done on chronic patients in psychiatric hospitals or nursing homes. Some investigators (Greenblatt, Stotsky, & DiMascio, 1968; Jeste, Potkin, Sinha, *et al.,* 1979; Siede & Muller, 1967) included only patients over 50, whereas others studied patients from different age groups. In most studies the neuroleptic-treated patients had received neuroleptics for at least several months. Jones and Hunter (1969) found a significantly higher prevalence of abnormal oral movements in the neuroleptic-treated group, although other types of movement disorders, such as tics and tremors, were also present in the non-drug-treated patients.

The two studies that did not find a significant difference in prevalence of dyskinesia between drug-treated and non-drug-treated patients—those of Demars (1966) and Brandon, McClelland, and Protheroe (1971)—suffer from some methodological shortcomings. Thus Demars's neuroleptic-treated patients were somewhat younger (mean age 53.4 years for men and 62.8 years for women) than his non-drug-treated patients (mean age 66.5 years for men and 70 years for women). The study by Brandon *et al.* (1971) has been criticized by Crane (1973b) for failure to mention severity of dyskinesia in the spontaneous dyskinesia group. A majority of patients in that group (75% of women and 50% of men) had clinical signs of dementia. The primary diagnoses in the organic mental syndrome group included Huntington's chorea, general paresis, epilepsy, and so forth. An accurate diagnosis of spontaneous dyskinesia among such patients is obviously subject to some error, especially in questionable or mild cases of dyskinesia.

---

[1]We excluded from this list a study by Faurbye, Rasch, Petersen, *et al.* (1964) since their definition of spontaneous dyskinesia seemed to us to be inaccurate. They defined "spontaneous dyskinesia" as dyskinesia in patients who had not received neuroleptics during the 1 month prior to the onset of the dyskinesia. This description is likely to include cases of persistent tardive dyskinesia whose symptoms continued for months after neuroleptics were withdrawn.

Table 2-1. Prevalence of Dyskinesia among Neuroleptic-Treated and Non-Neuro-leptic-Treated Psychiatric Inpatients

Investigators	Patients treated with neuroleptics		Patients not treated with neuroleptics		Comments
	n	Percentage with dyskinesia	*n*	Percentage with dyskinesia	
Demars (1966)	371	7	117	6.8	Non-neuroleptic-treated group about 10 years older
Degkwitz and Wenzel (1967)	766	17	525	1.3	
Siede and Muller (1967)	404	11.4	160	1.3	Elderly patients
Crane (1968a)	40	7.5	97	0	Men under 50 years in a Turkish hospital
Heinrich, Wage-ner, and Bender (1968)	554	17	201	3	
Greenblatt, Stotsky, and DiMascio (1968)	52	38.5	101	2	Elderly patients
Jones and Hunter (1969)	82	30.5	45	6.7	Patients over 40 years with abnormal mouth movements
Hippius and Lange (1970)	531	34.3	137	13.9	
Brandon, Mc-Clelland, and Protheroe (1971)	625	25.4	285	19.6	Criticized by Crane (1973b)
Crane (1973b)	926	17.1	46	2.2	
Jeste, Potkin, Sinha, *et al.* (1979)	88	23.9	198	4.5	Patients over 50 years
Bourgeois, Bouilh, Tignol, *et al.* (1980)	59	42.4	211	18	Elderly patients

When all 12 studies are taken together, the overall prevalence of dys-kinesia is 3.25 times greater in neuroleptic-treated than in non-drug-treated patients. It is necessary to add that dyskinesia among patients who had never received neuroleptics may have been due to various causes, such as ill-fitting dentures, senile chorea, or encephalitis. According to some neu-rologists, such as Baker (1969) and Altrocchi (1972), spontaneous orofacial dyskinesia not secondary to a known neurological disease is rare. Kline, who initially (1968b) questioned the existence of neuroleptic-induced persistent tardive dyskinesia, later concluded (Simpson & Kline, 1976) that it was common enough to make it "a matter of extreme importance."

There are two separate reports (not included in Table 2-1) of low prevalence of spontaneous dyskinesia among residents of homes for the elderly. Heinrich, Wagener, and Bender (1968) found dyskinesia in only 2 of the 110 such persons. Degkwitz's (1969) figures were 6 out of 750 men and 6 of 750 women (.8% each) who were not demented.[2]

Two other studies of abnormal involuntary movements in psychiatric patients are worth mentioning. Dincmen (1966) observed choreoathetoid movements in 3.4% of 1700 chronic patients from back wards of two state hospitals. He proposed the identification of a new syndrome called "chronic psychotic choreo-athetosis." Dincmen, however, did not mention whether his patients were receiving neuroleptics. It is possible that at least some of the patients showing those movements had tardive dyskinesia. Yarden and Discipio (1971) compared 18 newly admitted young schizophrenics who had choreiform or athetoid movements with 36 schizophrenic controls without such movements. A longitudinal study confirmed Kraepelin's finding—namely, patients with abnormal movements had poor prognosis, despite intensive treatment, in contrast to patients without choreoathetoid movements. This study thus lends further support to a distinction between drug-induced and non-drug-induced abnormal movements in schizophrenic patients. (As noted in Chapter 4, there is no evidence to suggest that the therapeutic response of tardive dyskinesia patients to neuroleptics is different from that of nondyskinetic patients.)

The evidence considered thus far permits one to conclude that the symptom complex that constitutes tardive dyskinesia is significantly more common in neuroleptic-treated patients than in comparable populations not treated with neuroleptics. It is, of course, possible to argue that neuroleptic-treated and untreated groups were not exactly comparable; otherwise, they would not have received different treatments. This argument may be valid, but can be countered by the fact that the tardive-dyskinesia-

---

[2]Another study (Delwaide & Desseilles, 1977) reporting a rather high prevalence of spontaneous dyskinesia among the elderly has one serious drawback: The authors merely mention that no neuroleptics were given at the time of the study; they give no information about past neuroleptic treatment in their subjects, 76% of whom were inpatients of a psychogeriatric unit.

like syndrome was uncommon in preneuroleptic years. Hence the higher prevalence of dyskinesia in the neuroleptic-treated patients is unlikely to be due to their primary psychiatric illness.

REVIEW OF EPIDEMIOLOGIC STUDIES
OF TARDIVE DYSKINESIA

Following reports by Schönecker (1957) and Sigwald *et al.* (1959), a large number of cases of tardive dyskinesia were reported in the 1960s. Until 1965, only three epidemiologic surveys appeared in the literature—namely, those by Uhrbrand and Faurbye (1960), Faurbye *et al.* (1964), and Hunter, Earl, and Thornicroff (1964). Since 1965, the number of such studies has increased considerably. Most of them have been cross-sectional studies of point prevalence—that is, the number of cases that existed at the specific time of the survey. A few investigators (Crane, 1968b, 1970; Jeste, Potkin, Sinha, *et al.,* 1979) have studied period prevalence—that is, the number of cases that existed during a period of time, such as a year. There are no large-scale longitudinal prospective studies of incidence or of lifetime prevalence of tardive dyskinesia.

Indirect methods of collecting epidemiologic data are less satisfactory than direct ones. Gibson (1979) sent questionnaires to other physicians to find out about their clinical experiences with patients with severe tardive dyskinesia. A low rate of return of such questionnaires results in a biased sample; also, the replies are often based on subjective impressions that may be colored by a few dramatic experiences. If interpreted cautiously, the questionnaire data may yield some useful clues. Crane (1968b, 1973b), who found a dramatic increase in the number of articles on tardive dyskinesia during the 1960s, suggested that tardive dyskinesia was becoming an increasingly common iatrogenic disorder.

SUGGESTIONS FOR FUTURE STUDIES

As the mean prevalence of both tardive dyskinesia and spontaneous dyskinesia is more than 1 in 200 persons (at risk), both the risk of drug-induced dyskinesia as well as the baseline risk may be considered high according to Jick's criteria (1977). In this situation a combination of long-term clinical trials and nonexperimental cohort studies is likely to be most helpful.

Good epidemiologic studies on tardive dyskinesia should have the following characteristics: (1) large, unselected or randomly selected patient populations; (2) diagnosis of tardive dyskinesia made by two or more clinicians and based on repeated examinations using standardized criteria; (3) assessment of severity of dyskinesia in a similar manner; (4) collection of all pertinent and reliable data; and (5) long-term follow-up of all patients. Studies using such a methodology would be helpful in comparing prevalence of dyskinesia among different treatment centers and also in judging annual incidence of this disorder.

PREVALENCE AMONG CHRONIC
PSYCHIATRIC INPATIENTS

There are many reports on prevalence of tardive dyskinesia among hospitalized, chronically ill psychiatric patients. These studies differ considerably in their methodology. To get a reasonably reliable estimate of prevalence of tardive dyskinesia, we selected those studies that met the following minimum requirements: (1) publication in recognized scientific journals or books in the English or German language; (2) some description of the original patient population that was screened for tardive dyskinesia; (3) study involving at least 50 patients in the total population; and (4) an apparently valid diagnosis of tardive dyskinesia based on clinical examination done by the investigators.

We found 37 studies that met these requirements (Table 2-2).[3] Whenever possible, we sought to reanalyze the data on prevalence of tardive dys-

---

[3]We excluded the following studies for specified reasons: (1) Hoff and Hofmann (1967) and Ettinger and Curran (1970) obtained figures for prevalence of tardive dyskinesia in the respective hospitals from the data provided by members of the staff in charge of various wards. This method is similar to, and therefore has all the disadvantages of, the questionnaire technique for collecting epidemiologic data, particularly in the absence of objective criteria for the assessment of tardive dyskinesia. (2) Eckman's (1968) method of diagnosing tardive dyskinesia is questionable. He mentions the following symptoms in three of his patients with tardive dyskinesia, whose clinical descriptions are provided. One patient had tremors, akathisia, convulsions, and weakness of arms; the second had tremors and akathisia; and only the third had oral dyskinesia. The first two patients' symptoms do not conform to those typical of tardive dyskinesia. (3) Roxburgh (1970) apparently restricted his diagnosis of tardive dyskinesia to severely debilitated cases and got a low prevalence figure of 1.7%. (4) Yagi, Ogita, Ohtsuka, *et al.* (1976) separated "acute dyskinesia" from persistent dyskinesia. They subdivided the latter into reversible and irreversible forms. However, they did not specify the features distinguishing between acute and persistent dyskinesia; also, the subtype of "rever-

kinesia in these studies so as to exclude patients whose diagnosis of tardive dyskinesia seemed questionable and to include only those patients whose dyskinetic symptoms were moderate to severe in intensity. Furthermore, we tried to separate neuroleptic-treated patients from those who had received either no neuroleptics or neuroleptics in very small total amounts in order to obtain a proper estimate of the prevalence of tardive dyskinesia among neuroleptic-treated patients. Table 2-2 summarizes the 37 studies in chronological order. It is apparent that there are differences in the prevalence rates reported. There are several possible reasons for such differences, which can be classified under methodological differences and population differences.

METHODOLOGICAL DIFFERENCES

Diagnostic Criteria

Many studies did not define the criteria for diagnosis of tardive dyskinesia. Overinclusive data are likely to inflate the figures of prevalence. Thus Faurbye *et al.* (1964) reported a prevalence of 26%. A careful look at their data shows that they included a number of patients with tremors, rigidity, and akathisia in their group of tardive dyskinesia patients. Hence we preferred to use the conservative estimate of 17 patients (out of 216 schizophrenics) who had the typical buccolingual masticatory triad to arrive at the prevalence figure of 7.9% among their patients. A possibility remains, however, that diagnostic differences may have contributed to some of the variance in the prevalence rates reported by different investigators.

---

sible persistent dyskinesia" sounds self-contradictory. (5) Frangos and Christodoulides (1975) computed overall prevalence of tardive dyskinesia among their inpatients and outpatients, but did not separate the two populations. (6) Simpson, Varga, Lee, *et al.* (1978) briefly screened the entire population of a state hospital for identifying cases with obvious dyskinesia. The investigators were careful to add that the prevalence of tardive dyskinesia would have been higher if they had examined all the patients more extensively. (This study, however, contains some useful analyses of data on psychotropic drug history.) (7) Kane, Wegner, Stenzler, *et al.* (1980) reported 4.6% prevalence of tardive dyskinesia in a combined population of inpatients and outpatients. However, a number of these patients had received minimal amounts of neuroleptics. Of the patients, 23.4% had been treated with neuroleptics for less than 3 months, and 13.7% had not received these drugs within the past year. As stated by the authors, the relatively short exposure of this population to neuroleptics is at least one explanation for the low prevalence rate found. As discussed later in this chapter, how a "neuroleptic-treated group" is defined influences the apparent prevalence rate.

Table 2-2. Prevalence of Tardive Dyskinesia among Chronic Psychiatric Inpatients

Investigators	Population	*n*	Percentage with tardive dyskinesia	Comments
Uhrbrand and Faurbye (1960)	Women treated with perphenazine	155	9.7	
Faurbye, Rasch, Petersen, *et al.* (1964)	Schizophrenic women	216	7.9	Patients with bucco-lingual masticatory triad
Hunter, Earl, and Thornicroff (1964)		450	2.9	Patients with severe persistent dyskinesia
Demars (1966)		371	7	
Turunen and Achte (1967)		480	5.6	
Degkwitz and Wenzel (1967)		767	10.3	Patients with moderate to severe tardive dyskinesia; another 6.6% had mild tardive dyskinesia
		499	22.8	Severity of tardive dyskinesia not mentioned
Crane and Paulson (1967)		182	13.2	
Siede and Muller (1967)	Elderly	404	11.4	
Paulson (1968a)		500	7	Patients with "conspicuous" persistent tardive dyskinesia
Heinrich, Wagener, and Bender (1968)		554	17	
Crane (1968a)	Men in United States "heavily" treated with neuroleptics	98	16.3	
	Men in Turkey "moderately" treated for mean 13 months	40	7.5	
Crane (1968c)	"Chlorpromazine study"	379	27.7	
Greenblatt, Stotsky, and DiMascio (1968)	Nursing home residents	52	38.5	
Jones and Hunter (1968)	Over 40 years of age	82	30.5	Patients with oral dyskinesia

(continued)

Table 2-2. (continued)

Investigators	Population	n	Percentage with tardive dyskinesia	Comments
Edwards (1970); also, Pryce and Edwards (1966)	Women	184	18.5	Patients with moderate to severe tardive dyskinesia; another 20.1% had mild or doubtful tardive dyskinesia
Dynes (1970)		1,200	8.6	Patients with oral dyskinesia
Lehmann, Ban, and Saxena (1970)		350	6.6	
Crane (1970)	"Trifluoperazine study"	127	26.8	
Hippius and Lange (1970)		531	34.3	
Brandon, McClelland, and Protheroe (1971)		625	25.4	
Kennedy, Hershon, and McGuire (1972)		63	41.3	Patients with moderate to severe tardive dyskinesia; another 20.6% had mild or doubtful tardive dyskinesia
Kinoshita, Inose, and Sakai (1972)	Japanese hospital	396	14.1	
Fann, Davis, and Janowsky (1972)		204	35.8	
Crane (1973b)		669	13	Patients with moderate to severe tardive dyskinesia; another 31.8% had mild tardive dyskinesia
Ogita, Yagi, and Itoh (1975)	Japanese hospital	123	17.9	
	French hospital	131	18.3	
Jus, Pineau, Lachance, et al. (1976a)		332	22.9	Patients with moderate to severe tardive dyskinesia; another 33.1% had mild tardive dyskinesia
Gardos, Cole, and LaBrie (1977b)		50	46	

Table 2-2. (continued)

Investigators	Population	*n*	Percentage with tardive dyskinesia	Comments
Mehta, Mallya, and Volavka (1978); also, Mehta, Mehta, and Mathew (1977)	Follow-up study	178	22.5	
Pandurangi, Ananth, and Channabasa-vanna (1978)	Indian patients hospitalized for 2 or more years	77	23.3	
Bell and Smith (1978)		1,329	26	Patients with definite tardive dyskinesia; another 14% had mild tardive dyskinesia
Smith, Oswald, Kucharski, *et al.* (1978); also Smith, Kuchar-ski, Oswald, *et al.* (1979)		293	30	Patients with moderate to severe dyskinesia
Jeste, Potkin, Sinha, *et al.* (1979)	Patients over 50 in a university hospital	88	23.9	Diagnosis of tardive dyskinesia based on specifically defined criteria; doubtful and mild dyskinesia excluded
Famuyiwa, Eccleston, Donald-son, *et al.* (1979)	Schizophrenic patients under 60 years of age	50	34	
Perris, Dimi-trijevic, Jacob-son, *et al.* (1979)		347	17.3	
Bourgeois, Bouilh, Tignol, *et al.* (1980)	Residents of a retirement home of a hospital	59	42.4	
Perényi and Aratō (1980)	Hungarian schizophrenic inpatients	200	23.5	Patients with mean AIMS rating of 2 or more; another 26% scored 1 on AIMS
Jeste and Wyatt (unpublished data)	State hospital	95	31.6	Patients with moderate to severe dyskinesia
TOTAL	(37 studies)	12,930	17.6	

Severity of Dyskinesia

Inclusion of cases of doubtful or mild dyskinesia may result in an unrealistically high prevalence rate, whereas selection of only severe cases may artificially lower the percentage of patients with dyskinesia. Bell and Smith (1978) noted that the prevalence of tardive dyskinesia in their 1329 patients would be 12% if only the severe cases were included, 26% if moderately severe cases were added, and 40% if patients with minimal symptoms of dyskinesia were included too. Smith (cited in Baldessarini *et al.*, 1980, p. 46) observed that the apparent prevalence of tardive dyskinesia was inversely related to the criterion of severity of dyskinesia as assessed by the score on the Abnormal Involuntary Movements Scale (AIMS). In all the studies where severity of dyskinesia was mentioned (e.g., Bell & Smith, 1978; Crane, 1973b; Degkwitz & Wenzel, 1967; Edwards, 1970; Jus, Pineau, Lachance, *et al.,* 1976a; Kennedy, Hershon, & McGuire, 1971), we have chosen the proportion of patients with moderate to severe dyskinesia and have excluded those with borderline or mild symptoms. Unfortunately, however, some other studies made no mention of symptom severity.

Type of Dyskinesia

Not all dyskinesia seen in psychiatric patients is tardive dyskinesia, nor is tardive dyskinesia necessarily an irreversible or incapacitating syndrome. Surverys done soon after withdrawal of neuroleptics may uncover a high proportion of withdrawal dyskinesias. In some patients, withdrawal dyskinesia may herald the onset of tardive dyskinesia, whereas in others it may be a readily reversible syndrome different from tardive dyskinesia. A follow-up may help differentiate between the two. A one-time survey of dyskinesia may make it difficult for the investigators to decide on the inclusion or exclusion of such cases. On the other hand, restricting the diagnosis of tardive dyskinesia to irreversible or incapacitated cases may result in an underestimation of the prevalence of tardive dyskinesia.

POPULATION DIFFERENCES

There is usually a higher prevalence of tardive dyskinesia among geriatric patients as compared to younger patients. (Table 2-2 specifies those studies that were done exclusively on elderly populations.) Women have a somewhat higher prevalence of dyskinesia than do men. (Studies done on one gender only are identified as such in Table 2-2.) Other variables, such as race, culture, and primary psychiatric diagnosis are not known to affect the prevalence of dyskinesia. It is necessary to separate neuroleptic-treated patients from those who had received either no neuroleptics or neuroleptics in very small amounts for a brief period. As noted earlier, the prevalence of spontaneous dyskinesia in the non-neuroleptic-treated population is low. Defining neuroleptic-treated patients as those who had received neuroleptics for at least 3 months in total amounts exceeding 100g equivalents of chlorpromazine, we found (Jeste, Potkin, Sinha, *et al.,* 1979) the prevalence of tardive dyskinesia to be 23.9% among our inpatients; the prevalence of dyskinesia was only 4.5% among these inpatients who had been treated with smaller amounts of neuroleptics or none at all. Even among neuroleptic-treated patients, the prevalence of tardive dyskinesia may be greater among those who received larger total quantities of these drugs (Chapter 4).

CHANGING EPIDEMIOLOGY

INCREASE IN REPORTED PREVALENCE

Combining all 37 studies published from 1960 through 1980 (Table 2-2), the overall weighted mean prevalence of tardive dyskinesia among chronically ill psychiatric inpatients treated with neuroleptics appears to be 17.6%. A careful look at the reports arranged in a chronological order shows, however, that the reported prevalence of dyskinesia has been on the rise during the past two decades (Table 2-3 and Figure 2-1). Combining the studies published within a decade, the overall weighted mean preva-

Table 2-3. Increasing Prevalence of Tardive Dyskinesia

Period	Number of studies	Total number of patients	Percentage with tardive dyskinesia
Through 1965	3	821	5.5
1966–1970	16	6,800	14.6
1971–1975	6	2,211	20.2
1976–1980	12	3,098	25.6
TOTAL (through 1980)	37	12,930	17.6

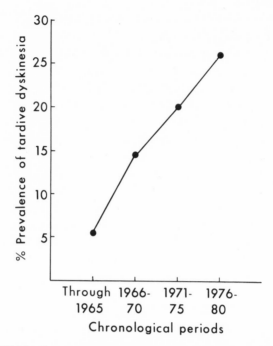

Figure 2-1. Weighted mean percentage prevalence of tardive dyskinesia among chronically ill psychiatric inpatients on neuroleptic treatment, based on 37 studies (Table 2-2) reported from 1960 through 1980.

lence of tardive dyskinesia among inpatients was 13.6% until 1970 (19 studies) and has jumped to 23.3% since 1971 (18 studies). Moreover, 14 of the last 18 studies found a prevalence exceeding 22%. The weighted mean prevalence in the 12 studies published during the past 5 years (1976 through 1980) has been 25.6%. One must first consider the possibility that this increase in reported prevalence may not be a real one, but may be merely an artifact of methodological and population differences. Various arguments for and evidence against such a possibility follow.

Argument 1

It may be argued that the apparent increase in prevalence is because of a heightened awareness of the condition. Whereas tardive dyskinesia could have been underdiagnosed in the earlier years, it may now be overdiagnosed as a result of the increasing publicity that this syndrome has received in recent years.

Probably the only direct way of testing this hypothesis would be by conducting prospective long-term studies of *incidence* (i.e., occurrence of new cases) of tardive dyskinesia in the same patient population by the same investigators using the same diagnostic criteria. We are not aware of any major published studies that were done on inpatients in this manner. Hence we have to rely on the following indirect evidence to answer Argument 1.

1. There have been eight reports since 1971 in which the diagnosis of tardive dyskinesia was explicitly restricted to patients with dyskinesia of moderate to severe intensity (Table 2-2). Doubtful and mild cases were specifically excluded. The overall weighted mean prevalence of tardive dyskinesia in these eight studies is 23.5%. It is likely that a number of these patients had persistent dyskinesia. This fact can be contrasted with a communication (cited by Schmidt & Jarcho, 1966) from the National Institutes of Health–National Clearinghouse for Mental Health Information (NCMHI) published in the early 1960s. It stated that there was nothing in the NCMHI document collection that referred to permanent movement disorders caused by phenothiazines.

2. Crane (1968c, 1970) reexamined the same patients at 6-month and 1-year follow-ups. He found an apparent increase in prevalence between the first and second examinations, which could be attributed to a heightened sensitiveness for detecting dyskinesia. There was, however, no further increase in prevalence between the second and third examinations. There is a limit to which awareness of a condition can be increased. It seems rather unlikely that among the researchers there has been a progressive and stepwise accentuation of diagnostic powers for detecting tardive dyskinesia all over the world during the past two decades, which could fully explain the rising prevalence seen in Figure 2-1.

3. Crane (1977) found that oral discussion of tardive dyskinesia and the publication of numerous articles on the subject had little impact on the prescribing practices of physicians, suggesting that there was no marked increase in the general awareness about this condition.

4. It may be argued that the cases of tardive dyskinesia diagnosed during the 1960s were those of persistent dyskinesia, whereas many of the cases being diagnosed now are those of early and reversible dyskinesia. We therefore compared the treatment response over the last 20 years (Chapter 10). The only treatment for tardive dyskinesia that has been reported throughout the past two decades has been neuroleptic withdrawal. Of all the patients in the studies published through 1970, 37.2% had symptom remission after withdrawal of neuroleptics for at least 3 months. The improvement rate among the patients from the studies published since 1971 was 42.3%. This difference between pre- and post-1970 reports is not significant. Other treatments (e.g., cholinergic drugs) were tried during the 1970s. We contrasted the treatment response through 1975 and since 1976. Of all the patients reportedly treated through 1975, 50.7% had improvement. This rate dropped to 41.7% among the patients in the studies published since 1976. Thus there is no indication that the cases of tardive dyskinesia that have been diagnosed in recent years are more reversible than those in the earlier periods.

5. If an increased awareness were responsible for the rising prevalence of tardive dyskinesia, then one might expect a similar increase in the prevalence of other long-term side effects of neuroleptics. Skin pigmentation and eye changes are thought to result from prolonged use of neuroleptics. In 1964 Greiner and Berry reported 70 cases of ocular and dermatologic complications of chronic treatment with chlorpromazine. Their article stirred considerable interest and was followed by a number of papers, editorials, and letters to the editors on that subject. Yet, the reported prevalence of eye and skin changes caused by neuroleptics has not increased dramatically. Appleton (1970) reviewed studies published during the 1960s; the overall weighted mean prevalence of ocular changes in patients receiving drug therapy was 29.1% (usually varying between 26% and 36% in different reports). In 1978 Ban found the prevalence of these changes to be from 20% to 35%. Similarly, the prevalence of skin pigmentation has remained at about 1%.

Argument 2

It may be contended that the increase in prevalence of tardive dyskinesia is due to the aging of patients during the last 20 years. Although this objection may be partly valid, it should be added that only 2 of the 18 studies published since 1971 have been done in selectively elderly populations.

Argument 3

The number of chronic psychiatric inpatients has been progressively decreasing since the mid-1950s. It may be argued that the patients who are currently in hospitals are generally sicker than the inpatients of the earlier decades. Furthermore, one report (Kucharski, Smith, & Dunn, 1980) suggested that patients with tardive dyskinesia might not be discharged as readily as those without dyskinesia, resulting in an inflated prevalence of the syndrome among inpatients. However, in recent studies the prevalence of tardive dyskinesia among outpatients receiving long-term neuroleptic treatment has usually been similar to that among the inpatients (Asnis, Leopold, Duvoisin, *et al.,* 1977; Chouinard, Annable, Ross-Chouinard, *et al.,* 1979; Smith, Kucharski, Eblen, *et al.,* 1979).

Comment

It therefore appears that the increase in the reported prevalence of tardive dyskinesia is not entirely an artifact. It is generally accepted that the length of neuroleptic therapy is one of the important factors in the etiology of tardive dyskinesia. Since the number of patients on long-term neuroleptic treatment has increased over the past two decades, so has the prevalence of tardive dyskinesia.

Two aspects of tardive dyskinesia should be stressed here. First, tardive dyskinesia is not synonymous with irreversible dyskinesia. As discussed in Chapters 3 and 10, tardive dyskinesia is reversible in a little over one-third of all patients. The rate of reversibility is likely to be higher among young patients than among elderly patients. Also, tardive dyskinesia is not necessarily a severe and disabling syndrome. Some patients may develop dyskinesia with relatively short-term use of neuroleptics, whereas others may not become dyskinetic in spite of prolonged intake of these drugs. Even in predisposed individuals, a "threshold" may have to be reached before the dyskinetic symptoms appear. It is possible to suggest that today, with the increasingly long-term use of neuroleptics, a higher proportion of patients than ever before are reaching that threshold. This may also mean that in the future, prevalence of tardive dyskinesia may not increase progressively, but may at some point reach a plateau. It is conceivable that such a plateau may have already been reached in the case of ocular and dermatologic complications of prolonged neuroleptic administration.

It is also useful to consider various changes that have occurred in psychopharmacologic practice during the last 20 years. Popularity of depot preparations, preference for once-a-day medication, concomitant use of high-potency neuroleptics (such as haloperidol) with antiparkinsonian agents, and resorting to high doses of certain neuroleptics—these have been some of the changes in drug treatment of schizophrenia. It is, of course, rash even to suggest that any of these changes might be directly responsible for the increasing prevalence of tardive dyskinesia. Indeed, the data on neuroleptic use collected by the IMS America, Ltd., Ambler, Pa., question a popular notion that increasing prevalence of tardive dyskinesia has paralleled increasing use of the so-called high-potency neuroleptics. These data, which are a measure of the outflow, from 1964 through 1978, of neuroleptic prescriptions from a representative panel of 800 retail pharmacies across the continental United States, show that the five most commonly prescribed neuroleptics have been two "low-potency" phenothiazines with predominantly sedative side effects (chlorpromazine and thioridazine) and three "high-potency" neuroleptics with predominantly acute extrapyramidal side effects (trifluoperazine, fluphenazine, and haloperidol). Whereas the combined mean annual number of prescriptions for chlorpromazine and thioridazine rose from 6.7 million in 1964–1965 to 14.5 million ten years later (1974–1975), that for trifluoperazine, fluphenazine, and haloperidol was almost unchanged (5.5 million in 1964–1965 and 6.22 million during 1974–1975). Hospital pharmacies, however, might show a different trend, particularly with regard to the use of long-acting intramuscular fluphenazine. Much more epidemiologic and experimental work is required before associating certain treatment practices with occurrence of tardive dyskinesia.

There are also other aspects of the changing epidemiology of tardive dyskinesia. The earlier stereotype of the typical candidate for tardive dyskinesia—an old, brain-damaged patient who has been hospitalized and treated for a number of years—is no longer exclusively valid. Tardive dyskinesia is now known to occur with a noticeable frequency in younger patients, non-brain-damaged subjects, and nonpsychotic patients (Klawans, Bergen, Bruyn, *et al.*, 1974) who have received neuroleptics.

To summarize, the overall weighted mean prevalence of tardive dyskinesia among chronically ill, neuroleptic-treated adult psychiatric inpatients during the past 5 years has been 25.6%. About two-thirds of them (i.e., 17% of the total) have persistent dyskinesia. Assuming that nearly one-fourth of these patients may have non-drug-related dyskinesia, the prevalence of persistent dyskinesia that may be attributable to neuroleptics is about 13%. How many of these patients have symptoms that are disabling is not known.

PATIENT- AND TREATMENT-RELATED VARIABLES

Differences among patient populations and treatment practices are at least partly responsible for differences in prevalence of tardive dyskinesia reported in different studies. Age, gender, and length and nature of neuroleptic treatment are among the variables influencing the prevalence of tardive dyskinesia. Other variables are considered in Chapter 4.

AGE

It is generally agreed that tardive dyskinesia is more common among the elderly than among younger patients. A number of studies (e.g., Demars, 1966; Edwards, 1979; Fann, Davis, & Janowsky, 1972; Hunter *et al.*, 1964) found that the mean age of tardive dyskinesia patients was higher than that of nondyskinetic patients. Table 2-4 compares prevalence of tardive dyskinesia in patients under 40 years with that in patients over 40 years, as reported in nine studies. The overall weighted mean prevalence of dyskinesia in patients over 40 is nearly three times that in younger patients. Except for two studies by Crane (1968c, 1970), which included patients up to age 56 only, the studies found prevalence of dyskinesia 1.5 to 22 times higher in patients over 40 than in patients under 40. Brandon *et al.* (1971), Crane and Paulson (1967), Degkwitz and Wenzel (1967), Fann *et al.* (1972), Jeste and Wyatt (1981), and Jones and Hunter (1969) noted that

Table 2-4. Distribution of Prevalence of Tardive Dyskinesia among Chronic Psychiatric Inpatients, by Age

Investigators	Patients under 40 years		Patients over 40 years	
	n	Percentage with tardive dyskinesia	*n*	Percentage with tardive dyskinesia
Degkwitz and Wenzel (1967)	255	5.5	512	22.7
Crane and Paulson (1967)	46	4.3	136	16.2
Crane (1968c)	116	20.7	263	30.8
Crane (1970)	49	24.5	78	28.2
Brandon, McClelland, and Protheroe (1971)	106	1.9[a]	806	26.2[a]
Fann, Davis, and Janowsky (1972)	29	17.2	175	38.9
Ogita, Yagi, and Itoh (1975)	44	0	87	27.6
	39	2.6	84	25
Perényi and Aratõ (1980)	71	16.9	129	27.1
Jeste and Wyatt (unpublished data)	28	14.3	67	38.8
TOTAL	783	9.7	2337	26.8

[a]Total prevalence for tardive dyskinesia and spontaneous dyskinesia.

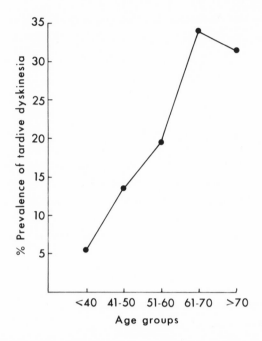

Figure 2-2. Weighted mean percentage prevalence of tardive dyskinesia among chronically ill psychiatric inpatients on neuroleptic treatment, based on studies done by Brandon, McClelland, and Protheroe (1971); Crane and Paulson (1967); Degkwitz and Wenzel (1967); Fann, Davis, and Janowsky, (1972); Jeste and Wyatt (1981); and Jones and Hunter (1969).

there was a progressive increase in prevalence of dyskinesia until age 70, after which there was no further significant increase.

Smith and Baldessarini (1980) also observed a similar relationship between age and prevalence of tardive dyskinesia. Figure 2-2 shows the weighted mean prevalence in various age groups, based on seven studies. It should be stressed that these were not prospective longitudinal studies of incidence of tardive dyskinesia with increasing age, but were quasi-longitudinal studies comparing prevalence in different age groups at the same time.

GENDER

Table 2-5 summarizes 20 studies on relative prevalence of tardive dyskinesia in men and women. These studies differ in their findings. Thirteen studies reported a higher prevalence in women. Crane (1968a) and Perényi

Table 2-5. Distribution of Prevalence of Tardive Dyskinesia among Chronic Psychiatric Inpatients, by Gender

Investigators	Men		Women	
	n	Percentage with tardive dyskinesia	*n*	Percentage with tardive dyskinesia
Hunter, Earl, and Thornicroff (1964)	200	0	250	5.2
Demars (1966)	166	4.8	205	8.8
Turunen and Achte (1967)	207	3.4	273	7.3
Crane and Paulson (1967)	66	15.2	116	14.7
Degkwitz and Wenzel (1967)	303	4.6	464	14
	193	20.7	306	24.2
Heinrich, Wagener, and Bender (1968)	228	12.3	326	20.2
Crane (1968a)	207	31	172	23.3
Jones and Hunter (1969)	13	7.7	69	34.8
Lehmann, Ban, and Saxena (1970)	168	4.2	182	8.8
Crane (1970)	62	27.4	65	26.1
Hippius and Lange (1970)	244	34.4	287	34.1
Brandon, McClelland and Protheroe (1971)	264	17.4	361	31.3
Kennedy, Hershon, and McGuire (1971)	32	25	31	58
Ogita, Yagi, and Itoh (1975)	70	17.1	53	18.9
Smith, Oswald, Kucharski, et. al (1978)	150	24.7	143	35.7
Jeste, Potkin, Sinha, et al. (1979)	27	22.2	61	24.6
Famuyiwa, Eccleston, Donaldson et al. (1979)	26	26.9	24	41.7
Perris, Dimitrijevic, Jacobson, et al. (1979)	213	9.4	134	29.8
Perényi and Aratō (1980)	100	31	100	16
Jeste and Wyatt (unpublished data)	25	24	70	34.3
TOTAL	2964	15.1	3692	20.6

and Aratō (1980) noted a higher prevalence in men. Crane (1970), Crane and Paulson (1967), Hippius and Lange (1970), Jeste, Potkin, Sinha, *et al.* (1979), and Ogita, Yagi, and Itoh (1975) found no difference in prevalence of dyskinesia between the two genders. Combining all 20 studies, the over-all weighted mean prevalence in women is about 41% higher than that in men. It is not clear whether the differences in the prevalence of dyskinesia between men and women are a result of certain biological characteristics of the two genders (e.g., brain neurotransmitter concentrations or the role of hormones) or merely reflect differences in treatment. Several groups of researchers (Degkwitz & Wenzel, 1967; Fann *et al.,* 1972; Simpson, Varga, Lee, *et al.,* 1978) noticed that women tended to receive longer or higher-dose psychopharmacologic treatment than men. (Whether women tend to have a more severe form of schizophrenia than men is uncertain.)

There are too few studies reporting prevalence of dyskinesia in differ-ent age groups by gender to allow one to determine differential effects of age on men and women in terms of development of tardive dyskinesia. It may be mentioned, however, that Smith, Oswald, Kucharski, *et al.* (1978) noted a linear increase in the prevalence of dyskinesia with age in women, whereas the prevalence decreased after the age of 70 in men (also see Bal-dessarini *et al.,* 1980, p. 50).

TREATMENT PRACTICES

Duration of neuroleptic therapy is one of the determinants of the preva-lence of tardive dyskinesia. Type of neuroleptic given, mode and frequen-cy of administration, daily dosage, drug-free periods, and other factors are discussed further in Chapter 4.

TARDIVE DYSKINESIA IN PSYCHIATRIC OUTPATIENTS

Initially, tardive dyskinesia was considered to be a rarity among psychiat-ric outpatients. Recent studies, however, have demonstrated this not to be the case. The number of studies on outpatients is, unfortunately, small. Also, such studies are even more difficult to evaluate than the studies on inpatients because of heterogeneous populations and variations in treat-ment practices, not to mention methodological aspects of the studies. One common, but frequently ignored, problem in outpatient studies is that of noncompliance. As many as 25% to 50% of outpatients may fail to take their medication (Blackwell, 1973). This makes it difficult to assess the exact proportion of patients on regular, long-term neuroleptic treatment. Besides, temporary noncompliance may result in withdrawal dyskinesia in some patients. The relationship of withdrawal dyskinesia to tardive dyskinesia is not yet clear.

Jeste, Olgiati, and Ghali (1971) found a low prevalence (4%) of tardive dyskinesia at the outpatient department of a hospital in Newark, N.J. Alexopoulos (1979) confirmed this finding at a nearby hospital that had a very similar outpatient department. The low prevalence in these two studies can be explained by the fact that those departments catered mainly to younger patient populations; also, the proportion of chronic schizophrenics on long-term neuroleptic treatment in the studies was relatively small. Similarly, Gardos, Samu, Kallos, *et al.* (1980) reported an absence of severe tardive dyskinesia in Hungarian schizophrenic outpatients who tended to receive electroconvulsive therapy in place of high-dose neuroleptic treatment. In contrast, Asnis *et al.* (1977), Chouinard, Annable, Ross-Chouinard, *et al.* (1979), and Smith, Kucharski, Eblen, *et al.* (1979) found a prevalence of over 30% in their outpatients on long-term neuroleptic treatment. As the community mental health programs expand, more and more of the patients who in the past would have been long-term inpatients are now returning to the community. An increasing prevalence of tardive dyskinesia among psychiatric outpatients is therefore to be expected. In one of the few studies on annual incidence of tardive dyskinesia, Gibson (1978a) followed 374 outpatients receiving depot fluphenazine or depot flupenthixol from 1974 to 1977. He observed a progressive increase in the number of patients with oral dyskinesia—from 7% in 1974 to 22% in 1977. Most of this increase was due to an increasing number of patients with mild dyskinesia. More studies of a similar type are needed.

SUMMARY

Dyskinesia occurs significantly more often in neuroleptic-treated than in non-neuroleptic-treated psychiatric patients. The overall prevalence of tardive dyskinesia among chronically ill psychiatric inpatients has jumped from about 13% between 1960 and 1970 to about 22% during the past decade and has reached a high of nearly 26% during the past 5 years. At least some of this increase is, in all probability, a real phenomenon. The risk of persistent dyskinesia that is attributable to neuroleptics is about 13%. The prevalence of dyskinesia increases progressively with age, at least until the age of 70, and is nearly three times more frequent in patients over 40 than in patients under 40. Tardive dyskinesia is a worldwide phenomenon, and its prevalence is influenced by neuroleptic usage. The epidemiology of tardive dyskinesia is changing. The earlier stereotype of an old, brain-damaged patient as a typical candidate for tardive dyskinesia is no longer exclusively valid. A noticeable frequency of tardive dyskinesia can be found in younger patients without apparent brain damage, nonschizophrenics, and outpatients treated with neuroleptics.

CHAPTER III

Clinical Manifestations and Diagnosis

ABNORMAL INVOLUNTARY MOVEMENTS: DIFFERENT TYPES

Phenomenologically, tardive dyskinesia is a movement disorder. It would therefore be useful to consider the various types of abnormal involuntary movements that are commonly encountered in clinical practice before discussing specific criteria for a diagnosis of tardive dyskinesia.

Of the different types of abnormal involuntary movements commonly encountered, the following are relevant to a discussion of tardive dyskinesia—tremor, chorea, ballismus, athetosis, dystonia, myoclonus, tic, mannerism, compulsion, and akathisia (Table 3-1). We should add that these are only symptoms and do not, by themselves, indicate specific disorders. Thus a tic may be a normal phenomenon or may be symptomatic of any one of a number of psychiatric and neurological diseases.

TREMOR

In Latin, "tremor" means shaking. A tremor is defined as a regular rhythmic movement of a part of the body, resulting from alternate contractions of agonist and antagonist muscles. (However, in certain tremors, such as the essential tremor, the agonist and antagonist muscles contract simultaneously.) The usual frequency is 3 to 12 per second, although occasionally it may be as high as 20 per second. The body parts most commonly

Table 3-1. Types of Abnormal Involuntary Movements

Type	Rhythmicity	Speed	Other features	Localization	Causes
Tremor	Present	Usually 3–12/sec	Fine or coarse	Fingers, toes, head, tongue	Psychological, drugs, alcohol, parkinsonism, encephalopathies
Chorea	Absent	Rapid, jerky	Quasi-purposive	Proximal parts of limbs, orofacial region	Huntington's disease, rheumatic fever, drugs, hysteria
Ballismus	Absent	Rapid, jerky	Usually unilateral, proximal, rotatory	Limbs	Hemorrhage into subthalamic nucleus, hysteria
Athetosis	Present	Slow	Sinuous; often coexists with chorea	Distal parts of limbs	Lesions of putamen
Dystonia	Absent	Slow	Painful	Axial muscles	Genetic disorders, encephalopathies, drugs, hysteria, tetanus
Myoclonus	Absent	Rapid, jerky	Sensory precipitation; may occur in sleep	Limbs	Certain genetic and acquired disorders, epilepsy
Tic	Present or absent	Variable	Apparently purposeful	Limbs, orofacial region; may be generalized	Psychological, Tourette's syndrome, encephalitis
Mannerism	Absent	Slow	Related to personality	Limbs, orofacial region, axial muscles	Psychological, encephalitis (?)
Compulsion	Usually absent	Usually slow	Purposeful, irresistible	Limbs, occasionally other areas	Psychological, encephalitis (?)
Akathisia	Absent	Variable	Feeling of inner restlessness	Limbs, axial muscles	Usually neuroleptics

affected by tremors include fingers, toes, head, and tongue. Tremors are usually classified into fine and coarse types. Fine tremors may result from conditions such as anxiety states, thyrotoxicosis, alcohol intoxication, and treatment with drugs such as lithium. Coarse tremors may be either static or action tremors. Static tremors occur while the affected part is at rest—for example, the pill-rolling tremor seen in Parkinson's disease and sometimes in elderly individuals. Action tremors are present during voluntary movements and may suggest cerebellar pathology. One specific type of coarse tremor is called "asterixis" or "flapping tremor." It consists of the sudden flapping of hand and arm, similar to that of a bird's wings, and is usually a manifestation of metabolic encephalopathy.

Neuroleptic-treated patients frequently exhibit fine tremors of fingers (parkinsonism) and occasionally of lips (rabbit syndrome). Neuroleptic-induced tremors are usually postural or action tremors rather than tremors at rest.

CHOREA

In Greek, "chorea" indicates dance. Chorea refers to nonrepetitive, quasi-purposive (i.e., movements may appear to be purposeful, but are not), rapid, and jerky movements involving proximal parts of limbs and sometimes the orofacial region. The movements are nonrepetitive in their site, frequency, and amplitude. The most common neurologic causes of chorea are Huntington's disease and Sydenham's chorea. Chorea can also be seen in a hysterical conversion reaction, may result from long-term use of neuroleptics or L-dopa, or may be a sign of intoxication with drugs such as lithium and tricyclic antidepressants.

BALLISMUS

The Greek *ballismos* means jumping about. "Ballismus" or "ballism" refers to sudden, wild, jerky, darting movements of arms and legs. Proximal location of movements and rotatory quality are characteristic of ballism. It may be restricted to one side of the body and is then called "hemiballismus" or "hemiballism." Hemorrhage into the subthalamic body of Luys leads to contralateral hemiballismus.

ATHETOSIS

The word "athetosis" is derived from Greek roots (*athetos* unfixed + *osis* condition). Neurologically, athetosis may be defined as a recurrent transition in posture between two extremes, such as pronation and supination. There is slow, sinuous, purposeless movement, usually involving distal parts of the extremities. Chorea and athetosis may coexist, in which case the condition is labeled "choreoathetosis."

DYSTONIA

Dystonia (Greek *dys* disturbed or abnormal + *tonos* tone), also called "torsion spasm," is a disorder of muscle tone. However, it frequently produces abnormal involuntary movements; hence it is considered here. The movements resulting from dystonia are often bizarre and grotesque and involve axial muscles such as those of the neck (torticollis), pelvis (tortipelvis), and trunk. The muscle spasms tend to be painful.

MYOCLONUS

"Myoclonus" (Greek *myo* muscle + *klonus* tumult) refers to a sudden, irregular contraction of a muscle or a group of muscles. If only a single muscle is involved, the part supplied by it may not move. When a muscle group is involved, a jerky movement (usually of a limb) results. Speed of movement, lack of rhythmicity, and precipitation by sensory stimuli such as a loud sound are distinguishing features of myoclonus (Adams & Victor, 1977). Myoclonus may be a symptom of petit mal epilepsy and is also seen in a number of neurologic disorders.

TIC

"Tic" (from French)) or habit spasm refers to a recurrent, apparently purposeful movement of a part of the body, resulting from spasmodic and coordinated contraction of related muscles. Like other involuntary movements considered in this section, a tic does not serve any practical function, although it may seem to do so. Tics may be psychogenic or may be a part of neurologic disorders such as Gilles de la Tourette's syndrome.

MANNERISM

A "mannerism" is a stereotyped involuntary (or semivoluntary) movement that is often peculiar to a person. Although mannerisms also occur in normal and neurotic subjects, bizarre and idiosyncratic mannerisms tend to be characteristic of schizophrenic patients. Mannerisms differ from most other abnormal involuntary movements in that they are less insistently repeated and are more in keeping with the subject's personality (Hinsie & Campbell, 1974).

COMPULSION

A "compulsion" is defined as an irresistible, stereotyped motor act that the person consciously wishes to avoid. It is often described as the motor equivalent of obsessive thinking. Unlike most other abnormal involuntary movements, compulsions are often purposeful and complex acts giving the appearance of volitional activity. Yet, they are not under conscious control of the subject. Compulsions may be psychogenic, although certain types of encephalitides may also predispose to them.

AKATHISIA

"Akathisia," sometimes spelled as "acathisia" or "akathizia," is a word of Greek origin (a absent + kathisis sitting). It refers to an inability to sit still, along with a feeling of inner restlessness. A common cause of akathisia is neuroleptic treatment. It is one of the acute or subacute extrapyramidal side effects of neuroleptics and responds to withdrawal or dose reduction of these drugs. Some patients seem to develop tolerance to this side effect with continued administration of neuroleptics. Antiparkinsonian drugs are not very effective in relieving akathisia.

FEATURES COMMON TO VARIOUS ABNORMAL INVOLUNTARY MOVEMENTS

Most of these movements are aggravated by emotional arousal and are reduced when the person is relaxed. Temporary voluntary control over the movements is commonly seen. With the exception of certain forms of myoclonus (e.g., palatal myoclonus), the movements are absent during sleep. Sedatives tend to suppress temporarily many types of abnormal movements. Coexistence of two or more kinds of abnormal involuntary movements in the same patient is common.

TYPES OF MOVEMENTS IN TARDIVE DYSKINESIA

Patients with tardive dyskinesia tend to have a number of abnormal movements. For scientific precision, it is necessary to separate the movements that constitute tardive dyskinesia from those that may be due to other factors. The term "dyskinesia" (Greek *dys* disturbed or abnormal + *kinesis* movement) refers to a distortion or defect of voluntary movements. Yet, in recent years that term has generally been restricted to certain types of abnormal involuntary movements, especially those induced by drugs. The movement disorders in neuroleptic-induced tardive dyskinesia are typically of the choreoathetoid type. Some patients undergoing prolonged neuroleptic treatment also develop tics, chronic dystonias, and akathisia. It is important to stress, however, that tremor, acute dystonia, myoclonus, mannerism, and compulsion are not to be included under the syndrome of tardive dyskinesia. Of course, patients with dyskinesia may have one or more of these other movement disorders (e.g., psychotic mannerisms or drug-induced tremors), but these movements should be considered as separate entities since their pathology, phenomenology, outcome, and treatment are different from those of tardive dyskinesias. Clinically, such a differentiation may sometimes be difficult; there is, however, a need to try to discriminate among different types of abnormal involuntary movements.

For example, a patient with both tardive dyskinesia and acute dystonia may have considerable improvement in dystonia with an antihistamine agent such as diphenhydramine (Nasrallah, Pappas, & Crowe, 1980). Unless the two disorders are distinguished, the clinician may wrongly conclude that the treatment had antidyskinetic effect. Glazer and Moore

(1980) described three patients with tardive dyskinesia who developed an acute extrapyramidal reaction to a single dose of intramuscular fluphenazine decanoate. This reaction, which included tremors, akathisia, and rigidity, subsided rapidly on administration of benztropine. Although benzotropine caused a drop in the AIMS score, the oral tardive dyskinesia was unchanged.

MANIFESTATIONS OF TARDIVE DYSKINESIA: A TOPOGRAPHICAL CLASSIFICATION

Following is a classification of the various manifestations of tardive dyskinesia according to their localization. (Figures 3-1 and 3-2 depict some of the manifestations of tardive dyskinesia.)

MOUTH, FACE, AND PHARYNX

Tongue

1. Fine vermicular contractions or tremor of intrinsic muscles of the tongue inside the oral cavity. There is no change in the position of the tongue inside the mouth.

2. Gross movements of (the extrinsic muscles of) the tongue inside the oral cavity. These may be rhythmic or choreiform, rolling or linear. The so-called bonbon sign refers to tongue movements producing a bulge in the cheek.

3. Protrusion of the tongue outside the oral cavity. This may be a repetitive, short-duration protrusion or a more prolonged one. The protruded part may include only the tip or a larger portion of the anterior half of the tongue. In the latter case, trauma and hypertrophy of the tongue may be seen. A sign that is more common in encephalitis lethargica than in tardive dyskinesia is referred to as the "fly-catcher's tongue." This consists of a very rapid and brief protrusion of a large portion of the anterior half of the tongue, resembling the sudden shooting out of an arm in hemiballismus.

Repetitive forward thrusting of tongue may result in a swallowing difficulty. Dysarthria is another complication.

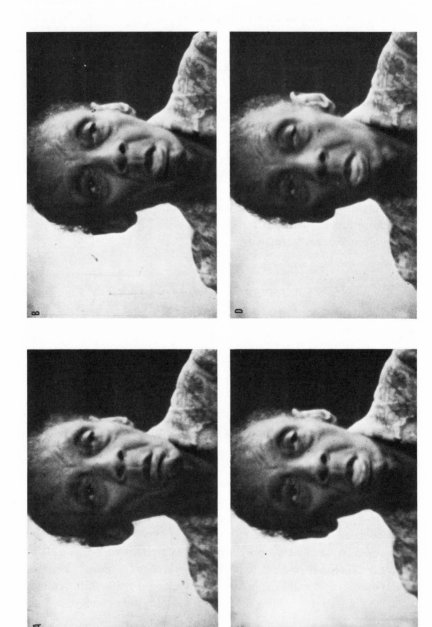

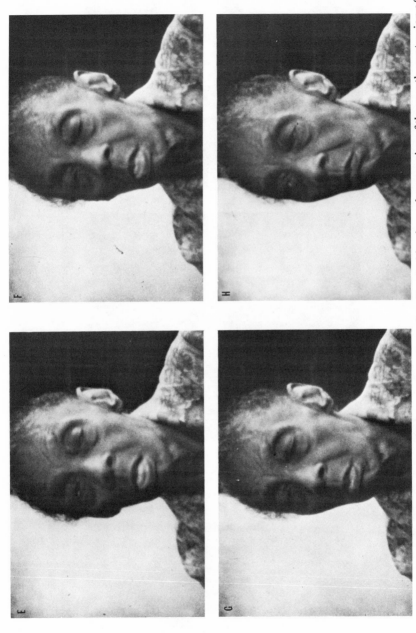

Figure 3-1. Serial pictures demonstrating certain manifestations of tardive dyskinesia, such as opening of the mouth, protrusion of the tongue, and blinking of the eyes.

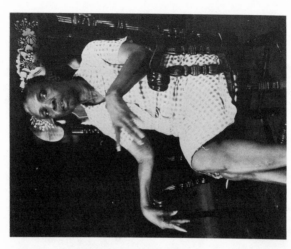

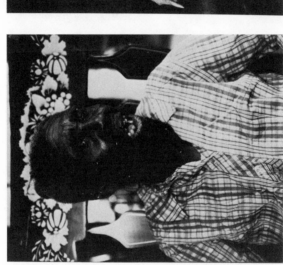

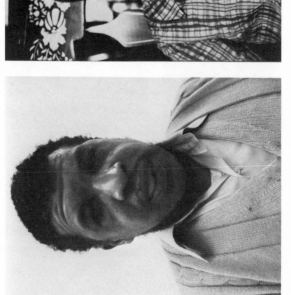

Figure 3-2. All these patients with tardive dyskinesia had a long history of neuroleptic treatment. (Left-hand photograph by Richard Jed Wyatt; middle and right-hand photographs by David K. Bauler.)

Jaw

1. Vertical movements—repetitive clenching of teeth, biting, opening and closing of mouth.

2. Horizontal movements from side to side.

3. Combined or complex movements—chewing.

Lips

1. Lower lip—pouting.

2. Both lips—clicking and smacking (sudden and audible parting of lips), puckering (as if a purse string running through the lips were pulled), licking, and sucking movements.

Other Facial Muscles

1. Eyes, eyelids, and eyebrows—blinking, blepharospasm (twitching or spasmodic contraction of orbicularis oculi), lifting of eyebrows.

2. Cheeks—retraction of angle of mouth, grimacing, puffing of cheeks, sucking movement.

3. Forehead—frowning.

Pharynx and Larynx

1. Grunting and other similar sounds.

2. Palatal dyskinesia.

UPPER EXTREMITIES

1. Choreiform movements of arm and forearm.

2. Athetoid movements of forearm, hand, and fingers.

3. Choreoathetoid movements involving a part of or the entire upper extremity.

4. Ballistic movements of arms.

LOWER EXTREMITIES

1. Toes—horizontal (spreading of toes), vertical (retroflexion), and combined movements. Occasionally, athetoid (slow, wave-like) movements of toes.

2. Foot and ankle—stamping movements, inversion and eversion of foot, lateral oscillations of ankle.

3. Leg and knee—stamping of leg, lateral movements of knee.

4. Entire lower extremity—stamping; shifting of weight from one extremity to the other; restless, fidgety movements. Rarely, sudden ballistic movements.

TRUNK AND AXIAL MUSCLES

Trunk

1. Rocking, oscillatory or twisting movements. These may involve variable portion of the trunk.

2. Respiratory irregularities and gastrointestinal symptoms such as retching and vomiting due to dyskinesias of diaphragm and intercostal and abdominal muscles.

Neck and Shoulder Girdle

1. Anteroposterior (nodding), lateral, or rotatory movements.

2. Movements resembling torsion dystonias (torticollis). Unlike true dystonias, these movements last for much shorter periods and are repeated more often. Also, pronounced rigidity and pain are not associated with these dyskinetic movements.

3. Raising or shrugging of shoulders.

Pelvic Girdle

1. Movements resembling torsion dystonias (tortipelvis), with characteristics similar to those of the movements described under "Neck and Shoulder Girdle."

2. Twisting or undulating movements seen on lying down, standing, or walking.

3. Gait disturbances—ataxic, broad-based, or spastic gaits.

The dyskinetic manifestations may be unilaterial or bilateral. Even when bilateral, they may be asymmetrical in intensity, being more pronounced on one side than on the other.

RELATIVE PREVALENCE OF DYSKINESIAS IN
VARIOUS PARTS OF THE BODY

Different parts of the body are involved in tardive dyskinesia with different frequencies. Tables 3-2 and 3-3 summarize studies of relative prevalence of dyskinesias in various parts of the body.[1] Not all the studies give prevalence figures for every area of the body. The overall weighted mean prevalence, however, is as follows: Of the patients diagnosed as having tardive dyskinesia, about 81% had abnormal orofacial movements, 51% had limb dyskinesias, and 23% had trunk and axial involvement. Thirty-three percent of all the patients had combined orofacial and limb dyskinesias. All the major regions of the body were affected in 11% of the tardive dyskinesia population.

A further breakdown by area shows that the tongue was the single most frequently involved part in tardive dyskinesia (56%). Abnormal involuntary movements of the lips were seen in 46% of the subjects, and jaw movements in 40%. Muscles of facial expression were involved in only 18% of the patients. Of the extremities, the upper limbs had dyskinesias more often (34%) than the lower ones (25%).

There are differences in the localization of dyskinesias in different patient groups. Age is an important variable in this respect. Orofacial dyskinesias are more common in the elderly as compared to younger patients, whereas the reverse is true for limb dyskinesias. We compared the localization of tardive dyskinesia in 54 patients over 50 years of age with that in 24 patients under age 50. We found that the involvement of the lips was three times as frequent in the older subjects as in the younger patients, possibly reflecting a contribution of edentulous state and dental problems to dyskinetic symptomatology. In contrast, upper extremities and limbs were affected about twice as often in the young as in the old. There were no major differences between the two groups in dyskinesias of other body parts.

To examine the specificity of localization of tardive dyskinesia, we

---

[1]Two possible problems in interpreting the results of such studies should be mentioned. First, the investigators often did not mention severity of symptoms in different regions. Second, an earlier notion that buccolingual masticatory dyskinesia was the "true" tardive dyskinesia may have biased the findings of some of the early studies in favor of a high prevalence of orofacial symptoms.

Table 3-2. Localization of Dyskinesias

Investigators	Number of patients	Percentage of patients with dyskinesias					Comments
		Orofacial	Limb	Trunk	Orofacial and limb	Total body	
Hunter, Earl, and Thornicroff (1964)	13	100	100	?	100	?	Elderly patients
Paulson (1968a)	33	75.8	57.6	18.2	36.4	3.0	Elderly patients
Jones and Hunter (1969)	33	75.8	51.5	?	39.4	?	Patients over 40 years
Yagi (1970)	7	85.7	42.9	0	28.6	?	
Itoh, Miura, Yagi, et al. (1971)	10	60	70	30	?	?	
McAndrew, Case, and Treffert (1972)	10	60	100	?	60	?	Children, 4–16 years
Kinoshita, Inose, and Sakai (1972)	56	100	7.1	0	7.1	0	
Karasuyama, Fujii, and Takahashi (1972)	32	100	34.4	3.1	34.4	3.1	
Polizos et al. (1973b)	34	2.9	100	100	2.9	2.9	Children (6–12 years) with withdrawal dyskinesia
Ogita, Yagi, and Itoh (1975)	24	100	29.2	25	29.2	?	French hospital
	22	100	31.8	27.3	31.8	?	Japanese hospital
Jeste (unpublished data)	54	94.4	48.1	14.8	42.6	24.1	Patients over 50 years
	24	79.4	83.3	20.8	58.3	16.7	Patients under 50 years
TOTAL	352	80.7	50.6	23.3	33.0	11.3	

Table 3-3. Prevalence of Dyskinesia in Orofacial Region and Limbs

Investigators	Number of patients	Percentage of patients with dyskinesias					
		Tongue	Jaw	Lips	Face	Upper extremities	Lower extremities
Faurbye, Rasch, Petersen, et al. (1964)	75	37.3	42.7	44	?	50.7	
Paulson (1968)	33[a]	33.3	66.7		?	48.5	21.2
Ogita, Yagi, and Itoh (1975)	46	95.7	100		?	4.3	26.1
Smith, Kucharski, Oswald, et al. (1979)	88	47.7	18.2	26.1	4.5	27.3	28.4
Jeste (unpublished data)	54[a]	66.7	64.8	71.4	29.6[b]	42.6	14.8
	24[c]	75	58.3	20.8	37.5[b]	79.2	37.5
TOTAL	320	55.9	46.1	17.5	34.3	34.3	24.9

[a]Only patients over the age of 50.
[b]Usually of mild intensity.
[c]Only patients under the age of 50.

studied the localization of other abnormal involuntary movements in 67 nondyskinetic psychiatric patients (45 over the age of 50, and 22 under age 50). These patients had received an average rating of 1 on the 0 to 4 AIMS, whereas the tardive dyskinesia patients mentioned earlier had been given a rating of 2 to 4. Hence the dyskinetic and nondyskinetic groups were not comparable in the mean severity of the abnormal involuntary movements. With this limitation, we found that the most common movement disorder in our elderly nondyskinetic population was involuntary lip movement due to denture problems, whereas facial tics, including eye blinking, were the most frequent abnormal involuntary movements in patients under 50. Tongue movements were the least common of the orofacial movements in the whole nondyskinetic group.

The relationship between increased blinking and tardive dyskinesia is uncertain. Stevens (1978) reported abnormalities of ocular movement, including increased spontaneous blinking and reduced reflex blinking in 34 of the 44 schizophrenic patients withdrawn from neuroleptics. She rightly concluded that it was not clear whether these abnormalities represented schizophrenic pathology or resulted from neuroleptic withdrawal. Casey, Gerlach, Magelund, *et al.* (1980) found no correlation between treatment-induced changes in severity of tardive dyskinesia and blink rates. A noticeable increase in spontaneous blinking in a neuroleptic-treated patient should arouse a suspicion of tardive dyskinesia (Karson, 1979), although elevated blink rates are neither necessary nor sufficient for diagnosing tardive dyskinesia.

It would thus seem that abnormal movements of the tongue, followed by those of the jaw and extremities, are the most specific among the frequent manifestations of tardive dyskinesia.

DIAGNOSTIC CRITERIA

For clinical, research, and medicolegal purposes, it is necessary to have a set of operational criteria for diagnosing neuroleptic-induced tardive dyskinesia. Following is a set of such criteria that we have found helpful. Further work is necessary to assess the relative value of each criterion for the diagnosis of tardive dyskinesia.

PHENOMENOLOGY

Nature of the Abnormal Movements

Dyskinesia may be defined as choreiform (i.e., nonrepetitive, rapid, jerky, quasi-purposive movements), or atheoid (i.e., continuous, slow, sinuous, purposeless movements), or rhythmic abnormal involuntary movements in certain areas of the body, which are reduced by voluntary movements of the affected parts and increased by voluntary movements of the unaffected parts.

Other Characteristics

The abnormal movements are aggravated by emotional arousal and reduced when the person is relaxed. They may be temporarily controlled by volitional effort. The movements are absent during sleep. (These characteristics are not specific to dyskinesias, but are shared by several other types of abnormal involuntary movements.)

Specific Localization of Neuroleptic-Induced Tardive Dyskinesia

One or more of the following three areas are affected in most cases: tongue, jaw, and extremities. Isolated involvement of other body parts (in the absence of dyskinesias of tongue, jaw, or extremities) is rare in tardive dyskinesia.

Movements To Be Excluded

Tremors, acute dystonias, myoclonus, mannerisms, and compulsions are not a part of the dyskinesia syndrome. Some of these involuntary movements may coexist with dyskinesias, but they need to be distinguished for clinical and research purposes.

HISTORY

Duration of Dyskinesia

The movement disorder should be present for at least 3 weeks before tardive dyskinesia can be diagnosed. Although the symptom severity may vary, the dyskinesia should be manifest continually over that period.

(Acute and withdrawal dyskinesias usually disappear within 1 to 3 weeks of removal of the treatment.)

Neuroleptic Treatment

The patient should have a history of treatment with neuroleptics for at least 3 continuous months.

Onset of Dyskinesia

The same movements should not have been present prior to treatment with neuroleptics. The dyskinesia should have appeared either while the patient was on neuroleptics or within a few weeks of neuroleptic withdrawal.

TREATMENT RESPONSE

1. Antiparkinsonian agents typically have no effect or even aggravate tardive dyskinesia.

2. Increasing the dose of a neuroleptic usually reduces intensity of dyskinesia. Dose reduction or withdrawal of neuroleptics tends to worsen the symptoms, at least temporarily.

3. Some catecholaminergic agents such as L-dopa and amphetamine aggravate tardive dyskinesia.

CONDITIONS TO BE RULED OUT AS THE PRIMARY CAUSE OF DYSKINESIA

The mere presence of the following conditions does not necessarily exclude a diagnosis of neuroleptic-induced tardive dyskinesia. It is imperative, however, to demonstrate that these other conditions are not primarily responsible for the given patient's dyskinesia. Ill-fitting dentures, use of drugs such as L-dopa or amphetamine, Huntington's chorea, Wilson's disease, and Sydenham's chorea are among the major causes of movement disorders that may mimic neuroleptic-induced tardive dyskinesia. Other conditions in differential diagnosis include heavy metal intoxication, liver and kidney damage, parathyroid disorders, Fahr's syndrome, and several other rare neurologic syndromes (Baldessarini *et al.,* 1980).

EARLY DIAGNOSIS

By the time moderate to severe tardive dyskinesia is diagnosed, the symptoms have usually been present for months or even years. The diagnostic criteria just described are useful in establishing a definitive diagnosis in doubtful cases and for research and medicolegal purposes. They may not, however, solve the problem of early diagnosis of tardive dyskinesia, which is of considerable importance in clinical practice. All the factors mentioned earlier that make the diagnosis of tardive dyskinesia difficult make its early diagnosis even more problematic. With one exception (Quitkin, Rifkin, Gochfeld, et al., 1977), there are no major long-term prospective studies of patients on chronic neuroleptic treatment that aimed at early detection of tardive dyskinesia.[2] Quitkin et al. observed dyskinesia from its inception in 12 psychiatric patients, the majority of whom were 20 to 40 years of age. The investigators reported that 8 of these 12 patients manifested only orofacial symptoms, whereas the other four had orofacial, limb, and trunk dyskinesias in varying combinations.

According to some, but not all, researchers, fine vermicular movements of the tongue inside the oral cavity are one of the earliest signs of tardive dyskinesia (*Physicians' Desk Reference,* 1982). Since there are no published follow-up reports on patients who presented only with fine vermicular tongue movements, the significance of this sign for early diagnosis of tardive dyskinesia has not been established. In spite of the limitations of the literature on this subject, the following suggestions may be helpful for facilitating early detection:

1. Any patient who has been on neuroleptics for at least several months may be at risk for developing tardive dyskinesia.
2. When such a patient begins to exhibit any abnormal involuntary movements of face, mouth, or limbs that were not present earlier, a possibility of dyskinesia may be considered.
3. Facial tics, abnormal jaw movements, fine worm-like movements of the intrinsic muscles of the tongue inside the mouth, increased frequency of blinking, and mild choreoathetoid movements of fingers or hands are probably some of the early signs of tardive dyskinesia. Onset of any of these abnormal movements suggests that tardive dyskinesia should be considered as a diagnostic possibility.

[2]Another study, by Kane, Struve, Woerner, *et al.* (1981), is still in progress.

The clinician should also be alert to some of the unusual signs that may herald tardive dyskinesia. These include (a) hyperkinetic dysarthria with motor speech breakdowns (Portnoy, 1979) and (b) respiratory dysfunction manifesting as irregular respiration or dyspnea (Ayd, 1979; Jackson, Volavka, James, *et al.*, 1980).

4. Temporary aggravation of symptoms on neuroleptic dose reduction and nonresponse to antiparkinsonian medications may be used for supporting the diagnosis of tardive dyskinesia.

5. To rule out other conditions that may produce similar symptoms, the steps discussed in the next section, "Differential Diagnosis," should be followed.

6. Management of dyskinesia after it is diagnosed is considered in Chapter 11.

DIFFERENTIAL DIAGNOSIS

Psychiatric patients on neuroleptic treatment manifest a number of abnormal involuntary movements. Hence the differential diagnosis of tardive dyskinesia becomes important. The diagnosis is relatively easy when a patient, being followed by the same clinician, gradually develops oral or limb dyskinesias with the characteristic features described earlier. When, however, a physician sees for the first time a psychiatric patient with a movement disorder, the differential diagnosis may be more difficult. A number of factors contribute to problems in the differential diagnosis of tardive dyskinesia, as follows:

1. There is no clinical or laboratory test that will establish or rule out tardive dyskinesia.

2. Gradual and painless evolution of the symptoms makes it difficult to date the onset of dyskinesia.

3. The patients themselves are often unaware of the dyskinesias (Alexopoulos, 1979).

4. The severity of the symptoms tends to fluctuate over a period of time.

5. Nondyskinetic movements such as mannerisms, tics, and drug-induced parkinsonism frequently coexist along with tardive dyskinesias in the same patients.

6. It may not always be easy to separate the contribution of neuroleptics to the production of oral dyskinesias from the contribution of other conditions, such as ill-fitting dentures.

7. The physician may be unaware of the long-term use of amphetamines or antihistamine drugs by the patient. These drugs are known to produce dyskinesias, too.

We suggest a sequential procedure to facilitate the differential diagnosis of tardive dyskinesia. When a clinician encounters a patient with abnormal involuntary movements, he or she should ask the following questions:

1. Does the patient have dyskinesia? The concomitant presence or absence of other movement disorders such as tremors and tics is of little relevance for this purpose.
2. Does any other disorder *fully* explain the etiology of the patient's dyskinesia? The mere presence of a dyskinesia-producing condition (e.g., denture problems) does not mean that such a condition is the sole cause of the abnormal movements in that subject.
3. If the dyskinesia is related (partly or entirely) to neuroleptic use, is it tardive dyskinesia? It is necessary to exclude acute and withdrawal dyskinesias, which are also associated with neuroleptic therapy.
4. What subtype of tardive dyskinesia does the patient have? Tardive dyskinesias may be clinically classified according to severity, symptom localization, and, most importantly, reversibility.

It must be added that this sequential procedure, which is useful for the diagnosis of tardive dyskinesia, is only a part of the total workup of the patient. There is hardly any patient with a sole clinical diagnosis of tardive dyskinesia. In all probability, the patient also has an underlying psychiatric or physical disorder for which he or she received neuroleptics. The patient may also have other side effects of neuroleptics and some possibly unrelated disorders (e.g., diabetes mellitus), which must be considered in the overall management of that patient. The outline that follows should therefore be taken as an important part, but not the whole, of the diagnostic workup.

DOES THE PATIENT HAVE DYSKINESIA?

Following is a brief description of some of the more commonly encountered nondyskinetic movement disorders that enter into the differential diagnosis of tardive dyskinesia. For obvious clinical reasons, we have classified these disorders according to the major abnormal involuntary movements with which the patients usually present themselves. Any of the conditions discussed may coexist with tardive dyskinesia. However, if any one or more of these nondyskinetic entities can explain the patient's movement disorder in its entirety, the patient does not have dyskinesia.

Tremors

Of the various causes of tremors, four conditions are more relevant to the present discussion: parkinsonism, rabbit syndrome, Wilson's disease, and cerebellar diseases. Each of these has a different presenting symptom.

Fine Tremors of Fingers at Rest in Parkinsonism. Parkinsonism is characterized by coarse (pill-rolling) tremor of the fingers (sometimes of the wrist and head, too) at rest, rigidity, postural abnormality, and diminished body movements (hypokinesia). The best known form of the disease is the idiopathic paralysis agitans, or Parkinson's disease, which usually begins in middle age. In other cases parkinsonism may be secondary to encephalitis, carbon monoxide or manganese poisoning, head injury, cerebrovascular disorders, or drugs.

In a patient with suspected tardive dyskinesia, the type of parkinsonism that is most likely to be seen is the neuroleptic-induced parkinsonism. It differs from Parkinson's disease in several respects. Neuroleptic-induced parkinsonism is associated with the more rapid tremor of the fingers seen during voluntary movement (rather than at rest); less rigidity; and quicker, greater, and more sustained response to anticholinergic medication than is the case with paralysis agitans. As a rule, the symptoms of parkinsonism remit on discontinuing neuroleptics (although exceptions to this rule have been reported) and sometimes even with continued use of neuroleptics. The absence of dyskinesias of the tongue, jaw, and limbs and improvement with anticholinergic therapy serve to distinguish parkinsonism from tardive dyskinesia.

Fine Tremor of Lips in the Rabbit Syndrome. Villeneuve (1972) first described this uncommon and late extrapyramidal side effect of neuroleptics. Its main symptom is rapid tremor of the lips, and occasionally of the jaw, resembling the movements of a rabbit's mouth while chewing. As suggested by Sovner and DiMascio (1977), this syndrome is related more to parkinsonism than to tardive dyskinesia. The rabbit syndrome responds favorably to anticholinergic agents and is reversible on removal of the neuroleptic. Clinically, the severity of tardive dyskinesia may be inversely correlated with that of the rabbit syndrome in the patients in whom the two disorders coexist. Absence of dyskinesias of the tongue, jaw (apart from tremor), and limbs, and symptom relief with anticholinergic drugs differentiate the rabbit syndrome from tardive dyskinesia.

Coarse Tremor of Upper Limbs in Wilson's Disease. Coarse "flapping" or "wing-beating" tremor of upper limbs and rigidity are the common presenting symptoms of Wilson's disease (hepatolenticular degeneration). Sometimes the tremor may resemble that in parkinsonism or in cerebellar diseases. Signs of liver disease (e.g., jaundice, ascites) accompany or follow the neurological manifestations. Wilson's disease, transmitted by an autosomal recessive gene, usually affects adolescents and young adults. An enzymatic disturbance in copper metabolism results in excessive deposition of copper in a number of tissues, including the liver, basal ganglia, certain other parts of the brain, and the cornea. Kayser–Fleischer (KF) ring (greenish brown pigmentation in the cornea at the sclerocorneal junction) seen on a slit-lamp examination is pathognomonic of Wilson's disease. When neurological signs are present, the KF ring is visible grossly, too. Decreased serum levels of ceruloplasmin (a copper-binding protein) and increased urinary excretion of copper and amino acids are other characteristics. Treatment with copper-chelating agents such as penicillamine offers symptomatic relief.

In young persons with suspected tardive dyskinesia, Wilson's disease can be ruled in or out by performing an ophthalmologic examination, liver function tests, and estimations of serum ceruloplasmin and urinary copper and amino acid levels.

Intention Tremor in Cerebellar Disease. A number of diseases affecting the cerebellum, such as tumors, demyelination (e.g., multiple sclerosis), and familial degeneration, are characterized by tremor of the hands, which is seen during movement and is absent at rest. Other cerebellar signs such as nystagmus, dysarthria, ataxia, dysmetrias, dysdiadochokinesia, and hypotonia are usually present, too. If cerebellar dysfunction is suspected, a thorough neurological evaluation, including computed tomography (CT), is indicated.

Other Causes of Tremor. Fine tremors of the fingers and hands are produced by anxiety states, alcoholism, hyperthyroidism, and drugs, including lithium and tricyclic antidepressants. Delirium tremens is associated with coarse tremors. Senile tremor is fine tremor affecting the lips, jaw, and head. These and other conditions causing tremors can usually be differentiated from tardive dyskinesia on the basis of history and physical examination.

Dystonias

These disorders of muscle spasm are characterized by slow, contorting movements of different body parts. Dystonia musculorum deformans is a disorder transmitted by an autosomal dominant or recessive gene. It becomes manifest by adolescence or even earlier and involves large muscle groups. Its course is progressive, and response to treatment is poor. Occasionally, dystonia musculorum deformans occurs sporadically in later life, without a positive family history, and may be nonprogressive.

In adults, dystonia may rarely occur in the absence of a positive family history.

Secondary dystonias may develop following infections, head injury, poisoning, or other affections of basal ganglia.

The dystonias most likely to be confused with tardive dyskinesia are neuroleptic-induced, acute orofacial dystonias.[3] Protrusion and retraction of the tongue may mimic lingual dyskinesia. The dystonia is, however, often painful. Usually the history shows acute onset following exposure to neuroleptics, especially the "high-potency" types, such as trifluoperazine and haloperidol. The involuntary movements are slow. Oculogyric crisis, torticollis, and tortipelvis are also present in a number of cases. Such dystonias respond dramatically to antihistaminic, muscle-relaxant, and anticholinergic medications. Spontaneous improvement following neuroleptic withdrawal is a rule. Thus phenomenology and response to treatment help to differentiate acute dystonias from dyskinesias. (Chronic or tardive dystonias may, however, form a part of the tardive dyskinesia syndrome and may have similar treatment-response characteristics.)

Myoclonus

The rapid, lightning-like jerks of myoclonus should usually present no difficulty in the differential diagnosis of dyskinesia. Certain forms of myo-

---

[3]Idiopathic orofacial dystonia (Meige's disease) usually has its onset in middle age, and is characterized by prolonged, symmetric, spasmodic contractions of orofacial muscles (Tolosa, 1981).

clonus, such as palatal myoclonus, occur during sleep, too. When myoclonus is a part of epilepsy, EEG abnormalities (usually polyspikes and waves) are present. Dyskinesias of the tongue, jaw, and lips are absent.

One condition in which myoclonus is a symptom that may create some diagnostic problem in cases of suspected dyskinesia is epilepsia partialis continua, or Kojewnikoff's epilepsy. Repeated abnormal movements of localized body parts, especially limbs, may superficially resemble dyskinesias. Careful observation (epilepsia partialis continua is monotonously rhythmic) and EEG will usually aid in settling the diagnosis.

Tics

Apparently purposeful tics, which result from coordinated activity of a number of related muscles, are often present in normal persons and also occur in persons with a variety of psychiatric and neurological disorders. Differentiating tics from dyskinesias is not difficult when the onset of tics has been known to precede the start of neuroleptic treatment. *De novo* appearance of tics in a patient receiving neuroleptics suggests a need to consider tardive dyskinesia as a diagnostic possibility. In such cases the clinician should apply various diagnostic criteria for tardive dyskinesia (described earlier). One example of a diagnostic difficulty is Gilles de la Tourette's syndrome with multiple and complex motor and vocal tics. Treatment of this disorder with haloperidol may, on rare occasions, produce tardive dyskinesia; hence Tourette's syndrome is discussed later under the section on primary causes of dyskinesia.

Mannerisms

Distinguishing between psychotic mannerisms and drug-induced dyskinesias is not always easy. As noted earlier, mannerisms are more consistent with an individual's personality and are often less stereotypically repeated than dyskinesias. Sometimes long-term observation and studying the response to medications may help in the differential diagnosis. If a reduction in neuroleptic dose aggravates the abnormal movements without influencing other psychopathology, or if anticholinergic drugs selectively worsen the movement disorder, the differential diagnosis would be in favor of tardive dyskinesia rather than mannerisms. In those few patients in whom it can be established definitely that the same movements had been present before neuroleptic therapy was initiated, the diagnosis of mannerisms would be favored.

Compulsions

A compulsive patient not only is aware of his or her movements, but also resists them consciously. Controlling these movements, however, produces almost unbearable anxiety, which is relieved only when he or she executes the act. These features, in addition to the patient's obsessive personality and the complex nature of the movements, aid in discriminating between compulsions and dyskinesia.

Akathisia

The subjective feeling of restlessness accompanying the inability to sit still is the distinguishing feature of neuroleptic-induced akathisia, unlike dyskinesia. Neuroleptic withdrawal almost always results in the disappearance of acute or subacute akathisia. Increasing the dose worsens akathisia, but often suppresses dyskinesia. (Sometimes, however, chronic akathisia seen in patients receiving long-term neuroleptic therapy has pharmacologic characteristics similar to those of other manifestations of tardive dyskinesia. In such cases akathisia may be considered an atypical variant of tardive dyskinesia.)

WHAT IS THE PRIMARY CAUSE OF THE PATIENT'S DYSKINESIA?

Once it is concluded that a patient has dyskinesia, the next step is to determine its main cause. This involves demonstrating not only that a dyskinesia-producing condition is present, but also that the condition is primarily responsible for the patient's movement disorder. Presented here are various conditions associated with dyskinesias, according to localization of symptoms in patients from different age groups.

Predominantly Orofacial Dyskinesias

Such dyskinesias are more frequent in the elderly than in the young.

In Children and Young Adults. Although abnormal involuntary movements of the orofacial region are not rare in younger patients, predominantly orofacial dyskinesias (which may mimic tardive dyskinesias) are uncommon. The condition to rule out in a young patient with prominent orofacial dyskinesias is the use of drugs. Of the various nonneuroleptic agents that may produce dyskinesias (Chapter 8), amphetamines and antihistamine drugs, taken for long periods, are most likely to be associated with such a movement disorder. A history of treatment with these agents should be sought, and, if positive, the drugs should be discontinued. In most instances the symptoms are readily reversible on medication withdrawal. Sometimes, patients with amphetamine dependence may deny a history of amphetamine abuse. If a clinician has reason to suspect that this may be the case, the possibility of amphetamine abuse should be thoroughly explored. Paper chromatography or the methyl orange test for detecting amphetamines in urine may be useful.

In the Middle-Aged and Elderly. Orofacial dyskinesias in this age group are not rare.

1. Denture or dental problems are probably the most common cause of nontardive oral dyskinesias in the elderly. In patients with dental problems or ill-fitting dentures, proper dental treatment results in alleviation of the oral dyskinesia (see Chapter 10). Usually, dyskinesias of dental origin are mild in intensity.

2. Lesions of the basal ganglia, including demyelination (as in multiple sclerosis), degeneration (e.g., Alzheimer's disease), neoplasms, and vascular pathology (e.g., arteriosclerosis), may result in orofacial dyskinesias, although this is quite uncommon.

3. Spontaneous persistent dyskinesias occurring in the absence of any known cause of such abnormal movements are rare (Altrocchi, 1972; Marsden, Tarsy, & Baldessarini, 1975). They are similar in appearance to the tardive dyskinesias, but tend to be mild in severity.

Limb Dyskinesias with or without Orofacial
and Trunk Involvement

A number of conditions can induce such abnormal movements, usually of the choreiform type.

In Children and Young Adults.
1. Sydenham's or rheumatic chorea (St. Vitus's dance) is thought to be a complication of rheumatic fever. It usually occurs between the ages of 5 and 15 and is characterized by choreiform movements of the limbs, face,

and trunk. In most cases the symptoms remit spontaneously within 3 to 6 weeks. Occasionally, mild choreiform movements may persist for several to many months. Other manifestations of rheumatic fever (polyarthritis, carditis, subcutaneous nodules, and erythema nodosum) may precede, accompany, or follow chorea. A form of Sydenham's chorea that occurs during pregnancy in young women is called "chorea gravidarum." Most of the laboratory tests (except for antistreptolysin-O titers) are normal during an episode of rheumatic chorea.

2. Gilles de la Tourette's syndrome is a rare, chronic disease afflicting children between 3 and 15 years of age (Shapiro, Shapiro, Bruun, *et al.,* 1978). It occurs three times as often in males as in females. There is frequently a family history of tics, compulsions, or Tourette's syndrome. Recently there have been case reports of Tourette's syndrome induced by long-term neuroleptic treatment (Kauffman, Jeste, Cutler, *et al.,* unpublished data; Klawans, Falk, Nausieda, *et al.,* 1978; Seeman, Patel, & Pyke, 1981; Stahl, 1980). The main symptoms are multiple motor and vocal tics and coprolalia (compulsive utterances of obscene words and phrases). The syndrome is believed to be associated with striatal catecholaminergic hyperactivity. Its relationship with brain damage is uncertain. The most effective treatment for symptom relief has been the use of a neuroleptic such as haloperidol; treatment with clonidine is also promising (Cohen, Detlor, Young, *et al.,* 1980).

Tourette's syndrome can be differentiated from other movement disorders because of its distinctive symptomatology. In early cases where the patient has only motor tics, the differentiation may be more difficult and may require a follow-up. On rare occasions, long-term use of haloperidol for Tourette's syndrome may lead to tardive dyskinesia (Mizrahi, Holtzman, & Tharp, 1980), and separating the latter from the motor manifestations of the original syndrome may be difficult. Careful documentation of various symptoms before and during the course of haloperidol therapy may aid in the early detection of tardive dyskinesia in these patients.

3. Hysterical conversion reaction is among the more common causes of dyskinesias in the young. Generally, such dyskinesias involve multiple parts of the body, tend to be more severe when the patient is attended to, and disappear when the subject is alone. The movements are often dramatic and bizarre and are sometimes grotesque; yet the patient rarely falls or gets injured because of the abnormal movements. A careful history usually reveals an unconscious motivation for the symptoms. Premorbid personality may or may not be hysterical—that is, characterized by traits such

as labile moods, self-centered attitude, attention-seeking tendency, low frustration tolerance, and excessive dependence. The symptoms are precipitated by stress, and removal of the stressful situation is likely to result in the disappearance of symptoms.

It is not uncommon to see hysterical overlay in patients with other movement disorders, including tardive dyskinesia. In such cases a dual diagnosis is warranted.

4. Malingering differs from hysteria in that it has a conscious motivation. In practice, however, the difference between hysteria and malingering is not clear-cut in all cases.

5. Hyperthyroidism occasionally manifests in the form of choreiform movements of limbs, along with other typical symptoms such as fine tremor of the hands, excessive sweating, anxiety, exophthalmos, and lid lag (Klawans, 1973). The thyroid is often enlarged, and thyroid function tests (e.g., serum protein-bound iodine, T_3 and T_4 levels) are abnormal. Diagnosis of hyperthyroidism is usually not difficult, provided that the possibility of hyperthyroid chorea is kept in mind.

6. Hypoparathyroidism has been reported, in isolated cases, to produce choreoathetoid dyskinesias. Hypoparathyroidism is usually secondary to accidental removal of parathyroids during thyroid surgery. The typical signs and symptoms include carpopedal spasm, numbness and cramps in the limbs, laryngeal stridor, and convulsions. Laboratory tests reveal hypocalcemia, hyperphosphatemia, absence of calcium in the urine, and increased calcifications on skull X ray. Hypoparathyroidism is a relatively rare, but easily diagnosable, cause of choreiform dyskinesias.

7. In Chapter 8, dyskinesias induced by nonneuroleptic drugs are discussed. Of such drugs, L-dopa is rarely used in younger patients. Amphetamines and antihistamine agents are likely to be implicated more often. Toxic amounts of tricyclic antidepressants or anticonvulsants may also induce choreoathetosis. A number of other drugs, such as the antimalarials, produce acute dyskinesias, which respond dramatically to drug withdrawal or to administration of anticholinergic and antihistamine agents. Obtaining a detailed medication history and then modifying the drug treatment accordingly will usually enable one to attribute a patient's dyskinesia to the likely offending agent.

8. Huntington's disease figures prominently in the differential diagnosis of tardive dyskinesia, especially when limb involvement is pronounced. Huntington's disease, or chronic progressive chorea, is transmitted by an autosomal dominant gene. The onset of symptoms may occur at any age, but is usually seen between 30 and 50 years. The characteristic twin features of this syndrome, chorea and dementia, may present simultaneously, or one (usually chorea) may precede the other. The abnormal movements are indistinguishable from those of dyskinesias induced by neuroleptics or L-dopa. The disease follows a slow, but progressively downhill, course and is usually fatal within 15 years of onset of symptoms. The only major palliative treatment is with neuroleptics such as haloperidol. Dopaminergic and anticholinergic drugs make the movements worse.

The movement disorder in Huntington's disease is similar to that in tardive dyskinesia in phenomenology[4] and in pharmacologic responses. The following characteristics of Huntington's disease should aid in its diagnosis: (a) family history of Huntington's disease, (b) presence of dementia, (c) slowly progressive downhill course, and (d) atrophy of caudate on pneumoencephalogram or CT scan. Sometimes, however, the differential diagnosis is difficult—for example, when the family history is unclear or unreliable or before dementia has become manifest. In such instances CT scanning and long-term follow-up would be warranted. Tardive dyskinesia is not associated with caudate atrophy on CT scans (Jeste, Wagner, Weinberger, et al., 1980). Also, the symptoms of tardive dyskinesia tend not to worsen progressively, but to fluctuate in severity or remain relatively stable over a period of years.

A different problem arises, however, when tardive dyskinesia develops in a patient with Huntington's disease who has been receiving chronic neuroleptic treatment (Buxton, 1976). This situation is similar to that seen with Tourette's syndrome. The use of neuroleptics may thus create a therapeutic dilemma. These drugs suppress many distressing symptoms of chorea, and yet may themselves produce dyskinesias *de novo*. Neuroleptic withdrawal or dose reduction may improve tardive dyskinesia in some patients, but is likely to aggravate the original choreic disorder. Switching to a different type of neuroleptic may be useful. Also, sedatives such as benzodiazepines may be helpful in the treatment of Huntington's disease patients who are difficult to manage.

9. Other diseases affecting basal ganglia may produce dyskinesias. Such disorders include encephalitides; neoplasms; vascular, degenerative,

---

[4]One interesting difference between the manifestations of the two disorders is in anomalies of conjugate ocular movements. Whereas impairment of optokinetic nystagmus has been reported in both conditions (Lipper, 1973), other disturbances, such as a disorder of upward gaze, reduced velocity of eye movements, and a fixed stare, have been described only in patients with Huntington's disease (Petit & Milbled, 1973).

or demyelinating diseases; collagen diseases, such as systemic lupus erythe-matosus; and metabolic encephalopathies, such as those resulting from liver diseases. It is not surprising that many types of lesions involving specific parts of the basal ganglia can produce dyskinesias. Historically, the best known of these has been von Economo's epidemic encephalitis lethargica, which has now become extinct. No new cases of this disorder have been reported during the past several decades.

When dyskinesia is accompanied by other neurological manifestations, or when the dyskinesia is becoming progressively more severe, a thorough evaluation is necessary to rule out the diseases of basal ganglia mentioned here.

In the Middle-Aged and Elderly. Some of the dyskinesia-producing disorders in this age group are similar to those in children and young adults. The three most important causes of non-neuroleptic-induced limb dyskinesia are as follows:

1. Huntington's disease.
2. Other diseases of basal ganglia. Degenerative and neoplastic diseases are more common in this age group than in younger subjects.
3. Nonneuroleptic drugs, especially L-dopa, used in the treatment of patients with Parkinson's disease. Differences between L-dopa-induced and neuroleptic-induced tardive dyskinesia are summarized in Chapter 8.

WHAT TYPE OF NEUROLEPTIC-INDUCED DYSKINESIA DOES THE PATIENT HAVE?

When it is found that neuroleptics have been at least partly responsible for the patient's dyskinesia, it does not necessarily mean that the patient has tardive dyskinesia. Neuroleptics can also produce acute dyskinesia and withdrawal-emergent dyskinesia, which differ from tardive dyskinesia in course and prognosis and probably in pathophysiology, too. Phenomenologically, however, all three types are similar.

Acute Dyskinesia

Dyskinesias that occur early in neuroleptic treatment have been known for a long time. They are comparable to other acute and subacute extrapyramidal syndromes caused by neuroleptics, namely, dystonia, akathisia, and parkinsonism. It is also worth noting that several nonneuroleptic drugs (e.g., antimalarial hydroxyquinolines) induce similar acute dyskinesias (see Chapter 8). With neuroleptics, the acute dyskinesias are less frequent than other acute extrapyramidal side effects. Ayd (1961) estimated their prevalence to be about 2.3%. They tend to remit quickly after neuroleptics are withdrawn or the dose is reduced; sometimes even continued administration of neuroleptics leads to the development of tolerance to acute dyskinesia. The symptoms also respond well to anticholinergic or antihistamine drugs. It is possible that nigrostriatal dopamine deficit or cholinergic excess may be responsible for this syndrome. There is as yet no evidence to show that patients who had acute dyskinesias are any more prone to develop tardive dyskinesia than patients without such a history.

Rapid onset of symptoms and quick response to neuroleptic withdrawal or to anticholinergic, antihistamine drugs should enable a clinician to differentiate acute from tardive dyskinesia.

Withdrawal-Emergent Dyskinesia

Neuroleptic withdrawal results in the development of dyskinesia in a variable proportion of patients. The incidence of withdrawal-induced dyskinesia is probably much higher in children (reported to be as high as 45% to 50%; Engelhardt, Polizos, & Waizer, 1975; Winsberg, Hurwic, & Perel, 1977) than in adults. As a rule, the dyskinesia disappears spontaneously within 1 to 3 weeks of stopping medication. The time course of withdrawal dyskinesia is similar to that of nigrostriatal, postsynaptic catecholamine receptor supersensitivity in animals, suggesting the possible pathophysiology underlying at least some types of withdrawal dyskinesia (see Chapter 5). Available clinical evidence does not indicate any definite relationship between withdrawal dyskinesia and tardive dyskinesia. Withdrawal-emergent dyskinesia remits spontaneously, or if neuroleptics are readministered. If the symptoms persist for at least several weeks after neuroleptic withdrawal or reinstitution, the diagnosis would be tardive dyskinesia rather than withdrawal dyskinesia.

Tardive Dyskinesia

After all the preceding conditions in the differential diagnosis are ruled out as being the principal cause of a patient's dyskinesia, a diagnosis of tardive dyskinesia is suggested. We must add, however, that the diagnosis of tardive dyskinesia is not made merely through a process of exclusion, but is also based on a demonstration of positive features of this syndrome. The specific diagnostic criteria for tardive dyskinesia were enumerated earlier.

WHAT SUBTYPE OF TARDIVE DYSKINESIA DOES THE PATIENT HAVE?

Tardive dyskinesia is not a single disease with uniform course, prognosis, and treatment. Hence subtyping a patient's tardive dyskinesia is important. This can be done in several ways, although the clinical and theoretical significance of some of the subtypes is not yet clear.

Subtyping according to Symptom Severity

There is no single method of assessing severity of dyskinesia that has both high reliability and validity. Gardos, Cole, and La Brie (1977a) have reviewed the subject of assessment techniques for tardive dyskinesia. They rightly point out that techniques using instrumentation (e.g., polygraphs) tend to have high reliability, but doubtful validity, since they do not distinguish between dyskinesia and nondyskinetic (including normal) movements. In contrast, subjective methods of rating, such as those employing rating scales, are more valid, but may have variable interrater reliability.

Probably the most satisfactory way of assessing intensity of dyskinesia is by using standardized rating scales. The two most widely used scales have been the AIMS, developed by the Psychopharmacology Research Branch of the National Institute of Mental Health, and Simpson's Rockland Research Institute Tardive Dyskinesia Rating Scale (Simpson, Lee, Zoubok, *et al.*, 1979) (see Appendix). Of these two, the AIMS has been employed more extensively; also, videotapes for training people to use the AIMS properly are available. The AIMS lists seven areas of the body and the more common abnormal movements in each area. Abnormal involuntary movements in each area are rated on a scale of 0 to 4. There is also a global rating of severity. With some experience, the AIMS can be employed with satisfactory reliability. It must be made clear that the AIMS is meant only for assessing intensity of all types of abnormal involuntary movements and not for distinguishing between tardive dyskinesia and other movement disorders. Hence clinical judgment must be used in differentially rating the severity of tardive dyskinesia and that of other concomitant abnormal movements.

The Simpson scale is a 34-item scale (although a 17-item, abbreviated scale is also available), with a provision for writing in idiosyncratic signs. Each item is given a score of anywhere from 1 to 6, and definitions of each scoring point are mentioned. Again, the interrater reliability of this scale is high when used by trained personnel. The scale includes certain signs, such as spasmodic torticollis, caressing of face and hair, and akathisia, which may not be a part of the tardive dyskinesia syndrome. Yet, this scale is, on the whole, more specific for tardive dyskinesia than is the AIMS.

Using a standardized scale, the clinician should try to judge the severity of the patient's dyskinesia either quantitatively or qualitatively (mild, moderate, or severe). The severity may change over a period of time; hence recording the symptom intensity on different occasions is useful. This procedure is also recommended for use in long-term follow-up of all patients on neuroleptics, whether or not they have tardive dyskinesia. Early detection of tardive dyskinesia, noticing relatively sudden changes in severity of dyskinesia, and assessing the patient's response to treatments are all facilitated by regular use of rating scales such as the AIMS or Simpson's scale, which take only a few minutes for completion.

Subtyping according to Symptom Localization

Barnes and Kidger (1979) suggested that orofacial dyskinesia and limb dyskinesia might be different entities, differing from each other in neuropathology, course, and treatment. According to these authors, orofacial dyskinesia represents the central component, and limb dyskinesia the peripheral component, of the tardive dyskinesia syndrome, and these two components may not always be related to each other. In support of such subtyping is the observation that limb dyskinesia is more common in younger patients, whereas the reverse is true for orofacial dyskinesia; also, it has been reported by several investigators (Bucci, 1971; Gardos & Cole, 1975; Jeste et al., 1977) that orofacial dyskinesia responds to treatment better than limb dyskinesia.

There are, however, other data that do not support the concept that the orofacial and limb dyskinesias are different entities. As noted earlier, about 80% of all tardive dyskinesia patients have orofacial manifestations, and 50% have limb involvement. Two-thirds of patients with limb dyskinesia also have orofacial symptoms. Thus clinically there is considerable overlap between the limb and orofacial dyskinesias.

To conclude, the clinical and theoretical implications of subtyping tardive dyskinesias according to topography of symptoms are uncertain.

Subtyping according to Course

The course of dyskinesia may be studied in relation to the neuroleptic therapy. Most studies show that continued administration of neuroleptics for months to patients with dyskinesia results in a temporary suppression of symptoms, but produces neither cure nor aggravation of dyskinesia (see Chapter 10). Withdrawal of neuroleptics for several months to several years has been found to reverse dyskinesia in 37% of the dyskinetic patients (Table 3-4). Thus there may be two subtypes of tardive dyskinesia: reversible and persistent. A third subtype, which we, and probably other clinicians, too, have encountered on occasion, but which has not been formally delineated, is intermittent dyskinesia.

Reversible Dyskinesia. It is often believed that the rate of reversibility of dyskinesia is positively correlated with the length of neuroleptic withdrawal. Table 3-4 shows, however, that this rate is highest (33.5%) during the first 3 months of neuroleptic discontinuance. Thus for research purposes, relief of symptoms within 3 months of neuroleptic withdrawal may be used as a test for reversibility of tardive dyskinesia, although for clinical purposes, the longer the withdrawal, the greater the chance of remission. It is not known whether readministration of neuroleptics results in a reinduction of dyskinesia or whether reversible dyskinesia is merely an early stage in the development of persistent dyskinesia. Our study (Jeste, Potkin, Sinha, *et al.,* 1979) showed that readministration of neuroleptics to eight patients with reversible dyskinesia did not reinduce dyskinesia during the 1-year follow-up. Similarly, we found no positive relationship between duration and persistence of dyskinesia. It is quite likely that a number of patients who respond to a variety of nonspecific treatments have reversible dyskinesia (see Chapter 10). Various factors that have been reported to be related to reversibility of tardive dyskinesia are discussed in Chapter 4. Biochemical and neuropsychological studies comparing patients with reversible and persistent dyskinesias are, however, lacking.

Intermittent Dyskinesia. We have observed a few patients who have had remissions and relapses of dyskinesia during the course of stable neuroleptic therapy. There was no obvious association between the appear-

Table 3-4. Treatment with Neuroleptic Withdrawal

Investigators	Length of withdrawal	Number of patients			Factors associated with persistent dyskinesia
		Improved	Not improved	Total	
Uhrbrand and Faurbye (1960)	.5–22 (average 5.6) months	8	12	20	Old age and brain damage
Haddenbrock (1964)	NS[a]	13	3	16	
Hunter, Earl, and Thornicroft (1964)	8–24 months	0	13	13	Brain damage
Faurbye, Rasch, Petersen, et al. (1964)	NS	NS ("most cases")	NS	109	
Pryce and Edwards (1966)	"Some months"	1	14	15	Brain damage
Demars (1966)	8.2 weeks (mean)	2	15	17	
Degkwitz and Wenzel (1967)	9 months	NS	NS ("most cases")	130	
Turunen and Achte (1967)	NS	10	16	26	Brain damage?
Paulson (1968)	3 months	0	33	33	Brain damage judged by abnormal EEG
Crane, Ruiz, Kernohan, et al. (1969)	10 weeks	18	16	34	Lower doses of neuroleptics before study (but not related to age, sex, or length of hospitalization).
Degkwitz (1969)	7–10 months	104	169	273	Old age and history of interrupted neuroleptic treatment (but not related to duration and dosage of drug therapy)
Edwards (1970)	2–12 (mostly 10–12) months	3	18	21	Brain damage
Dynes (1970)	6–12 months	0	10	10	Brain damage
Crane (1971b)	6–24 months	9	30	39	(Not related to age, sex, and length of hospitalization)

Study	Duration of treatment				Factors associated with reversibility
Hershon, Kennedy, and McGuire (1972)	13–22 (average 16) weeks	23	NS	NS	
Crane (1972b)	1–2 weeks	26	18	8	
	2 weeks twice	20	NS	NS	
Turek, Kurland, Hanlon, et al. (1972)	44 weeks	8	NS	NS	(Generally, worsening on withdrawing neuroleptics and improvement on reinstituting them)
	12 weeks twice	13	NS	NS	
	12 weeks	15	NS	NS	
Yagi, Ogita, Ohtsuka, et al. (1976)	Up to 2 years	14	4	10	Old age, brain damage, length of neuroleptic treatment, and duration of dyskinesia (but not related to sex, primary diagnosis, and type and dose of neuroleptics)
Quitkin, Rifkin, Gochfeld, et al. (1977)	Up to 4 months	11 (+1 with dose reduction)	1	10 (+1 with dose reduction)	Duration of dyskinesia
Alpert and Friedhoff (1978)	3 months	12	3	9	
Jeste, Potkin, Sinha, et al. (1979)	3 months or longer	18	8	10	Length of neuroleptic treatment and number of lengthy drug interruptions in the past
Itoh and Yagi (1979)	Less than 3 months	3	1	2	Old age
	Variable (up to 5 years)	14	5	9	
Jeste (unpublished data)	3 months or longer	14	10	4	Aging
TOTAL		631	399	232	

[a]NS = not stated.

ance or disappearance of dyskinesia and the patient's clinical status or therapeutic alteration. Gardos, Cole, and Sokol (1977) described patients whose dyskinesia underwent "very extensive fluctuations" in severity over time. The authors suggested that such "fluctuating" patients—who are probably similar to our intermittent dyskinesia patients—may be responsible for both false-positive and false-negative results in treatment studies and should preferably be excluded from drug trials. It would be useful to study such patients in a prospective, long-term fashion, with an eye on biochemical and other changes accompanying the fluctuations. It also remains to be seen whether patients with intermittent dyskinesia eventually develop persistent tardive dyskinesia.

Cutler, Post, Rey, et al. (1981) reported the occurrence of "state-dependent dyskinesia" in two rapidly cycling manic–depressive patients. The two patients, a 57-year-old woman and a 58-year-old man, had significantly greater dyskinesia during depression than during mania over several cycles. Tardive dyskinesia was most severe during the period of "switch" from mania into depression. It is worth mentioning that both patients, who had past histories of long-term, high-dose neuroleptic treatments, were drug free throughout the observation period of several months. Detailed studies of larger numbers of such patients are warranted.

Persistent Dyskinesia. This is one of the most serious complications of long-term neuroleptic treatment, since it does not respond to neuroleptic withdrawal or to most other available treatments. Although there have been relatively few studies on the course of dyskinesia over long periods in patients with persistent dyskinesia, the general impression is that there is often no marked worsening of the symptoms. A rapidly deteriorating course should suggest the possibility of a progressive brain disease and warrants a complete neurological workup and other medical evaluation. The following case history illustrates this point.

A 61-year-old chronic schizophrenic woman with a long history of neuroleptic treatment was referred because of severe dyskinesia involving the face, tongue, limbs, and trunk. The manifestations were typical of tardive dyskinesia. The patient's family and physician asserted, however, that the symptoms had begun only 2 or 3 months earlier and had rapidly become worse. A complete medical evaluation, including laboratory investigations, was suggested. This uncovered a carcinoma of the breast, with possible metastases in the brain. The patient died a few months later. Autopsy was refused.

In the majority of patients with persistent tardive dyskinesia, the symptoms remain fairly stable over a long period, although some fluctuations in severity do occur. It is necessary to add that "persistent" *does not* always mean "irreversible." We agree with Itoh and Yagi (1979) that dyskinesia may be called irreversible only after the symptoms have been found to persist for several years after discontinuation of neuroleptics.

Subtyping according to Biochemical–Pharmacologic Characteristics

Several investigators, such as Casey (1976) and Mackay and Sheppard (1979), have proposed the existence of distinct pharmacologic subtypes of tardive dyskinesia. Casey and Denney (1977) found that some patients responded to antidopaminergic or cholinomimetic drugs, whereas, paradoxically, others benefited from catecholamine agonists or anticholinergic drugs. Mackay and Sheppard (1979) suggested that the most pragmatic therapeutic approach to tardive dyskinesia might be to define a "pharmacological signature" for each patient in an acute dose study. This interesting idea deserves careful study in a large number of patients.

We believe that, if there are distinct pharmacologic subtypes of tardive dyskinesia, it may eventually be possible to predict them on the basis of biochemical tests. Thus patients with elevated noradrenergic activity may need treatment with drugs such as propranolol, whereas those with dopaminergic excess may respond well to specific dopamine antagonists. This is an area with considerable potential for valuable research.

Subtyping according to Other Characteristics

Tardive dyskinesia in the elderly is more often persistent than it is in younger subjects. Similarly, dyskinesia in the aged is usually orofacial, whereas that in the young frequently involves the limbs. Beyond these two facts, other differences between dyskinesias in the old and the young remain to be explored. Similarly, differences in dyskinesias according to primary psychiatric diagnosis (schizophrenia, affective disorders, organic mental syndrome, etc.) and to length of neuroleptic treatment necessary to induce dyskinesia are worth studying.

COMPLICATIONS

Severe or long-lasting tardive dyskinesia may result in a number of physical complications. On the other hand, even mild dyskinesia may lead to psychosocial problems in well-functioning patients.

PHYSICAL COMPLICATIONS

1. Dental and denture problems are among the common sequelae of oral dyskinesia. Abnormal movements of the tongue, jaw, and lips may produce loosening of natural or artificial teeth. Although it is true that ill-fitting dentures may contribute to oral dyskinesia, the reverse is also found in a number of cases.

2. Traumatic ulceration of the tongue, cheeks, and lips may result from involuntary movements of those parts against sharp teeth. The ulcers may become infected.

3. Hyperkinetic dysarthria has been described by Maxwell, Massengil, and Nashold (1970) and Portnoy (1979). Random and continual movements of the tongue and lips may produce muffled speech, which sometimes becomes unintelligible. The dysarthria may be characterized by intermittent voice breaks with arrests in expiration. There may also be changes in articulatory posturing, omission of sibilants, and marked fluctuations in oral diadochokinesia.

4. Swallowing disorders secondary to dyskinesias of the tongue and pharynx are not rare, although they are infrequently diagnosed. Massengil and Nashold (1969) conducted a cinefluorographic analysis of the swallowing pattern in three dyskinetic patients and found a pronounced tongue thrust interfering with swallowing. A frame-by-frame tracing of the Rugar bolus showed that the tongue, instead of completing its normal upward and backward motion as in normal swallowing, repeatedly jutted forward. This made it difficult for the bolus to move from the oral cavity into the pharyngeal area.

5. Impairment of the physiological optokinetic nystagmus was detected in 9 out of 12 dyskinetic patients by Lipper (1973). The clinical significance of this finding in patients with tardive dyskinesia is uncertain.

6. Respiratory disturbances in patients with tardive dyskinesia have been reported by Ayd (1979), Casey and Rabins (1978), Jackson *et al.* (1980), and Weiner, Goetz, Nausieda, *et al.* (1980). Such disturbances usually take the form of shortness of breath at rest and irregularities in respiratory rate, depth, and rhythm, accompanied by involuntary grunting, snorting, and gasping noises. Signs of cardiopulmonary disease, such as orthopnea, cyanosis, and edema, are absent. The only abnormality found on laboratory tests is respiratory alkalosis.

7. Severe gastrointestinal dyskinesia that required hospitalization was described by Casey and Rabins (1978). Persistent vomiting, aerophagia, episodic retching, and paroxysmal contraction and distension of the abdominal wall associated with irregular respiration were thought to be gastrointestinal components of the tardive dyskinesia syndrome. The patient, who also had orofacial, limb, and trunk dyskinesia, improved considerably with haloperidol treatment.

8. Weight loss may occur among patients with severe dyskinesia, but is probably not common. Gardos, Cole, and Sokol (1977) reported significant negative correlations between body weight and severity of tardive dyskinesia in two patients followed longitudinally. However, a 2-year follow-up study of 253 patients revealed no characteristic or persistent weight changes associated with tardive dyskinesia, even in patients with severe dyskinesia (Smith, Dunn, & Burke, 1980).

9. Reduced life expectancy was reported by Mehta, Mallya, and Volavka (1978), who found that significantly more dyskinesia patients were dead at the end of a 5-year follow-up period than matched controls. The mean age of patients in each group was 72.3 years. Of the 35 patients in each group, 19 dyskinetic patients and 12 controls had died by the time of the follow-up. In another preliminary study, Kucharski, Smith, and Dunn (1979) did not find such an association between tardive dyskinesia and mortality.

10. Falls and injuries due to gait disturbances may occur.

PSYCHOSOCIAL SEQUELAE

Embarrassment resulting from the obvious abnormal movements of the various body parts can and does produce psychosocial problems, especially for outpatients. Even mild dyskinesia may produce anxiety, guilt, shame, and anger and may lead to severe reactive depression. Since the dyskinesia is a social and occupational handicap, it often produces functional deficits and stigmatization. Kucharski *et al.* (1980) found that inpatients with higher AIMS scores were not discharged as readily as those with lower ones. One possible explanation for this phenomenon, which was observed across all age groups, could be that tardive dyskinesia hindered rehabilitation efforts and community acceptance of the patients. Loss of job skills and self-care skills is particularly noticeable among young men with dyskinesia. Baldessarini (1981) reports one suicide, one instance of paranoid psychosis in a formerly neurotic patient, and one case of psychotic depression that were attributable to tardive dyskinesia.

CHAPTER IV

Etiology

Tardive dyskinesia results from long-term drug-treatment. Yet, only a certain proportion of patients so treated develop tardive dyskinesia. It is apparent that a number of variables related both to the drug treatment and to the individual patient play a role in the etiology of this disorder.

Treatment-related variables include (1) length of neuroleptic treatment, (2) amount of neuroleptic intake, (3) type of neuroleptic, (4) drug-free periods, (5) polypharmacy, (6) antiparkinsonian drugs, (7) other drugs, (8) hospitalization, and (9) physical treatments.

Patient-related variables include (1) age, (2) gender, (3) constitutional predisposition, (4) dental state, (5) primary psychiatric illness, (6) susceptibility to other extrapyramidal side effects, and (7) race and eye color.

TREATMENT-RELATED VARIABLES

LENGTH OF NEUROLEPTIC TREATMENT

On analyzing data with discriminant function analysis, Gardos, Cole, and La Brie (1977b) and Jeste, Potkin, Sinha, *et al.* (1979) found that duration of neuroleptic treatment was a significant discriminator between dyskinetic and nondyskinetic patients. In a cross-cultural comparison of psychiatric inpatients from Turkey and the United States, Crane (1968a) observed a markedly higher prevalence of tardive dyskinesia in the American patient population, which had received neuroleptics for a much longer period than the Turkish patients.

It may seem surprising that a number of investigators (Brandon *et al.,*

1971; Demars, 1966; Jus *et al.*, 1976b; Kennedy *et al.*, 1971; Mallya, Jose, Baig, *et al.*, 1979; Simpson, Varga, Lee, *et al.*, 1978) have reported a lack of a significant positive relationship between tardive dyskinesia and length of neuroleptic administration. There are at least two possible explanations for this apparent discrepancy. First, constitutionally susceptible individuals may develop dyskinesia with neuroleptic use for relatively short periods, whereas nonpredisposed patients may remain free of dyskinesia despite longer treatment with these drugs. Second, the prevalence of tardive dyskinesia may not rise linearly with the duration of drug treatment. For example, Crane (1974) reported that the prevalence of dyskinesia in his patients was not related in a simple, direct manner to the length of neuroleptic intake. Moderate and severe dyskinesia was more frequent in patients who had been treated for 6 to 8 years than in those who had received shorter or longer courses of treatment. This finding lends support to the notion that factors other than the length of neuroleptic administration contribute to the etiology of tardive dyskinesia. It may also indicate that the number of patients with dyskinesia became smaller among patients treated for more than 8 years when compared to patients treated for 6 to 8 years—possibly a result of remission of dyskinesia in some patients (spontaneous or treatment-related) or deaths (or disappearance from the study population for other reasons) of some patients with dyskinesia.

In an interesting analysis, Siede and Muller (1967) observed that their organic mental disorder patients with tardive dyskinesia had a history of neuroleptic therapy ranging from 6 months to 3 years. In contrast, the "nonorganic" patients with dyskinesia had been treated for 3 to 10 years. A number of investigators (Chouinard & Jones, 1979; Hale, 1974; Moline, 1975; Stimmel, 1976) have reported cases in which the symptoms of dyskinesia developed within a few months of starting neuroleptics. These findings are consistent with the notion of constitutional susceptibility to tardive dyskinesia in some patients.

In summary, the interaction of the length of treatment with other variables such as constitutional predisposition may be more crucial than the duration of drug use per se. Several questions with considerable clinical relevance remain unanswered. Do different types of neuroleptics have to be administered for the same length of time before dyskinesia manifests in a given proportion of patients taking the particular drugs? Is it possible that persons who have not developed dyskinesia after some years of drug treatment will never develop this complication? It has been suggested that reversible dyskinesia develops earlier in the course of neuroleptic therapy and that with continued treatment it becomes persistent (Faurbye, 1970; Hollister, 1975). This suggestion is unproven, but needs to be explored further.

AMOUNT OF NEUROLEPTIC INTAKE

Daily Dose

Demars (1966), Jus *et al.* (1976b), and Lehmann *et al.* (1970) reported that the average daily or monthly amount of neuroleptics that the patients with tardive dyskinesia had received in the past was similar to or lower than that received by patients without dyskinesia.

Total Intake[1]

Crane (1968a, 1974), Heinrich *et al.* (1968), Lehmann *et al.* (1970), and Pryce and Edwards (1966) found a significant positive association between the total amount of neuroleptics ingested and the prevalence of tardive dyskinesia. On the other hand, Brandon *et al.* (1971), Jus *et al.* (1976b), Mallya *et al.* (1979), Simpson, Varga, Lee, *et al.* (1978), and Smith *et al.* (1978) failed to observe such a relationship between neuroleptic amount and tardive dyskinesia.

Kennedy *et al.* (1971) reported that in male patients tremor of the oral region was associated with a high total dose, whereas choreiform dyskinesia in the same region was significantly associated with a low total dose. Crane *et al.* (1974) and Smith *et al.* (1978) found a positive correlation between the severity of tardive dyskinesia and the maximum dose of neuroleptics that the patients had received, but not between the score and the total neuroleptic intake. Siede and Muller (1967) computed neuroleptic intake in dyskinetic patients with and without organic mental disorder. The intake was higher among patients without brain damage.

The differences in the findings of various investigators outlined here are similar to those seen earlier with regard to length of treatment. The complex interaction of neuroleptic treatment with other factors, especially constitutional susceptibility, is probably one reason for the discrepancy in

---

[1]Hargreaves and Gaynor (1980) have recently proposed a preliminary statistical model for assessing the risk of tardive dyskinesia in terms of prescribed dosage and other factors.

the results. It is also possible that, given the same amount of a neuroleptic, some patients may develop much higher blood levels than others (Jeste *et al.*, 1979) and may be at a greater risk for developing tardive dyskinesia.

Current Dose

Most investigators (Fann *et al.*, 1972; Kennedy *et al.*, 1971; Pandurangi *et al.*, 1978; Simpson, Varga, Lee, *et al.*, 1978) found that the prevalence or severity of tardive dyskinesia was not related to the current daily dose of neuroleptics. Bell and Smith (1978) observed no difference in prevalence of dyskinesia between patients on or off neuroleptics at the time of rating. Crane obtained varying results in his studies. Crane and Paulson (1967) reported that the prevalence of dyskinesia was highest (about 21%) among 48 patients who were then taking no neuroleptics, whereas none of the 26 patients receiving neuroleptics in daily doses equivalent to more than 600 mg of chlorpromazine had dyskinesia. In two subsequent studies, Crane (1968c, 1970) observed that tardive dyskinesia was most frequent (especially in patients over 40 years of age) among those who were receiving higher daily doses of phenothiazines. In a multifactorial analysis, Crane (1974) found no significant correlation between current dose and prevalence of tardive dyskinesia. When the effects of age and current dose were averaged, dyskinesia became significantly related to maximum dose. When the maximum dose or duration of neuroleptic therapy was held constant, current dose levels became inversely related to tardive dyskinesia.

The relationship between current neuroleptic dose and tardive dyskinesia is obviously complicated. High daily doses may increase drug toxicity and thus contribute to a greater prevalence of dyskinesia. On the other hand, neuroleptics may suppress symptoms of dyskinesia so that currently drug-free patients might have a higher prevalence of dyskinesia.

TYPE OF NEUROLEPTIC

Neuroleptics can be classified on the basis of their propensity to cause acute side effects. It is generally agreed that sedative and autonomic side effects are more common with aliphatic and piperidine types of phenothiazines, whereas the piperazine group of phenothiazines and butyrophenones are more likely to induce extrapyramidal reactions such as dystonias. Attempts to define the risk of long-term side effects have been less successful. Neuroleptic-induced ocular pigmentation is usually thought to be a result of the chronic, high-dose intake of thioridazine, although cases of ocular pigmentation associated with the use of other neuroleptics have also been reported. So far it has not been possible to determine the relative risk of tardive dyskinesia associated with different kinds of neuroleptics.

Faurbye *et al.* (1964), Heinrich *et al.* (1968), Jus *et al.* (1976b), Kennedy *et al.* (1971), Mallya *et al.* (1979), Pandurangi *et al.* (1978), Perris *et al.* (1979), and Simpson, Varga, Lee, *et al.* (1978) reported that the prevalence of tardive dyskinesia could not be correlated with the use of any specific neuroleptics. We found only one large-scale survey in which the prevalence of tardive dyskinesia among patients treated with individual neuroleptics was computed. Faurbye *et al.* (1964) noted that 47 out of the 185 patients treated with chlorpromazine (25.4%) had developed dyskinesia and that 12 out of 62 treated with perphenazine (19.4%), 10 out of 74 treated with thioridazine (13.5%), 4 out of 21 treated with prochlorperazine (19.1%), and 2 out of 15 treated with haloperidol (13.3%) had tardive dyskinesia. Some of these patients, however, had received more than one neuroleptic in the past.

It is often difficult to attribute tardive dyskinesia in a patient to a specific drug. Few psychiatric patients are treated with a single neuroleptic over a period of years. In a patient who has received several neuroleptics (and other types of treatments), it may be impossible to decide which neuroleptic caused the dyskinesia. The difficulty is compounded by the fact that most of the clinical studies of tardive dyskinesia have been retrospective; the time of onset of dyskinesia in individual patients is therefore uncertain. A survey of the drugs that the patients are currently receiving may not be particularly helpful in determining an association between specific neuroleptics and tardive dyskinesia, since the dyskinesia may have existed for a long period prior to the survey and may be unrelated to the current drug therapy. For example, we (Jeste, Rosenblatt, Wagner, *et al.*, 1979) found that the majority of elderly female inpatients with tardive dyskinesia were, at the time of our study, receiving thioridazine. The records revealed that the patients had been given a number of other neuroleptics in the past. The present thioridazine treatment primarily reflected the ward physician's preference for that drug in the management of geriatric subjects. In some cases there was evidence from the patients' charts that the signs of dyskinesia had preceded the use of thioridazine in those patients.

Some investigators believe that tardive dyskinesia is rare when certain neuroleptics such as reserpine or clozapine are used. There is no strong clinical basis to support this belief. Degkwitz (1969), Sigwald *et al.* (1959), Simpson, Varga, Lee, *et al.* (1978), and Uhrbrand and Faurbye (1960) have described dyskinetic patients who had been treated with reserpine either alone or in combination with other drugs. Reserpine and clozapine have not been prescribed as frequently as phenothiazines or butyrophenones in psychiatric practice. There has been at least one report of aggravation of tardive dyskinesia with clozapine treatment (Doepp & Buddeberg, 1975). A number of new neuroleptics, which were initially claimed to have a low risk of inducing tardive dyskinesia, were later found to be as likely to produce dyskinesia as the older drugs. Probably all neuroleptics, when given in equivalent amounts and for similar periods to similar patients, carry a comparable risk of causing tardive dyskinesia.

Recently there have been several articles indicating that the use of depot fluphenazine may be associated with a particularly high prevalence of tardive dyskinesia (Chouinard, Annable, Ross-Chouinard, *et al.,* 1979; Gardos *et al.,* 1977; Smith *et al.,* 1978). In a prospective study of the incidence of tardive dyskinesia, Gibson (1978a) followed 374 outpatients receiving depot fluphenazine or flupenthixol. Prior to the beginning of this study, the patients had received oral neuroleptic medication (including fluphenazine or flupenthixol) for a mean of 10 years. They were then placed on intramuscular injections of either of these depot preparations. Over a 3-year follow-up period, the proportion of patients with tardive dyskinesia jumped from 8% to 22%, although in three-fourths of the cases the symptoms of dyskinesia were mild. Fluphenazine and flupenthixol were equally involved in the increased prevalence of tardive dyskinesia. Later, Gibson (1979) reported the results of a questionnaire survey on the incidence of severe choreiform tardive dyskinesia (generalized body chorea with or without abnormal movements of the lower face or tongue) among patients treated by psychiatrists in England and Wales. On the basis of the amounts of different neuroleptics prescribed in those regions during a 1-year period, Gibson gave the following figures for the overall incidence of severe choreiform dyskinesia: 1 out of 230 patients treated with depot flupenthixol, 1 out of 400 patients treated with depot fluphenazine, and 1 out of 1800 patients (or 1 out of 900 schizophrenics) treated with oral neuroleptics.

It is difficult to interpret definitively these studies suggesting that depot fluphenazine and flupenthixol may be associated with a significantly higher prevalence of tardive dyskinesia than other neuroleptics. At least three related factors must be considered. First, most of the patients in these investigations had received other neuroleptics, too. As mentioned earlier, it is not possible in such cases to attribute dyskinesia to a specific neuroleptic. Second, the selection of patients for treatment with depot preparation may introduce bias in comparing patients on different neuroleptics. Third, the amount of neuroleptic actually consumed may be much higher following parenteral fluphenazine administration than after oral neuroleptic use because of differences in patient compliance as well as in drug absorption. Blood neuroleptic levels tend to be relatively low in patients chronically treated with oral neuroleptics (Rivera-Calimlim, Gift, Nasrallah, *et al.*, 1978), probably because of alterations in gastrointestinal absorption of the drugs (Adamson, Curry, Bridges, *et al.*, 1973). This may not happen when the depot preparations are administered parenterally, so that the patients may continue to have high blood (and possibly brain) concentrations of neuroleptics (Gibson, 1978a).

It is also worth noting that in some studies treatment with other types of neuroleptics has been found to correlate significantly with tardive dyskinesia. Gardos, Cole, and La Brie (1977b) and Jeste, Potkin, Sinha, *et al.* (1979) reported a significantly greater intake of sedative or low-potency-type neuroleptics (such as thioridazine or chlorpromazine) by dyskinesia patients as compared to nondyskinesia patients. Gerlach and Simmelsgaard (1978) observed that haloperidol treatment was followed by higher scores on a dyskinesia scale (probably withdrawal dyskinesia + tardive dyskinesia) than was treatment with thioridazine or clozapine. Any simple interpretation of these results is premature.

To summarize, all neuroleptics probably have a similar propensity to produce tardive dyskinesia. Several recent studies indicate that the use of depot fluphenazine (or flupenthixol) may be associated with an increased prevalence of tardive dyskinesia, although the data published so far do not permit us to make any definitive conclusions on this point.

DRUG-FREE PERIODS

Since persistent tardive dyskinesia results from long-term administration of neuroleptics, it may be logical to expect that frequent and prolonged interruptions in drug treatment would reduce the incidence of dyskinesia (Ayd, 1970; Crane, 1972a). The American College of Neuropsychopharmacology–Food and Drug Administration (FDA) Task Force (1973) gave two reasons for recommending such drug interruptions. First, discontinuing neuroleptics may unmask latent dyskinesia in some patients and thus permit an early diagnosis of the syndrome. The relationship of withdrawal dyskinesia to persistent tardive dyskinesia is, however, unclear (see Chapter 3). Second, drug interruptions may afford some protection against the long-term hazards of neuroleptics, especially persistent tardive dyskinesia.

Several investigators have studied, retrospectively, the possible contribution of drug-free periods to the prevalence of persistent dyskinesia. It is notable that, to our knowledge, no published study has found a significantly lower prevalence of persistent dyskinesia among patients on interrupted drug treatment as compared to patients on continuous treatment. Degkwitz (1969) reported that persistent dyskinesia occurred more frequently in patients who had a history of frequent interruptions in treatment. Crane (1974) observed that the dyskinesia and nondyskinesia groups did not differ from each other in continuity of drug regimens (defined as taking the medication at least 90% of the time). Jus *et al.* (1976b) studied four variables related to drug interruptions (mean total duration of drug-free period, mean number of drug-free intervals, and mean duration and mean standard deviation (SD) of the durations of drug-free intervals) in five groups of patients (patients on any neuroleptics; patients on high-potency neuroleptics, such as the piperazine type of phenothiazines; patients on low-potency neuroleptics, such as aliphatic and piperidine derivatives of phenothiazines; patients on multiple neuroleptics; and patients on neuroleptics and antiparkinsonian agents). The researchers compared, on each of the four drug-interruption-related variables, patients with and without dyskinesia from each of these five groups. Of the 20 comparisons, only one yielded a statistically significant difference. The mean duration of intervals without high-potency neuroleptics was shorter in the dyskinesia group (17 months) than in the nondyskinesia group (23 months). By definition, the patients could have received low-potency neuroleptics during these intervals without high-potency neuroleptics. Since 1 out of 20 comparisons could be statistically significant by chance alone, the finding could have been overstressed.

We (Jeste, Potkin, Sinha, *et al.,* 1979) studied three groups of patients —those with persistent dyskinesia, those with reversible dyskinesia, and those without dyskinesia. The persistent dyskinesia group had a significantly greater number of drug-free periods of 2 months each and a significantly greater percentage of drug-free time since onset of neuroleptic treatment than the groups with reversible dyskinesia and without dyskinesia. The persistent dyskinesia patients also had significantly longer neuroleptic treatment and longer duration of psychiatric illness than the patients with reversible dyskinesia and without dyskinesia.

Since some of these variables were likely to be correlated with one another (e.g., the length of treatment may often be a function of the duration of illness), we conducted a multivariate (discriminant function) analysis to determine the relative independent contribution of each variable to the result. The variable that best separated the groups of persistent and reversible dyskinesias (which did not differ significantly from each other in age, gender, or primary psychiatric diagnosis) was the number of prolonged (i.e., of 2 months each) drug interruptions. This variable correctly classified 76% of all dyskinetic patients into reversible and persistent groups. The mean (± SD) number of prolonged drug interruptions was 5.6 ± 1.4 for the persistent dyskinesia group and 2.1 ± 1.8 for the reversible dyskinesia group. (In the nondyskinetic patients, that number was 1.6 ± 1.8.) We argued that the association between the number of neuroleptic-free periods and persistent dyskinesia might be indirect and that some intervening variables, such as length of neuroleptic treatment, primary psychiatric illness, or presence of parkinsonism and other side effects, might be responsible for both the drug interruptions and the persistent dyskinesia. Further statistical analysis showed, however, that the length of neuroleptic treatment and the number of drug interruptions appeared to make somewhat independent contributions to the persistence of tardive dyskinesia. Also, there was no significant positive correlation between the number of prolonged drug-free periods and primary psychiatric diagnosis, parkinsonism, and other side effects of the drugs. Since we took into account only those drug-free periods that preceded the diagnosis of tardive dyskinesia, they were not a result of a conscious decision to stop the drugs to treat dyskinesia. We found no difference in the apparent reasons for drug interruptions in the patients with persistent and reversible dyskinesias.

Our study indicated two possibilities: (1) There were some unidentified variables that led to drug interruptions as well as to persistent dyskinesia, and (2) frequent and prolonged interruptions in the course of long-term neuroleptic therapy increased the likelihood of persistent dyskinesia in patients who were otherwise predisposed (for unknown reasons) to develop tardive dyskinesia. A possible neurophysiological basis for the second theory is suggested by the phenomenon of "kindling" (recently reviewed by Post, 1980). Goddard (1972) and Post and Kopanda (1976) have reported that repeated intermittent administration of electrical or chemical (e.g., cocaine, lidocaine, fluoroethyl, pentylenetetrazol) stimulation results in sensitization, or kindling. On the other hand, continuous or massed stimulation retards kindling and produces tolerance. In a clinical study, Ballenger and Post (1978) found that the severity of alcohol withdrawal symptoms increased progressively over years of alcohol use in a stepwise manner. The investigators suggested that repeated periods of alcohol abstinence might have served as stimuli for the kindling of subcortical structures. It is tempting to postulate that, in our patients, repeated lengthy drug interruptions might have had a kindling effect on the nigrostriatal system and thus favored the development of persistent dyskinesia in predisposed individuals. There is, however, no experimental evidence so far to support or rule out a kindling effect of intermittent administration of neuroleptics.

There are at least three published studies of the effects of drug holidays on animal models of tardive dyskinesia. (The relevance of the animal models to the clinical syndrome of tardive dyskinesia is discussed in Chapter 9). It is interesting that none of these studies found salutary effects of drug interruptions. Weiss and Santelli (1978) reported that monkeys who did not develop dyskinesias with daily administration of neuroleptic did so when switched to intermittent treatment. We (Jeste, Stoff, Potkin, *et al.,* 1979) observed no reduction in behavioral supersensitivity to *d*-amphetamine in rats who were given intermittent haloperidol compared with the animals who received the drug daily. Bannet, Belmaker, and Ebstein (1980) reported a similar finding in mice, using a biochemical measure (^{3}H-spiroperidol binding) of supersensitivity.

In summary, the contribution of drug interruptions to the prevention of persistent tardive dyskinesia is, at best, uncertain. In predisposed individuals, prolonged and lengthy drug-free periods do not decrease, and may even increase, the chances of development of persistent tardive dyskinesia (Degkwitz, 1969; Jeste, Potkin, Sinha, *et al.,* 1979). Indeed, Simpson (1980) has suggested that the increased prevalence of tardive dyskinesia among certain groups of patients with affective disorders may be related to these patients' intermittent treatment with neuroleptics (during psychotic episodes only). This is not to suggest that drug interruptions produce persistent dyskinesia, but only to indicate a need for an open mind and further research on this issue. There are no large-scale data on a possible relationship between shorter drug-free periods (e.g., drug-free weekends) and prevalence of tardive dyskinesia. Yet, it is worth noting that McCreadie, Dingwall, Wiles, *et al.* (1980) found that switching patients from continuous fluphenazine treatment to intermittent administration (four times a day) of pimozide resulted in an increased incidence of tardive dyskinesia.

POLYPHARMACY

Bell and Smith (1978) found that the prevalence of moderate to severe tardive dyskinesia was somewhat higher (15.1%) in patients receiving, at the time of the rating, two or more neuroleptics as compared to the prevalence in patients receiving one neuroleptic (11.6%). Current administration of neuroleptics may, however, be unrelated to the production of dyskinesia. Regarding past use of polypharmacy, Demars (1966) and Simpson, Varga, Lee, et al. (1978) reported that this variable did not differentiate between dyskinesia and nondyskinesia groups. There is thus little evidence to suggest that polypharmacy increases the risk of tardive dyskinesia, although it is possible that specific drug combinations might be more hazardous in this respect.

ANTIPARKINSONIAN DRUGS

One biochemical theory of tardive dyskinesia (see Chapter 5) states that this syndrome is associated with nigrostriatal dopamine–acetylcholine imbalance, with relative underactivity of the cholinergic system. The most convincing clinical evidence in favor of this hypothesis has been the aggravation of tardive dyskinesia by antiparkinsonian (anticholinergic) agents such as trihexyphenidyl, benztropine, biperiden, procyclidine, and orphenadrine (Chapter 10), which are commonly used to treat or even prevent neuroleptic-induced parkinsonism. Whether these drugs themselves produce, or at least predispose, to neuroleptic-induced persistent tardive dyskinesia is, however, doubtful.

 Kiloh, Smith, and Williams (1973) and Klawans (1973) were among the first to suggest that antiparkinsonian drugs might cause tardive dyskinesia. Kiloh, Smith, and Williams (1973) reported three cases of tardive dyskinesia presumably induced by anticholinergic drugs. All of their patients (over the age of 50), had, however, been treated with neuroleptics, and antiparkinsonian drugs seemed to aggravate the dyskinesias (orofacial in two patients, limb dyskinesia in one), probably induced by neuroleptics. Birket-Smith (1974) presented six cases of dyskinesia (involving mouth and face in all cases, limbs in two) that appeared to have been caused by antiparkinsonian agents; none of the patients had received neuroleptics. In all the cases, the dyskinesia disappeared within 1 to 6 weeks of discontinuing the offending drugs. Recently, Warne and Gubbay (1979) published a case report of tardive dyskinesia induced by anticholinergic drugs. To our knowledge, antiparkinsonian (anticholinergic)-drug-induced persistent tardive dyskinesia is a rarity.

We found ten epidemiologic studies in which a possible relationship between the use of antiparkinsonian agents and the prevalence of tardive dyskinesia was explored. It is quite striking that only two of these studies (Mallya *et al.*, 1979; Perris *et al.*, 1979) found a significant association between the two. Mallya *et al.* (1979) observed that their 28 patients with tardive dyskinesia had been treated with antiparkinsonian drugs longer (34 vs. 18 months) and in larger amounts (4.5 vs. 1.6 g) as compared with 28 matched controls. Perris *et al.* (1979) reported that a significantly larger number of dyskinesia patients (18 of 18) had received antiparkinsonian drugs as compared to matched controls (12 of 18). The two groups, however, did not differ significantly in the total amount of those drugs consumed. The investigators noted a significant positive correlation ($r = .51$) between severity of dyskinesia and amount of anticholinergic agents. Kennedy *et al.* (1971) and Pandurangi *et al.* (1978) reported that dyskinesia prevalence was unrelated to a history of antiparkinsonian drug use. Crane (1974) noted that an apparent positive association between antiparkinsonian drug administration and tardive dyskinesia was probably misleading, since the antiparkinsonian drug use seemed to be a function of the intensity of treatment with neuroleptics. When most factors related to overall drug therapy were averaged, tardive dyskinesia was no longer found to be correlated with antiparkinsonian drug intake. Bell and Smith (1978), Gardos, Cole, and La Brie (1977b), Jeste, Potkin, Sinha, *et al.* (1979), Jus *et al.* (1976b), and Simpson, Varga, Lee, *et al.* (1978) concluded that the prevalence and severity of tardive dyskinesia were unrelated to the mean total amount or duration of administration of antiparkinsonian agents.

Thus the published data offer little support for the assertion that antiparkinsonian drugs significantly increase the prevalence of tardive dyskinesia. This fact also argues against the theory of a primary cholinergic system pathology in the etiology of tardive dyskinesia. It is worth noting that prolonged treatment of Parkinson's disease patients with anticholinergic agents has not been known to pose any serious risk of persistent tardive dyskinesia. It is true that antiparkinsonian drugs often aggravate pre-existing dyskinesia; it is possible that they do so indirectly by increasing catecholaminergic activity in the nigrostriatal region.

OTHER DRUGS

A number of drugs other than neuroleptics have been reported to cause dyskinesias in some patients. These are discussed in Chapter 8.

HOSPITALIZATION

A direct relationship between length of hospitalization and tardive dyskinesia is questionable. Crane (1970) and Greenblatt *et al.* (1968) reported that the prevalence of tardive dyskinesia was not related to length of hospitalization. In another study of Turkish and American patients, Crane (1968a) found that dyskinesia prevalence was proportional to the length and amount of neuroleptic therapy and unrelated to hospitalization. None of the 97 Turkish patients who had prolonged institutionalization, but minimal drug treatment, had developed tardive dyskinesia. In contrast, 3 out of 40 Turkish patients "moderately" treated with neuroleptics, and 16 of 98 American patients "heavily" treated with these drugs, had tardive dyskinesia.

Some other studies have shown a positive relationship between length of hospitalization and prevalence of tardive dyskinesia; it is, however, not clear whether the differences in the length of institutionalization between patients with and without dyskinesia primarily reflected differences in age or duration of neuroleptic treatment. Thus Pandurangi *et al.* (1978) observed that tardive dyskinesia was significantly more common in patients hospitalized for more than 2 years. It seems, however, that in their patient population the dyskinesia patients who had been hospitalized for less than 2 years also had neuroleptic treatment for less than 2 years, whereas those with longer institutionalization had proportionately longer drug therapy. Simpson, Varga, Lee, *et al.* (1978) found a slight, but statistically significant, difference between the mean duration of hospitalization of the dyskinesia group (21.4 years) and that of the total hospital population (19.5 years). It is interesting to note that there was an even greater difference in the mean ages of the two groups—64.8 years versus 59.0 years. Brandon *et al.* (1971), Crane (1968c), Fann *et al.* (1972), and Lehmann *et al.* (1970) reported that dyskinesia was more common in chronically hospitalized patients. The differences they observed were usually present only in certain subgroups of patients—for example, in elderly patients or in women. Moreover, the possible confounding effects of related variables such as age and duration of drug administration on prevalence of dyskinesia were not considered. In a separate study, Smith *et al.* (1978) noted that the length of hospitalization tended to be directly proportional to the patients' ages.

Recent reports (see Chapter 2) showing that tardive dyskinesia is as prevalent among outpatients as it is among inpatients argue against the suggestion that tardive dyskinesia is related, in some direct manner, to institutionalization per se.

PHYSICAL TREATMENTS

Early reports (e.g., Hunter *et al.*, 1964; Uhrbrand & Faurbye, 1960) indicated that tardive dyskinesia patients had not only long-term neuroleptic treatment, but also physical treatments such as electroconvulsive therapy (ECT) and leukotomy in a number of instances. This raised a possibility that these somatic therapies might predispose to tardive dyskinesia by causing brain damage. Indeed, Uhrbrand and Faurbye (1960) ascribed several cases of tardive dyskinesia to ECT itself. We now consider various studies on the relationship between physical treatments and tardive dyskinesia.

Electroconvulsive Therapy

Brandon *et al.* (1971), Degkwitz and Wenzel (1967), Demars (1966), Edwards (1970), Heinrich *et al.* (1968), Pandurangi *et al.* (1978), Perris *et al.* (1979), and Pryce and Edwards (1966) found no association between tardive dyskinesia and history of ECT. Simpson, Varga, Lee, *et al.* (1978) observed that only one-half as many patients (9 out of 40) with dyskinesia had ECT as controls (17 out of 40). Although Uhrbrand and Faurbye (1960) attributed dyskinesia in four of their patients to ECT, a causal relationship between ECT and dyskinesia was unclear. These four patients were over the age of 55, and all had been treated with neuroleptics for longer than 6 months. Faurbye *et al.* (1964) and Lehmann *et al.* (1970) reported a higher prevalence of tardive dyskinesia in patients who had received ECT, and Gardos, Cole, and La Brie (1977b) noted that ECT was one of the significant discriminators between dyskinesia and nondyskinesia groups. We should, however, consider the fact that ECT is usually administered (at least in the Western countries) only to a selected minority of patients and that the latter are also likely to have received intensive drug therapy.

Interestingly, ECT has also been tried as a treatment for tardive dyskinesia (Chapter 10).

Leukotomy

Brandon *et al.* (1971), Demars (1966), Faurbye *et al.* (1964), Pryce and Edwards (1966), Simpson, Varga, Lee, *et al.* (1978), and our own studies revealed no association between leukotomy and tardive dyskinesia. Only one survey (Perris *et al.*, 1979) found a significantly greater prevalence of tardive dyskinesia among lobotomized patients. Of the ten lobotomized patients in that series, eight had dyskinesia.

Insulin Coma Treatment

Heinrich *et al.* (1968) and Simpson, Varga, Lee, *et al.* (1978) noticed no relationship between tardive dyskinesia and history of insulin coma treatment. Lehmann *et al.* (1970) observed a higher prevalence of dyskinesia in patients treated with insulin or ECT, whereas Degkwitz and Wenzel (1967) found a lower prevalence of dyskinesia among insulin-treated patients. Brandon *et al.* (1971) also reported a significantly lower prevalence of tardive dyskinesia in patients with a history of insulin treatment, although most of the subjects in the latter group were under 50 years of age.

Summary

There is little satisfactory evidence to implicate physical treatments such as ECT, leukotomy, and insulin coma in the etiology of tardive dyskinesia. It is also notable that dyskinesia was not reported as a complication of these treatments prior to the introduction of neuroleptics in psychiatry, although somatic therapies had been a common form of treatment of psychiatric patients since the late 1930s.

PATIENT-RELATED VARIABLES

AGE

Aging and Prevalence of Dyskinesia

It was stated in Chapter 2 that the prevalence of tardive dyskinesia among psychiatric inpatients seemed to increase with age. The prevalence is three times greater in patients over 40 years than in patients under 40. A review of the relevant literature by Smith and Baldessarini (1980) showed a strong linear correlation between age (in the age group of 40 to 70 years) and both the prevalence and severity of tardive dyskinesia. There was also a strong inverse correlation between rates of spontaneous remission of tardive dyskinesia and age. (A possible relationship between aging and localization of tardive dyskinesia is discussed in Chapter 3.)

One possible criticism of a causal relationship between aging and tardive dyskinesia is that the older patients may have had longer neuroleptic treatment than the younger patients. This criticism may not be valid, however, since a number of the studies did not observe a significant difference in the length of neuroleptic treatment between dyskinesia and nondyskinesia groups. Indeed, Jus *et al.* (1976b) reported that age at onset of treatment was the most significant variable distinguishing between the two groups. Our own study at Saint Elizabeth's Hospital, Washington, D.C., corroborates the significant association between dyskinesia and older age at onset of the treatment. It is also probable that older individuals may develop tardive dyskinesia with smaller total amounts and shorter total duration of neuroleptic treatment when compared to younger patients. Prospective clinical studies are needed to test this hypothesis. It is worth noting, too, that several investigators have reported a higher prevalence of spontaneous dykinesia in geriatric populations than in younger populations (Brandon *et al.*, 1971; Degkwitz, 1979; Faurbye *et al.*, 1964).

Possible Mechanisms

Elderly persons usually have an increased susceptibility to adverse drug effects. A number of possible reasons for this fact have been suggested (Hollister, 1979; Verwoert, 1976). The following factors deserve special consideration.

Peripheral or Pharmacokinetic Mechanisms. Absorption, metabolism, and excretion of drugs are often altered, which results in their increased accumulation in the elderly. We (Jeste, De Lisi, Zalcman, *et al.*, 1981) found threefold higher serum neuroleptic levels in patients over 50 years as compared to younger patients receiving comparable doses of similar neuroleptics.[2] Although there is no evidence for increased absorption of neuroleptics, other peripheral mechanisms may possibly account for such a difference in serum levels of neuroleptics. Hypoalbuminemia causing reduced protein binding and increased concentrations of unbound drug, and liver and kidney damage producing impaired metabolism and excretion of neuroleptics may be among such mechanisms.

Central Mechanisms. Neuronal damage, changes in the number of receptors, and reduced efficiency of homeostatic or compensatory mechanisms may all conceivably increase the risk of neurological side effects in the aged. There is little doubt that significant neuronal loss in various areas of the brain, including the nigrostriatal system, accompanies the aging process. It has been proposed that a loss of presynaptic, dopaminergic neurons may result in denervation supersensitivity of postsynaptic receptors in the basal ganglia. The available data, however, question this seemingly attractive hypothesis. Makman, Ahn, Thal, *et al.* (1979) and Weiss, Greenberg, and Cantor (1979) have presented biochemical evidence for selective decreases in the number of biogenic receptors as well as in the receptor capacity to develop supersensitivity with aging in animals. Schöcken and Roth (1977) have reported a reduction in the number of β-adrenergic receptors with age in man.

We need to consider the possibility that the neuronal damage in the nigrostriatal system of the aged may involve alteration of presynaptic mechanisms (e.g., diminished reuptake; Pradhan, 1980), which may predispose to the development of tardive dyskinesia. It is interesting to note that Tanner and Domino (1977) reported enhanced effects of *d*-amphetamine (with predominantly presynaptic action), but not of apomorphine (presumed to be a postsynaptic receptor agonist) in aged gerbils. Smith and Leelavathi (1980) found increased response to both drugs in older

[2]Recently, Yesavage, Becker, Werner, *et al.* (1982) reported a positive correlation (Pearson's $r = .43$; $p < .05$) between age and serum levels of thiothixene following an orally administered acute single test dose (20 mg) of the drug.

rats; they, however, did not rule out the possibility that the peripheral metabolism of apomorphine might have been altered in the old animals.

Impaired capacity of homeostatic or compensatory mechanisms is to be expected in the geriatric patients. The nature of such mechanisms has not been fully explored.

Other Factors. Various physical diseases (e.g., arteriosclerosis) that accompany old age may, in unknown ways, predispose to complications such as tardive dyskinesia. Also, the elderly patients are likely to receive polypharmacy for their different ailments. Some of these drugs, such as anticholinergic and antihistaminic agents, may potentiate tardive dyskinesia. The aged might be getting higher doses of a neuroleptic because of misinterpretation of prescribing directions on the physician's or the patient's part. Local factors, such as ill-fitting dentures, may also contribute to oral dyskinesia.

GENDER

Chapter 2 enumerated 20 studies comparing the prevalence of tardive dyskinesia in the two genders. The reported overall mean prevalence of dyskinesia was about 41% higher in women than in men.

Several investigators have tried to study a possible interaction between age and gender as a determinant of the prevalence of tardive dyskinesia. Smith *et al.* (1978) observed, among inpatients, a linear increase in the prevalence of dyskinesia with age in women, but a curvilinear relationship in men. Women had a significantly higher prevalence of tardive dyskinesia than men only in the age groups of 70 to 79, and 80 and above. In a subsequent study of outpatients, the same group of researchers (Smith, Kucharski, Eblen, *et al.,* 1979) found a linear increase in the prevalence of dyskinesia with age in both genders, although the positive relationship with age was somewhat attenuated among older men. A different team of investigators – namely, Bell and Smith (1978) – reported a lack of a statistically significant interaction between age and gender as a contributory factor to the prevalence of dyskinesia. In another article, Smith, Kucharski, Oswald, *et al.* (1979) noted that female inpatients tended to have more severe dyskinesia than male inpatients. By contrast, Chouinard, Annable, Ross-Chouinard, *et al.* (1979) observed more severe forms of tardive dyskinesia among male outpatients.

It is fair to conclude that, although tardive dyskinesia may be somewhat more frequent in women than in men, gender seems to play a much smaller role than age as a determinant of the prevalence of dyskinesia. Furthermore, it is not clear whether any observed differences in the prevalence of dyskinesia in the two genders are a result of possible biological characteristics of the genders (such as brain neurotransmitter concentrations or role of hormones—see Chapter 5) or merely reflect differences in treatment. For example, Degkwitz and Wenzel (1967) found that women had been treated with higher doses of more potent neuroleptics and had also received antiparkinsonian medications more often than had men. Laska, Varga, Wanderling, et al. (1973) and Sheppard, Collins, Fiorentino, et al. (1969) reported that women were more likely to be treated with multiple drugs (polypharmacy) and with higher doses. Jones and Hunter (1969) and Simpson, Varga, Lee, et al. (1978) noticed that the duration of neuroleptic treatment was significantly longer in female than in male patients. Fann et al. (1972) observed that women tended to have longer hospitalization than men.

To summarize, the relationship between gender and prevalence of tardive dyskinesia is as yet poorly understood.

CONSTITUTIONAL PREDISPOSITION

Tardive dyskinesia occurs in some patients who have had relatively brief or low-dose neuroleptic treatment, while it may not develop in other, apparently similar patients despite long-term, high-dose therapy. This suggests a likelihood of constitutional predisposition to tardive dyskinesia. Susceptible individuals may manifest dyskinesia on receiving relatively small total amounts of the drugs, whereas individuals with constitutional resistance may not have this disorder even after taking relatively large total quantities of the medications. The nature of the presumed constitutional predisposition to tardive dyskinesia is uncertain. Several possibilities, which are not mutually exclusive, exist.

Biochemical Individuality

Williams (1956) was probably the first to use this term, suggesting that each person has his or her characteristic biochemical makeup. Although biochemical predisposition to some psychiatric illnesses is most likely present, its existence and precise nature are often difficult to demonstrate. We found significantly lower platelet and lymphocyte monoamine oxidase (MAO), higher plasma dopamine β-hydroxylase (DBH) activities, and higher serum neuroleptic levels in a subgroup of patients with tardive dyskinesia as compared to controls matched for age, gender, primary psychiatric illness, hospitalization, and length of neuroleptic treatment (Chapter 5). It is tempting to suggest that certain disturbances in central dopaminergic and noradrenergic functions and in peripheral metabolism of neuroleptics might increase susceptibility to neuroleptic-induced tardive dyskinesia, at least in a subgroup of patients. Obviously, much further work is necessary before assuming such a causal relationship between observed biochemical differences and development of tardive dyskinesia.

Genetic Predisposition

A number of extrapyramidal disorders, such as Huntington's disease, dystonia musculorum deformans, and, sometimes, Gilles de la Tourette's syndrome, are transmitted genetically. The role of hereditary factors in the etiology of drug-induced extrapyramidal disorders is more difficult to prove. Myrianthopoulos, Kurland, Kurland, *et al.* (1962) conducted a survey to determine hereditary susceptibility to neuroleptic-induced parkinsonism. They screened 728 relatives of 59 neuroleptic-treated patients with parkinsonism and 777 relatives of 67 neuroleptic-treated patients without parkinsonism. The researchers found 13 cases of Parkinson's disease among relatives of patients with neuroleptic-induced parkinsonism in contrast to only 3 cases of Parkinson's disease among relatives of controls. This difference between the two groups was statistically significant, indicating a possibility of genetic predisposition to neuroleptic-induced parkinsonism. Eldridge (1970) suggested that phenothiazine-induced unmasking of acute dystonia might be used as a screening test for the heterozygous state in families of patients with torsion dystonias (which are sometimes transmitted genetically).

So far little work has been done to explore the possibility of hereditary susceptibility to tardive dyskinesia. Jacob Brody (1981) of the National Institutes of Health, Bethesda, Md., studied six pairs of twin patients (four monozygotic and two dizygotic) on long-term, high-dose phenothiazine treatment. He found that the specific type of neurological side effect was not determined genetically, since identical twins appeared to develop distinctly different patterns of reaction.[3]

Psychological Factors

Levinson, Malen, Hogben, et al. (1978) examined the role of certain psychological factors in susceptibility to chlorpromazine-induced acute extrapyramidal symptoms. Of the three measures studied, namely, premorbid social competence, field, and self–object differentiation, only the first turned out to be a good predictor of the predisposition to acute extrapyramidal symptoms. The investigators reported that premorbid asocial schizophrenics were more likely to develop such side effects as compared to schizophrenics with high premorbid social competence. We are not aware of any such published studies on the role of psychological factors in predisposition to tardive dyskinesia.

DENTAL STATE

Involuntary stereotyped movements of the mouth—lips, jaw, and tongue —are not rare among elderly persons without teeth or with ill-fitting dentures. Sutcher, Underwood, Beatly, et al. (1971) proposed that loss of teeth (with the rich supply of nerve endings within them) or inadequate dento-oral prosthesis might result in confusing proprioceptive input from the stomatognathic system into the thalamus and the extrapyramidal system. The consequent oral dyskinesia represents searching movements of the buccolingual masticatory muscles in an attempt to find clues to orient the mandible and oral structures in space.

A possible association between edentulous state or ill-fitting dentures and tardive dyskinesia has been studied by several investigators. Brandon et al. (1971), Edwards (1970), and Pryce and Edwards (1966) found a

---

[3]We recently studied 50-year-old female schizophrenic quadruplets with a long-term history of neuroleptic treatment. Only one of the four patients had definite tardive dyskinesia (Jeste, Cutler, De Lisi, et al., unpublished data). The only published evidence so far suggesting a contribution of genetic factors to the development of tardive dyskinesia is a report of the presence of the syndrome in two schizophrenic brothers treated with neuroleptics (Weinhold, Wegner, & Kane, 1981).

much higher percentage of edentulous patients in the tardive dyskinesia group as compared to the group without dyskinesia. Brandon *et al.* (1971), however, noted that if the edentulous and denture groups were combined, the prevalence of tardive dyskinesia in women over 50 years was the same as that for women with natural teeth. The researchers concluded that patients with facial dyskinesia tended to have difficulty in retaining their dentures in their mouths because of continual movements of the tongue, jaw, and lips. Thus ill-fitting dentures may not necessarily contribute to the development of orofacial dyskinesia, but could also be a consequence of the dyskinesia.

In our own study of elderly patients, we found that an edentulous state or ill-fitting dentures per se hardly ever produced severe dyskinesia. Kennedy *et al.* (1971) and Pandurangi *et al.* (1978) reported the lack of a significant correlation between the state of dentition and tardive dyskinesia. It seems that local factors such as dental problems may play a small role in the development or aggravation of orofacial dyskinesia; they are, however, not sufficient to lead to severe dyskinesia, and sometimes they may be a result of the dyskinesia itself.

PRIMARY PSYCHIATRIC ILLNESS

As Table 6-3 shows, there is no relationship between tardive dyskinesia and primary psychiatric illness. Dyskinesia has been observed frequently among neurotic patients, patients with psychosomatic disorders, and those with major affective disorders, who have received long-term neuroleptic treatment. If the overall prevalence of tardive dyskinesia is highest among chronic schizophrenics, it is mainly because that group is most likely to have been treated with neuroleptics in greater amounts and for prolonged periods.

Beginning with Sigwald *et al.* (1959), a number of authors (Allen & Stimmel, 1977; Davis, Berger, & Hollister, 1976; Evans, 1965; Faurbye *et al.*, 1964; Klawans *et al.*, 1974; Rosenbaum, Niven, Hanson, *et al.*, 1977) described tardive dyskinesia among nonschizophrenic and non-brain-damaged patients. Davis, Berger, and Hollister (1976) and Rosenbaum *et al.* (1977) were struck by a relatively high prevalence of tardive dyskinesia among patients with a primary affective disorder, especially depression. While screening patients with tardive dyskinesia, the investigators observed that a majority of these patients had been treated for depression with neuroleptics and other treatments. These researchers postulated that depression, with the associated disturbances in central catecholamine and acetylcholine functions, may predispose to the development of tardive dyskinesia. Whether or not this is true, there certainly does not seem to be a direct relationship between schizophrenia and tardive dyskinesia.

Degkwitz (1969) and Hippius and Lange (1970) reported a positive correlation between severity of psychotic symptoms and that of tardive dyskinesia. Degkwitz noticed this relationship on withdrawal of neuroleptics. Here it is necessary to consider the possibility that the stress of psychotic relapse itself might aggravate the symptoms of tardive dyskinesia. In our studies we have not found any significant correlation between severity of schizophrenic symptoms and degree of dyskinesia. Crane (1968a) also noted a lack of association between severity of psychosis and that of dyskinesia in his Turkish and American patients. On the other hand, Cutler *et al.* (1981) noticed that the severity of dyskinesia in two of their manic–depressive patients seemed to be related to the intensity of depression. Heinrich *et al.* (1968), and Jeste, Potkin, Sinha, *et al.* (1979) did not observe any significant relationship between prevalence of tardive dyskinesia and duration of primary psychiatric illness.

Chouinard and Jones (1980) proposed that chronic neuroleptic treatment induces supersensitivity in the nigrostriatal, mesolimbic, and tuberoinfundibular dopamine systems and produces tardive dyskinesia, supersensitivity psychosis, and hyperprolactinemia, respectively. Most other investigators, however, have not found a significant positive association between tardive dyskinesia and the other two conditions.

To summarize, the overall data do not suggest a consistent relationship between tardive dyskinesia and primary psychiatric illness (type, subtype, symptoms, severity, therapeutic response to neuroleptics, etc.).

SUSCEPTIBILITY TO OTHER EXTRAPYRAMIDAL SIDE EFFECTS

Crane (1972b) suggested that tardive dyskinesia was more likely to develop in patients with neuroleptic-induced parkinsonism than in those not exhibiting that side effect. The logic behind this hypothesis was that persons with "labile" extrapyramidal systems might develop parkinsonism early in the course of neuroleptic therapy, and tardive dyskinesia with continued treatment. Since parkinsonism usually develops within a few days or weeks of starting neuroleptics, its occurrence could serve as an early indicator of the risk of dyskinesia in a particular patient. Unfortunately, there are several problems in testing Crane's hypothesis; also, the evidence supporting it is not strong.

Difficulties in testing Crane's hypothesis include the following:

1. Certain neuroleptics (e.g., trifluoperazine, haloperidol) are more likely to induce parkinsonism than others (such as thioridazine, mesoridazine) in the same subjects, although all of these drugs probably have a similar propensity to produce tardive dyskinesia.
2. Prophylactic use of antiparkinsonian agents makes it difficult to decide whether a patient might have developed parkinsonism.
3. Patients with parkinsonism are usually treated with antiparkinsonian drugs. The latter themselves have been claimed by some investigators to increase the likelihood of dyskinesia (Klawans, 1973).
4. A reliable retrospective history of parkinsonism is often difficult to obtain since many patients develop tolerance to this side effect within a few months.
5. Appearance of tardive dyskinesia may coincide with disappearance of parkinsonism. The two disorders are presumed to be biochemical opposites (see Chapter 5).
6. Withdrawal of neuroleptics may result in improvement in parkinsonism and simultaneous appearance of dyskinetic symptoms (Crane, 1972b; Crane & Naranjo, 1971). The latter may merely represent withdrawal dyskinesia and may be different from tardive dyskinesia.

Degkwitz (1969), Degkwitz and Wenzel (1967), Jeste, Potkin, Sinha, *et al.* (1979), Jus *et al.* (1976a), and Pandurangi *et al.* (1978) found no correlation between tardive dyskinesia and presence or severity of parkinsonism. Demars (1966) noted that the two syndromes rarely occurred together, and Chouinard, De Montigny, and Annable (1979) observed an inverse relationship between total scores for parkinsonian symptoms and for dyskinesia. In contrast, Heinrich *et al.* (1968) reported that pharmacogenic parkinsonism occurred frequently in patients with tardive dyskinesia.

To summarize, there is no satisfactory evidence to support the notion that the occurrence of parkinsonism in a patient indicates his or her increased susceptibility to tardive dyskinesia.

OTHER FACTORS

Race

Simpson (1973) reported that all three of his patients who developed tardive dyskinesia with relatively small total amounts of neuroleptics were of Eastern European Jewish extraction. He suggested a possible parallel with dystonia musculorum deformans, which is more common in Eastern European Jews and which often becomes symptomatic when the patients are challenged with small amounts of neuroleptics. Mehta and Itil (1973) failed to find any such association between prevalence of dyskinesia and race in their patients. Tardive dyskinesia has been observed in all races and in patients from different backgrounds. It is possible that some racial subgroups may be at a greater risk of developing this complication than others. Some investigators have found Parkinson's disease to be more prevalent among the caucasian than among other races. Whether this difference is related to the pigmentation in the substantia nigra is unknown. It may be interesting to explore the relative risks of tardive dyskinesia in patients from various genetic–racial backgrounds.

Eye Color

Brandon *et al.* (1971) reported an interesting observation. The prevalence of tardive dyskinesia as well as that of spontaneous dyskinesia among men was significantly greater in patients with blue eyes (42 out of 216) than in those with brown and intermediate eye color (19 out of 200). Such a difference was not apparent among women. The researchers thought that the association of dyskinesia with eye color probably indicated a genetic or constitutional predisposition to develop dyskinesia among men with blue eyes. A later study by Gardos, Sokol, Cole, *et al.* (1976) could not confirm the postulated relationship between blue eyes in men and tardive dyskinesia. Seven out of 30 blue-eyed men had tardive dyskinesia, as compared to 21 out of 66 men with brown or intermediate eye color.

SUMMARY

A large number of variables related both to treatment and to individual patients are involved in the etiology of tardive dyskinesia. Length or total amount of neuroleptic administration, aging, and constitutional predisposition are among the most important factors in the etiology of the disorder. These and other variables interacting in a complex manner lead to the induction of tardive dyskinesia in some patients.

CHAPTER V

Biochemical Theories

INTRODUCTION

Neuroleptics are presumed to exert their principal clinical effects by acting on the central neurotransmitter systems, especially the catecholaminergic systems. It is therefore natural that biochemical theories of tardive dyskinesia should abound. The most popular hypothesis states that tardive dyskinesia results from postsynaptic dopamine receptor supersensitivity in the nigrostriatal system. According to a number of researchers, cholinergic and γ-aminobutyric acid (GABA)-ergic mechanisms also play an important role in the pathophysiology of tardive dyskinesia. At present there is little direct evidence to confirm or rule out any of these biochemical theories.

The physiology and pathology of neurotransmitter systems in the basal ganglia are discussed in this chapter, with particular reference to the possible involvement of these mechanisms in the pathogenesis of tardive dyskinesia. Studies of endocrine function and neuroleptic metabolism in patients with dyskinesia are also discussed. At the end of the chapter, we present a critical overview of biochemical studies of tardive dyskinesia.

DOPAMINE

$$HO{-}\underset{HO}{\overset{}{\bigcirc}}{-}CH_2\text{-}CH_2\text{-}NH_2$$

PHYSIOLOGY OF THE DOPAMINERGIC SYSTEM

Synthesis of Dopamine

The dietary precursors of dopamine are phenylalanine and tyrosine. Phenylalanine is one of the essential amino acids; that is, it cannot be synthesized *de novo* by the human body and therefore has to be consumed from an external source. Milk and other protein-rich foods provide the normally required amounts of phenylalanine in the diet. This phenylalanine is converted in the liver into tyrosine (which may also come directly from the diet) through the action of the enzyme phenylalanine hydroxylase. Tyrosine enters the bloodstream, crosses the blood–brain barrier, and is selectively taken up by the dopaminergic neurons. Here it is hydroxylated to dihydroxyphenylalanine (DOPA), which is then decarboxylated to dopamine. Tyrosine hydroxylase is the rate-limiting enzyme in the formation of dopamine. The synthesized dopamine is stored in vesicles in the presynaptic neuron. Stimulation of the dopaminergic neuron results in the release of dopamine from the granules into the synaptic cleft. Dopamine then acts on the specific receptors located on the postsynaptic neurons. This leads to a chain of events presumably associated with release of successive "messengers" (such as cyclic AMP [cAMP]) and altered polarization of the neuron. When stimulation of the presynaptic neuron ends, release of dopamine into the synapse and its subsequent action on the postsynaptic neuron ceases, and the postsynaptic neuron returns to a state of repolarization.

Metabolism of Dopamine

There are two principal enzymes involved in the metabolism of dopamine — namely, MAO, located inside the presynaptic neuron, and catechol-*O*-methyltransferase (COMT), present mostly in the synaptic cleft. The MAO oxidizes dopamine to 3,4-dihydroxyphenylacetic acid (DOPAC), and the COMT methylates dopamine to 3-*O*-methyltyramine. When both enzymes metabolize dopamine, the product is homovanillic acid (HVA). Dopamine released into the synapse may either be metabolized by COMT or be taken back (reuptake) into the presynaptic neuron and then oxidized by MAO. Homovanillic acid and DOPAC are the principal metabolites of dopamine. They are removed relatively quickly from the brain and the cerebrospinal fluid (CSF) into the bloodstream and primarily excreted into the urine.

Localization of Dopamine Neurons

Three dopamine pathways have received considerable attention:

1. Nigrostriatal—Axons arise from cell bodies in the substantia nigra
   and terminate in caudate nucleus and putamen, which are parts of
   the corpus striatum. This pathway is presumably involved in functions of the extrapyramidal system.
2. Mesolimbic—Axons originate from cell bodies situated dorsal to
   the interpeduncular nucleus and terminate in the nucleus accumbens septi and olfactory tubercle of the mesolimbic system, which
   is concerned with emotional behavior.
3. Tuberoinfundibular or hypothalamic–hypophyseal—Cell bodies
   in the arcuate nucleus of the hypothalamus give rise to axons, which
   terminate in the median eminence. This tract probably controls the
   secretion of hypothalamic trophic hormones and also influences
   the release of pituitary hormones—mainly prolactin and growth
   hormone.

Dopamine neurons have been shown to be present in the cerebral cortex and the retina, too. Commissiong, Gentleman, and Neff (1979) have
also demonstrated the presence of an uncrossed nigrospinal dopaminergic
pathway. It may be a spinal counterpart of the extrapyramidal system in
the brain.

Dahlström and Fuxe (1964, 1965) identified specific dopaminergic
cell groups in the rat brain. Voogd and Huijzen (1979) have described
these cell groups in a synopsis of the central nervous system. Table 5-1
summarizes localization of eight dopaminergic cell groups (A_8 through
A_{15}). Of these, A_8 through A_{10} are mesencephalic, A_{11} through A_{14} are di-
encephalic, and A_{15} is telencephalic. Nigrostriatal pathways originate from
A_8 and A_9 cells, mesolimbic pathways from A_{10} cells, and tuberoinfundibular pathways from A_{12} cells.

Multiple Receptors for Dopamine

A considerable amount of research in recent years, reviewed by Kebabian
and Calne (1979), and more recently by Costall and Naylor (1981), suggests that at least two distinct categories of dopamine receptors can be
identified on the basis of biochemical and pharmacologic criteria. These
have been called "D_1 and D_2 receptors." Stimulation of D_1 receptors in-

Table 5-1. Localization of Monoaminergic Cell Groups

Cell group	Localization
Noradrenergic	
A_1	Around nucleus of lateral funiculus
A_2	Dorsolateral to hypoglossal nucleus
A_3	Dorsal to inferior olivary nucleus
A_4	Beside superior cerebellar peduncle
A_5	Around facial and superior olivary nuclei
A_6	Locus ceruleus
A_7	Ventral pontine portion of lateral reticular formation
Dopaminergic	
A_8	Mesencephalic reticular formation
A_9	Pars compacta of substantia nigra
A_{10}	Ventral tegmental area
A_{11}	Dorsal hypothalamic periventricular region
A_{12}	Infundibular nucleus
A_{13}	Zona incerta
A_{14}	Between A_{13} and A_{15}
A_{15}	Olfactory bulb
Serotonergic	
B_1	Nucleus raphes pallidus
B_2	Nucleus raphes obscurus
B_3	Nucleus raphes magnus
B_5	Nucleus raphes pontis
B_6 and B_8	Superior central nucleus of Bechterew
B_7	Nucleus dorsalis raphes

creases the synthesis of cAMP through the action of a specific dopamine-sensitive adenylyl cyclase. In contrast, D_2 receptors show no such cyclase linkage. Phenothiazines are equipotent in blocking both types of receptors. However, haloperidol, molindone, pimozide, sulpiride, tiapride, and oxiperomide are presumed to be more potent in blocking D_2 than D_1 receptors. It has been suggested that D_1 receptors might be involved in the pathophysiology of schizophrenia, and D_2 in tardive dyskinesia ("Editorial," 1979). At present this is still a speculative hypothesis.

Earlier, Klawans (1973) proposed that two populations of dopamine neurons in the caudate (one facilitated and the other inhibited by dopamine) respond differentially to neuroleptics. Evidence for this theory is rather weak (Tarsy & Baldessarini, 1977).

Measurement of Central Dopaminergic Activity

In humans, there is no direct and reliable way of measuring dopaminergic activity in the brain. Dopamine in the CSF and blood has rarely been measured in the past. Measurement of CSF-HVA is a commonly used method for judging dopaminergic activity. Since HVA is cleared relatively quickly from the CSF into the bloodstream, probenecid may be administered to block the outflow of the acid metabolites in the CSF by way of choroid plexus and thus to raise the concentration of these metabolites. Probenecid also reduces the renal excretion of HVA. Olsson and Roos (1968) suggested that the rate of rise in the concentration of HVA and 5-hydroxyindoleacetic acid (5-HIAA) in the brain and CSF after probenecid may be an indicator of the rate of synthesis and turnover of dopamine and 5-hydroxytryptamine, respectively, in the brain. Significantly lower than normal levels of CSF-HVA after probenecid in patients with Parkinson's disease (Olsson & Roos, 1968) are in accordance with the demonstrated nigrostriatal dopamine deficiency in this disease. Bowers, Moore, and Tarsy (1979) noted that, since the caudate nucleus formed a major part of the boundary of the lateral ventricle, CSF studies might be especially useful in diseases involving the striatum. These investigators measured CSF-HVA as an indicator of presynaptic dopamine turnover, and CSF-cAMP as a possible index of dopamine receptor activity in the brain.

Table 5-2 summarizes the findings on CSF-HVA in various conditions. It is interesting to note that CSF-HVA is low in several conditions associated with abnormal involuntary movements, including hyperthyroidism (Klawans, 1973, p. 93), but not in Gilles de la Tourette's syndrome (Van Woert, Jutkowitz, Rosenbaum, et al., 1976).

DISTURBANCES OF DOPAMINERGIC FUNCTION

Table 5-3 summarizes the presumed disturbances of dopaminergic function in various conditions. It must be added that direct evidence of specific pathology of the dopaminergic system is available only in one disease process—Parkinson's disease. Several studies have convincingly demonstrated a loss of dopamine neurons in the nigrostriatal system in patients with Parkinson's disease (see Hornykiewicz, 1976). The evidence for dopaminergic hyperactivity in schizophrenia (reviewed by Matthysse, 1978, and

Table 5-2. CSF-HVA Concentrations in Various Conditions

Condition	CSF-HVA
Parkinson's disease	↓[a]
Neuroleptic-induced parkinsonism	↓ or N[b]
Huntington's disease	↓
Dystonia musculorum deformans	↓
Hyperthyroidism[c]	↓
Gilles de la Tourette's syndrome	↑[d]
Senile dementia	↓
Schizophrenia	Variable
Acute treatment with neuroleptics	↑
Chronic treatment with neuroleptics	N or ↑
Neuroleptic-withdrawal-emergent dyskinesia	↓ or N
Tardive dyskinesia	↓, N, or ↑

[a]↓ = lower than controls.
[b]N = normal.
[c]Klawans, Shenker, Weiner, *et al.* (1973).
[d]↑ = higher than controls.

Table 5-3. Presumed Disturbances of Dopaminergic Function

Condition	Site of disturbance		
	Mesolimbic	Nigrostriatal	Hypothalamic
Schizophrenia	↑[a]	N[b]	N
Parkinsonism	N?	↓[c]	N?
Neuroleptic action	↓	↓	↓
Tardive dyskinesia	N	↑	N
Hyperprolactinemia	N	N	↓
L-Dopa action	↑	↑	↑
Huntington's disease	N	↑	N
Gilles de la Tourette's syndrome	N	↑	N

Note. Direct evidence for such presumed disturbances is usually lacking, as in schizophrenia. We must also add that this table is based on generalizations that may not apply to all the patients having a particular disorder. For example, it is possible that catatonic schizophrenics may have increased dopaminergic activity in the nigrostriatal system, too, and patients with Huntington's disease or Gilles de la Tourette's syndrome suffering from psychosis may have dopaminergic hyperactivity in the mesolimbic area.

[a]↑ = increased.
[b]N = normal.
[c]↓ = decreased.

Meltzer, 1979) is indirect and is essentially based on our knowledge of the mechanism of action of drugs that reduce (neuroleptics) or increase (dopaminergic drugs) the symptoms of schizophrenia. There are sufficient experimental data to allow one to conclude that most neuroleptics, such as phenothiazines, act by blocking dopamine receptors, whereas d-amphetamine and L-dopa, which aggravate symptoms of schizophrenia, increase dopaminergic activity (mainly at the presynaptic level). It should be stressed that there is no satisfactory evidence of a generalized dopaminergic overactivity in schizophrenia.

IS THERE DOPAMINERGIC OVERACTIVITY IN TARDIVE DYSKINESIA?

The evidence suggesting an excessive dopaminergic activity in tardive dyskinesia is indirect:

1. Dopaminergic agents such as L-dopa and amphetamine aggravate symptoms of tardive dyskinesia (Chapter 10).
2. Dopamine-depleting (e.g., reserpine, tetrabenazine) and dopamine-blocking (e.g., phenothiazines, butyrophenones) neuroleptics are the most effective suppressors of tardive dyskinesia (see Chapter 10).
3. Withdrawal of neuroleptics usually results in an initial worsening of the symptoms of tardive dyskinesia.
4. Dopaminergic drugs (e.g., L-dopa and ergolines) given to patients with Parkinson's disease produce dyskinesias that are phenomenologically similar to neuroleptic-induced tardive dyskinesia.
5. Dyskinesias induced by L-dopa, as well as those occurring spontaneously in Huntington's disease and Gilles de la Tourette's syndrome, are reduced by neuroleptics and aggravated by several dopaminergic agents. All these movement disorders are presumed to be associated with nigrostriatal dopaminergic hyperactivity.
6. Anticholinergic drugs tend to aggravate or have little effect on tardive dyskinesia. The symptoms of parkinsonism (idiopathic and drug-induced) respond to drugs in a manner opposite to that of tardive dyskinesia—that is, they are reduced by anticholinergic agents and dopaminergic drugs and are aggravated by neuroleptics. Parkinson's disease is known to be associated with a nigro-

striatal deficit of dopamine (and, hypothetically, a consequent increase in cholinergic functioning). It is therefore believed that tardive dyskinesia may be associated with nigrostriatal dopaminergic hyperactivity.

Limitations of the Hypothesis of Dopaminergic Overactivity in Tardive Dyskinesia

There are four basic limitations. First, there is as yet no direct evidence, in antemortem or postmortem studies, of excessive dopaminergic function in patients with tardive dyskinesia. It may be added, however, that there have been few large-scale and well-conducted studies that sought such evidence. The various studies on the CSF have not found consistent changes in the concentrations of dopamine metabolites in dyskinetic patients (Table 5-4).

Second, there is little indication of a generalized overactivity of dopaminergic systems in tardive dyskinesia. Various researchers (Asnis, Sachar, & Langer, 1979; Cohen, Cooper, & Altshul, 1979; Ettigi, Nair, Cerbantes, et al., 1976; Jeste, Neckers, Wagner, et al., 1981; Meltzer, Goode, Fang, et al., 1976; Pandye, Garver, Tamminga, et al., 1977; Tamminga, Smith, Pandye, 1977) did not find any significant difference between dyskinesia patients and matched controls in the prolactin and growth hormone concentrations in the blood, reflective of the tuberoinfundibular dopamine activity. Similarly, there does not appear to be any consistent correlation between the presence or severity of dyskinesia and mesolimbic dopaminergic pathology as (possibly) suggested by schizophrenic symptomatology. Despite case reports of the so-called tardive or supersensitivity psychosis (Chouinard & Jones, 1980), development or aggravation of schizophrenia-like psychosis with prolonged neuroleptic treatment is an exception rather than a rule. There is little clinical evidence that occurrence of tardive dyskinesia in previously nonpsychotic patients is accompanied by development of psychosis.

Third, Matthysse (1978) and others have aptly pointed out that response to drugs may not necessarily indicate central pathogenesis of a disease. Thus patients with Parkinson's disease were successfully treated for years with anticholinergic drugs. Yet, we now know that the primary pathology in this disease is not an excess of acetylcholine, but rather a deficiency of dopamine (in the nigrostriatal system). Similarly, the hyperdopaminergic state (dopamine receptor supersensitivity?) in Huntington's dis-

Table 5-4. Studies of Monoamine Metabolites in the CSF

Investigators	Number of dyskinetic patients	Controls	Findings
Pind and Faurbye (1970)	8	From literature (Olsson & Roos, 1968)	HVA and 5-HIAA levels increased after probenecid, similar to the controls. High levels in both groups?
Chase, Schnur, and Gordon (1970)	6	5 schizophrenics treated with neuroleptics	HVA (and 5-HIAA) levels lower in dyskinetic patients and in patients with drug-induced parkinsonism.
Chase (1973)	8	Patients with various neurological diseases	HVA levels after probenecid lower than normal controls. Response to haloperidol also low in 6 dyskinetic patients. Lowest values in parkinsonian patients.
Curzon (1973)	7	None	HVA and 5-HIAA similar to controls.
Gerlach, Thorsen, and Fog (1975)	7	None	Haloperidol reduced dyskinesia, increased HVA. Clozapine did not affect dyskinesia, but reduced HVA and 5-HIAA.
Roccatagliata, Albano, and Besio (1977)	4	None	Trazadone reduced dyskinesia, increased HVA, reduced 5-HIAA.
Winsberg, Hurwic, and Perel (1977)	3 children with withdrawal-emergent dyskinesia	3 children without withdrawal-emergent dyskinesia	Lower HVA and 5-HIAA levels after probenecid in dyskinetic children; cAMP not different from controls.
Bowers, Moore, and Tarsy (1979)	11	26 schizophrenic and 19 depressed patients	HVA similar to controls; cAMP significantly lower compared to schizophrenic controls, but similar to depressed patients.
Nagao, Ohshimo, Mitsunobu, *et al.* (1979)	12	15 chronic schizophrenics (nondyskinetic)	HVA, MHPG, 5-HIAA, cAMP, and cGMP similar to controls. Sodium valproate or cyproheptadine reduced dyskinesia, reduced HVA, and increased cAMP and cGMP. Patients with drug-induced tremor (parkinsonism) had lowest HVA and 5-HIAA levels.

ease (inferred on the basis of drug response) is probably a consequence of a severe decrease in the levels of GABA in the basal ganglia. It is therefore possible that the putative dopaminergic overactivity in tardive dyskinesia may be secondary to another biochemical disturbance.

Fourth, a coexistence of the symptoms of parkinsonism and tardive dyskinesia would not be expected on the basis of this theory. A number of studies have shown, however, that there is often no inverse correlation between the severity of the two syndromes in the same patients (Degkwitz, 1969; Degkwitz & Wenzel, 1967; Jeste, Potkin, Sinha, *et al.,* 1979; Jus *et al.,* 1976a; Pandurangi *et al.,* 1978).

We can conclude that an excess of dopaminergic activity in the nigrostriatal system in tardive dyskinesia is suggested by pharmacologic response, but has not yet been demonstrated directly. It is also possible that there are several subtypes of this syndrome and that dopaminergic hyperactivity may be associated with only certain subtypes.

POSSIBLE MECHANISMS FOR DOPAMINERGIC OVERACTIVITY IN TARDIVE DYSKINESIA

Dopaminergic overactivity can conceivably result from functional disturbances (with or without structural pathology) at three levels: presynaptic, synaptic, and postsynaptic. The most popular hypothesis suggests postsynaptic receptor supersensitivity in tardive dyskinesia. There is little work on synaptic pathology in this syndrome.

Postsynaptic Receptor Supersensitivity

"Supersensitivity" may be defined as a decrease in the amount of the agonist required to elicit a given biological response (Langer, 1975). It is the opposite of "tolerance" (defined as an increase in the amount of a substance required to produce a given response); therefore supersensitivity has also been called "reverse tolerance." It is worth noting that supersensitivity is an observable phenomenon and does not necessarily imply any specific pathophysiological mechanism.

Langer (1975), who reviewed the extensive literature on denervation supersensitivity, notes that the increased responsiveness of a surgically denervated organ to specific agonists was known to the nineteenth-century physiologists. Until recently, most of the experimental work on denervation supersensitivity involved the peripheral nervous system. In 1961 Stavraky described supersensitivity to acetylcholine following lesions of the afferent pathways in the central nervous system. Ungerstedt (1971) provided probably the first direct demonstration of central catecholaminergic denervation supersensitivity. By unilateral injections of 6-hydroxydopamine into the brain, he produced a specific destruction of the catecholamine neurons in the nigrostriatal system (on the injected side) in rats. The denervated side showed a markedly heightened response to dopamine agonists, L-dopa, and apomorphine. This work has been confirmed many times since Ungerstedt's publication (see Tarsy & Baldessarini, 1974). According to Langer (1975), the relatively gradual evolution of supersensitivity and the increased responsiveness to apomorphine (presumed to be a specific postsynaptic dopamine receptor agonist with little presynaptic dopamine stimulant action) suggest that such supersensitivity is postsynaptic.

Most of the neuroleptics are believed to block the effect of dopamine on postsynaptic receptors. Long-term neuroleptic administration may thus be expected to produce prolonged blockade of dopamine receptors (Figure 5-1). This situation is likened to a chemical denervation of those receptors produced by 6-hydroxydopamine. It is therefore logical to hypothesize that long-term use of neuroleptics also results in a supersensitiv-

Figure 5-1. Postsynaptic dopamine (DA) receptor supersensitivity hypothesis.

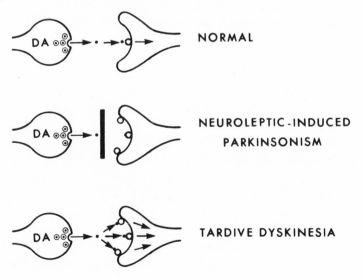

NORMAL

NEUROLEPTIC-INDUCED
PARKINSONISM

TARDIVE DYSKINESIA

ity of dopamine receptors. In Chapter 9, we have summarized animal studies indicating that chronic treatment with neuroleptics followed by their discontinuation results in an increased responsiveness to dopamine agonists. Here, too, the temporal course of development of supersensitivity and the heightened response to apomorphine suggest that the supersensitivity may be primarily postsynaptic.

Possible mechanisms for postsynaptic receptor supersensitivity include increased sensitivity of the available receptors and an increase in the number of receptors. The presence of the former mechanism has not yet been demonstrated convincingly, although it cannot be ruled out. A study involving labeling of dopamine receptors with tritiated dopamine and haloperidol in rat brain (Snyder, 1976) provided support to the hypothesis that an increase in the amount or number of functional receptors is responsible for postsynaptic dopaminergic supersentivity following long-term use of neuroleptics. The investigators observed an increase in the binding of the labeled ligands following either an injection of 6-hydroxydopamine into the substantia nigra or prolonged administration of neuroleptics. The increase in the binding sites correlated positively with the degree of behavioral supersensitivity to apomorphine seen in the same animals. It is reasonable to believe, although not yet proven, that the binding sites represent functional dopamine receptors.

Thus there is strong experimental evidence to support the hypothesis of postsynaptic dopamine receptor supersensitivity following chronic neuroleptic treatment in animals. Next, it is necessary to see if there is clinical evidence of such receptor supersensitivity in patients with tardive dyskinesia and other related disorders.

Clinical Evidence of Dopamine Receptor Supersensitivity. Langer (1975) and Sharpless (1975) have reviewed supersensitivity-like phenomena in the central nervous system. Clinical examples of such phenomena include the following:

1. Parkinson's disease and L-dopa—It has been suggested that the loss of presynaptic dopaminergic neurons in the substantia nigra in Parkinson's disease results in denervation supersensitivity of the postsynaptic receptors of the caudate and putamen. This supersensitivity may be an important reason for the efficacy of L-dopa in Parkinson's disease (Langer, 1975) and even for the L-dopa-induced dyskinesias. Although this is an attractive hypothesis, there

is as yet no satisfactory evidence to support it. Indeed, the absence of dyskinesias either early in the course of the disease (Tarsy & Baldessarini, 1977) or early during the L-dopa treatment argues against the L-dopa-induced dyskinesias being primarily a result of denervation supersensitivity. It is likely that L-dopa treatment itself induces postsynaptic receptor supersensitivity (see Chapter 8).

2. Drug-withdrawal syndromes—According to Sharpless (1969), disuse supersensitivity may be responsible for the phenomena of tolerance and withdrawal syndromes seen with some centrally acting drugs. In view of the numerous experiments suggesting the occurrence of postsynaptic dopaminergic supersensitivity following prolonged neuroleptic administration in animals, it is probable that at least some cases of neuroleptic-withdrawal-emergent dyskinesias may be a result of receptor supersensitivity.

3. Epilepsy—Sharpless (1975) and Stavraky (1961) mentioned the possible contribution of supersensitivity to the pathophysiology of epilepsy. Damage to certain neurons may lead to supersensitive postsynaptic receptors that overreact to stimuli, the consequence being a seizure. This theory may be particularly applicable in the case of the so-called reflex or sensory precipitation epilepsy (e.g., musicogenic epilepsy secondary to a temporal lobe lesion).

It is apparent that the possibility of postsynaptic receptor supersensitivity playing a role in certain central nervous system disorders exists, although direct clinical evidence to prove it beyond reasonable doubt is lacking.

Investigators have tried different approaches to testing dopamine receptor supersensitivity in tardive dyskinesia.

1. Clinical association with history of neuroleptic-induced parkinsonism—Nigrostriatal dopaminergic hypofunctioning (clinically manifested by symptoms of parkinsonism) might be expected to predispose to the development of postsynaptic receptor supersensitivity (which, according to the hypothesis, manifests as tardive dyskinesia). Although Crane (1972b) found a significant association between tardive dyskinesia and a past history of drug-induced parkinsonism, several other studies (see Chapter 4) failed to detect such an association. It is, of course, possible that parkinsonism and tardive dyskinesia might involve different types of dopamine receptors.

2. Response to receptor agonists—If tardive dyskinesia were caused by postsynaptic receptor supersensitivity, we might expect to see worsening of dyskinesia with drugs such as apomorphine and bromocriptine. There is, however, little evidence to indicate aggravation of tardive dyskinesia with apomorphine (Carroll, Curtis, & Kokmen, 1977; Meltzer *et al.*, 1976; Tolosa, 1978a) or bromocriptine (Pöldinger, 1978; Ringwald, 1978). These drugs were sometimes given in doses as high as 6 mg of apomorphine (Carroll *et al.*, 1977) and 32 mg of bromocriptine (Ringwald, 1978), and it is unlikely that their action was restricted to the inhibitory autoreceptors[1]; in all probability, they acted on postsynaptic receptors, too. In contrast, aggravation of tardive dyskinesia by amphetamine and L-dopa, which act presynaptically, is a well-known phenomenon (see Chapter 10).

   3. CSF studies—CSF-HVA concentrations have been used as an index of presynaptic dopaminergic activity, and CSF-cAMP concentrations as an indicator of postsynaptic dopamine receptor functioning. If tardive dyskinesia were associated with postsynaptic dopamine receptor supersensitivity, one might expect to find elevated CSF-cAMP and lowered CSF-HVA, the latter indicating diminished presynaptic activity, which might predispose to, or be a compensatory consequence of, postsynaptic supersensitivity. Studies summarized in Table 5-4 do not support the supersensitivity hypothesis. Bowers *et al.* (1979) observed significantly lower CSF-cAMP in dyskinetic patients compared to schizophrenic controls, whereas Nagao, Ohshimo, Mitsunobu, *et al.* (1979) found no difference in cAMP between the two groups. Winsberg *et al.* (1977) also concluded that cAMP did not appear to be involved in withdrawal-emergent dyskinesias in children.

   Studies of CSF-HVA levels in tardive dyskinesia patients have yielded conflicting results. Bowers *et al.* (1979), Curzon (1973), and Nagao *et al.* (1979) noted that the dyskinesia patients had CSF-HVA levels similar to those of the nondyskinetic psychiatric patients. Chase (1973) and Chase, Schnur, and Gordon, (1970) reported lower CSF-HVA in their patients with dyskinesia. It seems, however, that two of their eight patients had very high HVA concentrations, while the other six had low values. Pind and Faurbye (1970) compared the CSF-HVA levels in their dyskinetic patients with those of the controls from the study by Olsson and Roos (1968) and found no difference between the two groups. As noted by Bowers *et*

---

[1]It is postulated that apomorphine and bromocriptine, when administered in small doses, act on presynaptic autoreceptors. Stimulation of these autoreceptors is presumed to result in inhibition of dopamine synthesis and release.

al. (1979), however, those control values were probably too high. Furthermore, the mean age of the controls (77.3 years) was significantly higher than that of the patients of Pind and Faurbye (53.5 years). Gottfries, Gottfries, Johansson, *et al.* (1971) have reported a significant positive correlation between age and CSF-HVA level. Therefore it seems that the dyskinetic patients of Pind and Faurbye had high CSF-HVA concentrations. In sum, there has been no consistent pattern of CSF-HVA in the reported studies of patients with tardive dyskinesia. Individual patients may have low, normal, or high concentrations. Interestingly, Winsberg *et al.* (1977) obtained lower CSF-HVA in children with withdrawal-emergent dyskinesias as compared to children without such dyskinesia.

The CSF data have considerable limitations. It is possible that only a subgroup of dyskinesia patients with low CSF-HVA may have postsynaptic dopaminergic supersensitivity.

4. Receptor supersensitivity and old age—The receptor theory fails to explain the increased prevalence of tardive dyskinesia in the elderly. Makman *et al.* (1979) demonstrated a decrease in the number of functional monoamine receptors in old animals, whereas Weiss, Greenberg, and Cantor (1979) found a reduced capacity of the aged tissues to increase the number of receptors in response to the lowering of neurotransmitter input.

Summary. Prolonged treatment of animals with neuroleptics produces postsynaptic dopamine receptor supersensitivity. There is, however, no satisfactory clinical evidence that this mechanism is responsible for tardive dyskinesia. Of course the available data do not rule out the possibility of such supersensitivity in certain subtypes of dyskinesia, particularly the relatively short-lived withdrawal-emergent dyskinesias. We agree with Baldessarini (1979) and others that the postsynaptic receptor supersensitivity may be too short-lived to explain persistent tardive dyskinesias. Other mechanisms are likely to be involved.

Presynaptic Overactivity

Increased synthesis or reduced reuptake of dopamine, reduced activity of MAO, and subsensitivity of presynaptic inhibitory autoreceptors for dopamine are among the principal mechanisms that may cause presynaptic dopaminergic·overactivity. Another possible mechanisms is the phenomenon of neuronal "sprouting" following partial neuronal lesions in animals, produced electrolytically or by 6-hydroxydopamine injection. The clinical significance of this last phenomenon is uncertain (Baldessarini & Tarsy, 1978).

Normally, when the concentration of dopamine in the synapse exceeds a certain threshold, a feedback mechanism becomes operative, resulting in diminished release and increased reuptake of dopamine. Breakdown of this self-inhibitory feedback system is the primary cause of presynaptic overactivity (Langer, 1975). Although Trendelenburg (1963) called it "presynaptic supersensitivity," most of the presynaptic mechanisms may not involve supersensitivity (i.e., increased responsiveness to a given concentration of an agonist). Hence "presynaptic overactivity" may be a preferable term.

Carlsson and Lindqvist (1963) first demonstrated enhanced turnover of dopamine following neuroleptic administration in animals and suggested that this was probably a feedback response to neuroleptic-induced postsynaptic dopamine receptor blockade. Such an increase in dopamine turnover has been found to be a short-lasting response. Continued administration of neuroleptics leads to the lowering of dopamine synthesis and release in corpus striatum (Scatton, Garret, & Julou, 1975). It is conceivable that in some patients a reduction in presynaptic dopaminergic activity may not occur despite prolonged neuroleptic therapy. These patients (possibly with structural damage to the presynaptic neurons) may be at risk for developing tardive dyskinesia. The high CSF-HVA levels and low CSF-cAMP concentrations reported in some patients with tardive dyskinesia (Table 5-4) support a likelihood of presynaptic dopaminergic overactivity in subgroups of dyskinesia patients.

Tolerance or subsensitivity of presynaptic autoreceptors that inhibit synthesis and release of dopamine may cause enhanced dopaminergic functioning. However, little is known so far about the contribution, if any, of such a mechanism to the development of tardive dyskinesia.

Peripheral MAO and DBH Activities in Tardive Dyskinesia. Our studies (Jeste, Phelps, Wagner, *et al.,* 1979; Jeste, De Lisi, Zalcman, *et al.,* 1981; Jeste, Kleinman, Potkin, *et al.,* 1982) suggest that a sizable subgroup of patients with tardive dyskinesia is associated with low platelet and lymphocyte MAO activities and high plasma DBH activity (Figures 5-2 through 5-4). Seventeen schizophrenic women over 50 years of age had significantly lower platelet MAO activity (mean $\pm$ *SEM,* 25.3 $\pm$ 1.9 nmol/mg/h) than a control group (34.7 $\pm$ 1.9 nmol/mg/h) matched for

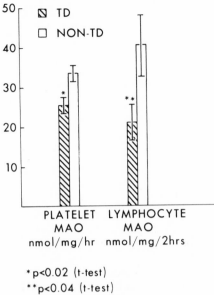

*p<0.02 (t-test)
**p<0.04 (t-test)

Figure 5-2. Platelet and lymphocyte MAO activities in matched female patients with and without tardive dyskinesia (TD).

Figure 5-3. Plasma DBH activity in female schizophrenic patients with and without tardive dyskinesia (TD).

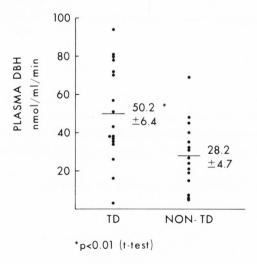

*p<0.01 (t-test)

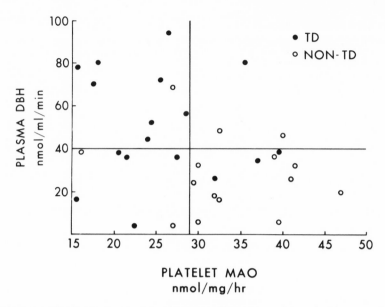

Figure 5-4. Distribution of female schizophrenic patients with and without tardive dyskinesia (TD) according to platelet MAO and plasma DBH activities.

gender, primary psychiatric diagnosis, mean age, length of hospitalization, and duration of neuroleptic treatment. A study of lymphocyte MAO activity in 8 patients from each group showed that the dyskinetic patients had significantly lower values (21.1 ± 4.7 nmol/mg/2 h) than the controls (40.3 ± 7.5 nmol/mg/2 h). A comparison of plasma DBH activity in all 17 patients from each group revealed that the patients with tardive dyskinesia had significantly higher plasma DBH activity than the controls (50.2 ± 6.4 vs. 28.2 ± 4.7 nmol/min/ml).

Using mean platelet MAO and plasma DBH activities for the total population as cutoff points, we divided the patients into four groups: low MAO/low DBH, low MAO/high DBH, high MAO/low DBH, and high MAO/high DBH. The distribution of dyskinetic versus nondyskinetic patients into these four groups differed significantly. Eight of the 9 patients in the low MAO/high DBH category were dyskinetic, whereas only 3 of the 13 patients in the high MAO/low DBH group had dyskinesia. There was, however, no significant correlation between MAO and DBH activities in individual patients. A 1-year biochemical follow-up showed high correlation (intraclass correlation coefficient .79 for MAO, .80 for DBH) between enzyme values in 1979 and 1980. Despite changes in neuroleptic medication in some patients during the year, dyskinetic patients still had significantly lower platelet MAO and higher plasma DBH activities than controls. Preliminary results of another study (unpublished data) suggest that the low MAO/high DBH patients with tardive dyskinesia also had high plasma renin activity, an indicator of increased catecholaminergic (especially noradrenergic) function. Recently we have replicated the finding of low platelet MAO and high plasma DBH activities in dyskinetic patients in a population of men under 50 years.

These results suggest that at least a subgroup of tardive dyskinesias is associated with peripheral indices of increased catecholaminergic (and perhaps, mainly noradrenergic) activity. It is unclear whether the biochemical findings are a result, a risk factor, or a mere accompaniment of tardive dyskinesia. The relationship between peripheral and central enzyme activities is also uncertain.

Freedman, Roffman, and Goldstein (1973) and Lieberman, Freedman, and Goldstein (1972) reported increased plasma DBH activity in Huntington's disease, which shares several features with tardive dyskinesia. These investigators also observed significantly reduced plasma DBH activity in untreated patients with Parkinson's disease, which is in some ways an opposite of tardive dyskinesia. Two studies on the use of DBH inhibitors in the treatment of dyskinesias had encouraging results. Viukari and Linnoila (1977) found fusaric acid useful in patients with tardive dyskinesia, and Birket-Smith and Andersen (1973) observed reduction in L-dopa-induced dyskinesias with disulfiram.

In sum, there are some peripheral indications of differences in activities of catecholaminergic enzymes between a subgroup of dyskinetic patients and controls. The significance of these findings is not yet clear.

Other Data. The concept of presynaptic hyperactivity is not new. Schelkunov (1967) was probably the first to show that prolonged neuroleptic treatment followed by medication withdrawal in animals resulted in catecholaminergic hyperactivity. He considered several mechanisms that might be responsible for this effect, including increased synthesis and turnover of catecholamines. Robbins and Fischbach (1971) reported that chronic disuse of the rat soleus neuromuscular junction resulted in increased presynaptic transmitter release. Morphine-induced supersensitivity to dopamine may be a central presynaptic phenomenon (Lomax, 1977). Engel, Liljequist, and Johannessen (1976), Seeman and Lee (1975), and

Smith *et al.* (1978) showed significant presynaptic effects with neuroleptic use in animals. The possibility of presynaptic overactivity in tardive dyskinesia was mentioned by Baldessarini and Tarsy (1978), Carlsson (1970), and Korczyn (1972).

Summary. Presynaptic mechanisms that may result in dopaminergic overactivity do exist. These may play an important role in at least certain subgroups of patients with tardive dyskinesia. They have not received the attention they deserve and need to be studied more carefully. Particularly interesting in this respect are the findings of low platelet and lymphocyte MAO and high plasma DBH in patients with tardive dyskinesia. We agree with Sharpless (1975) that, in our present preoccupation with receptor processes, we may be overlooking disturbances in presynaptic functions.

NOREPINEPHRINE (NORADRENALINE)

PHYSIOLOGY

Norepinephrine is synthesized from dopamine in the noradrenergic neurons. The enzyme that catalyzes this reaction is DBH. The major end products of metabolism of norepinephrine are vanillylmandelic acid (VMA) and 3-methoxy-4-hydroxyphenylglycol (MHPG), formed by the combined actions of MAO and COMT, and normetanephrine, formed by methylation of norepinephrine by COMT. Measurement of urinary[2] and CSF levels of MHPG is often used as an index of central noradrenergic function; VMA levels primarily reflect the activity of the peripheral sympathetic nervous system.

Peripherally, norepinephrine is present in the adrenal medulla and in the sympathetic nervous system. In the brain there are two principal pathways containing noradrenergic cells:

---

[2]A recent study by Blombery, Kopin, Gordon, *et al.* (1980) suggests, however, that only about 20% of the urinary MHPG is derived from the brain, and therefore urinary MHPG should not be used as a valid index of brain norepinephrine metabolism.

1. Ventral—Cell bodies in the brain stem give rise to axons that terminate in the hypothalamus and limbic system, including the nucleus accumbens septi. Some axons descend to end in the spinal cord.
2. Dorsal—Cell bodies in the locus ceruleus give rise to axons that go in different directions and terminate in cerebral cortex, hippocampus, and cerebellum.

Table 5-1 summarizes locations of seven (A_1 through A_7) specific noradrenergic cell groups (Dahlström and Fuxe, 1964, 1965; Voogd & Huijzen, 1979). Central noradrenergic functioning is believed to be associated with regulation of psychomotor activity, certain affective states, and reward behavior.

Norepinephrine–Dopamine Interrelationship

Central noradrenergic mechanisms probably act synergistically with the striatal dopaminergic system, at least with respect to locomotor activity. Hornykiewicz (1976) suggests that norepinephrine sets up the sensitivity of those neuronal systems on which dopamine acts in regulating locomotor activation, although the exact site in the brain for such an interaction is not yet known. In support of this hypothesis, Hornykiewicz offers pharmacologic evidence. For example, DBH inhibitors, which inhibit the synthesis of norepinephrine from dopamine, tend to reduce locomotor excitation caused by catecholaminergic agents such as L-dopa; direct norepinephrine agonists such as clonidine can then restore the locomotor effects of L-dopa. Norepinephrine function is also linked to 5-hydroxytryptamine mechanisms (discussed later).

PATHOLOGY OF THE NORADRENERGIC SYSTEM

There is considerable indirect evidence to indicate that primary affective disorders (depression and mania) are associated with pathophysiology of the noradrenergic system. Although Parkinson's disease is a dopamine deficiency disease, norepinephrine concentrations are also reduced in the nucleus accumbens septi (and other limbic–hypothalamic structures) and probably contribute to the symptom of akinesia (Hornykiewicz, 1976). L-Dopa, the most widely used drug in the treatment of Parkinson's disease, increases turnover of dopamine as well as norepinephrine.

Plasma DBH activity, which sometimes parallels noradrenergic function, is higher than normal in patients with Huntington's disease and lower than normal in untreated patients with Parkinson's disease (Lieberman *et al.*, 1972). Although the "dopamine hypothesis" has been the most popular biochemical theory of schizophrenia, there are now impressive data to suggest that central noradrenergic overactivity may also be present in at least a subtype of schizophrenia (Carlsson, 1979; Farley, Price, McCullough, *et al.*, 1978; Kleinman, Bridge, Karoum, *et al.*, 1979; Lake, Sternberg, van Kammen, *et al.*, 1979).

Many drugs that act on the dopamine system also act directly on the noradrenergic mechanisms, and vice versa. Amphetamine and L-dopa stimulate both systems. Although neuroleptics are often considered to be specific dopamine antagonists, they also exert norepinephrine-blocking action to a variable extent (Peroutka & Snyder, 1980). There is no correlation between the dopamine-blocking and norepinephrine-blocking effects of individual neuroleptics (Pletscher & Kyburz, 1976). Different investigators have reported that the blockade of α-noradrenergic receptors by neuroleptics may be relevant to the sedative action (Fuxe, Hokfelt, & Ungerstedt, 1970), extrapyramidal effects (Anden & Grabowska-Anden, 1980), or therapeutic effects (Robinson, Berney, Mishra, *et al.*, 1979). Using cerebellar Purkinje cell as a model neuronal system, Freedman (1977) and Marwaha, Hoffer, Geller, *et al.* (1981) found that the antipsychotic actions of fluphenazine and haloperidol might be related to interference with noradrenergic effects.

On the other hand, there is no significant correlation between antipsychotic potency of various neuroleptics and noradrenergic receptor blockade. Pletscher and Kyburz (1976) noted that, among the six neuroleptics they studied methiothepin was the least potent and pimozide the most potent in enhancing the turnover of norepinephrine in rat brain. If the potency of methiothepin in this respect were taken as 1, that of haloperidol would be 6, clozapine 18, thioridazine 27, chlorpromazine 35, and pimozide 140. The equivalent doses of these drugs for antipsychotic efficacy in man follow a different order (Table 1-1).

NOREPINEPHRINE AND TARDIVE DYSKINESIA

Most of the arguments supporting the hypothesis of dopaminergic overactivity in tardive dyskinesia can also be applied to advancing an hypothesis of noradrenergic hyperactivity in this syndrome. Some drugs that produce similar dyskinesias (e.g., amphetamine) are norepinephrine stimulants, too. Also, drugs that best suppress these dyskinesias (neuroleptics) block noradrenergic receptors in addition to dopamine receptors. Our findings of low platelet and lymphocyte MAO and high plasma DBH and renin activities in a subgroup of tardive dyskinesia patients may indicate enhanced noradrenergic activity in these patients. Also compatible with this hypothesis is a study (described later in this chapter under "Neuroleptic Metabolism") suggesting an association between tardive dyskinesia and high serum levels of sulforidazine, the most potent of thioridazine metabolites in binding to α-noradrenergic receptors. Reports of successful treatment of tardive dyskinesia with noradrenergic antagonists such as the DBH inhibitor, fusaric acid (Viukari & Linnoila, 1977), the β-adrenergic receptor blocker, propranolol (Bacher & Lewis, 1980; Kulik & Wilbur, 1980; Moreira & Karnio, 1979) and the presynaptic noradrenergic inhibitor, clonidine (Freedman, Bell, & Kirch, 1980), are consistent with the possibility of a noradrenergic contribution to the pathogenesis of tardive dyskinesia.

We think that investigators have so far paid much less attention to the role of norepinephrine in tardive dyskinesia, whereas they have studied the dopaminergic system more extensively. In view of the suggestion that norepinephrine sets up the sensitivity of those neural systems on which dopamine acts and thus controls locomotor activity (Hornykiewicz, 1976), much more work on noradrenergic involvement in tardive dyskinesia is warranted.

ACETYLCHOLINE

$$(CH_3)_3N^+\text{-}CH_2CH_2\text{-}O\text{-}\overset{O}{\overset{\|}{C}}\text{-}CH_3$$

PHYSIOLOGY

Choline is the precursor of acetylcholine. The synthesis of acetylcholine occurs as follows:

Acetyl coenzyme A		Acetylcholine
+	(Choline acetyltransferase)	+
Choline	$\longrightarrow$	Coenzyme A

Choline can be formed by successive methylations of ethanolamine in liver. It is then transported by the blood to the brain (Cooper, Bloom, & Roth, 1978).

The breakdown of acetylcholine is catalyzed by cholinesterases. The resulting products of the hydrolysis are choline and acetic acid. Cholinesterases are of two principal types: True or specific acetylcholinesterase (present in tissues, including neurons) catabolizes acetylcholine faster than other choline esters, whereas pseudocholinesterase or nonspecific cholinesterase (found in the serum) hydrolyzes other choline esters (e.g., butyrylcholine) more rapidly than acetylcholine.

Acetylcholine is present in the peripheral as well as the central nervous system. Brain stem and corpus striatum are relatively rich in acetylcholine content.

Dopamine–Acetylcholine Balance in the Basal Ganglia

There is presumed to be a reciprocal relationship between dopaminergic and cholinergic activities in the basal ganglia. The evidence for this hypothesis is both clinical and experimental.

The clinical evidence includes the following:

1. Parkinson's disease, which is known to be associated with a severe nigrostriatal dopamine deficiency, shows significant syptomatic improvement with dopaminergic (e.g., L-dopa) as well as anticholinergic (e.g., trihexyphenidyl) drugs. On the other hand, the symptoms are aggravated by antidopaminergic and cholinergic agents.
2. There is a striatal cholinergic deficit in the brains from patients with Huntington's disease (Hornykiewicz, 1976). Dopamine-blocking drugs such as the neuroleptics produce a suppression of chorea, whereas dopaminergic agents aggravate the movement disorder in Huntington's disease.

The evidence gleaned from animal behavior experiments is as follows:

1. Stereotypy and locomotor excitation induced by dopaminergic drugs such as amphetamine and methylphenidate are considered to be due to striatal and mesolimbic dopaminergic stimulation, respectively. These effects are blocked by cholinergic drugs and enhanced by anticholinergic agents (Arnfred & Randrup, 1968).
2. Cools, Hendricks, and Korten (1975) studied the behavioral effects of injections of various drugs (haloperidol, dopamine, atropine, and carbachol) into the caudate nuclei of rhesus monkeys.

The investigators concluded that striatal dopamine and acetylcholine counteracted the effects of each other with respect to the process involed in the generalization of seizures.

3. Both neuroleptics and cholinergic drugs produce catalepsy in animals. Anticholinergic agents inhibit neuroleptic-induced catalepsy (Scheel Krüger, & Randrup, 1968).

4. Costall, Naylor, and Olley (1972) and Ungerstedt, Butcher, Butcher, *et al.* (1969) reported that unilateral injections of neuroleptics or cholinergic drugs into the caudate nucleus produced circling ipsilateral to the side of the injection; on the other hand, similar injections of dopaminergic or anticholinergic agents led to circling contraleteral to the side of the injection.

In the area of microiontophoretic studies, Bloom, Costa, and Salmoiraghi (1965) observed that dopamine applied microiontophoretically to individual neurons of the caudate nucleus of the cat produced depression of the spontaneous firing rate of most of the neurons, whereas acetylcholine caused facilitation of most cells.

All of these data suggest a dopamine–acetylcholine balance in the basal ganglia, in which both neurotransmitters exert mutually antagonistic effects. On the basis of this hypothesis, dopaminergic and anticholinergic drugs might be expected to have qualitatively similar effects, whereas dopamine inhibitors and cholinomimetic compounds would exert similar actions. Clinical experience as well as recent experimental work, however, point to the somewhat simplistic nature of this theory. In a review of the dopamine–acetylcholine interaction, Tarsy (1977) has referred to a number of clinical, animal behavioral, and physiological data that do not fit the hypothesis of dopamine–acetylcholine seesaw.

Recent work on the possible mechanisms of dopamine–acetylcholine interaction has uncovered some interesting leads. In cats immobilized by gallamine, systemic administration of oxotremorine (a cholinergic drug) or perfusion of the caudate nucleus with acetylcholine enhances release of striatal dopamine (Bartholini & Stadler, 1975). In contrast, anticholinergic compounds such as atropine reduce striatal dopamine turnover (Bartholini & Pletscher, 1971). These findings suggest that striatal dopaminergic neurons receive a cholinergic excitatory input. In similar perfusion experiments, the release of acetylcholine in the caudate nucleus is increased by dopamine-blocking neuroleptics and reduced by dopamine agonists (Stadler, Lloyd, Gadea-Ciria, *et al.,* 1973). This observation indicates an inhibitory effect of dopamine on striatal cholinergic neurons. Thus, whereas acetylcholine facilitates dopaminergic activity, dopamine inhibits cholinergic neurons in the striatum. Studies by Bunney and Aghajanian (1976a) suggest acetylcholine-dopamine interaction at the level of substantia nigra, too.

Possible Mechanism of Doapmine-Acetylcholine Interaction in the Basal Ganglia

Figure 6-2 shows the hypothesized interactions of these two neuronal systems with each other and with GABA'ergic neurons in the basal ganglia. Dopaminergic neurons originating in the substantia nigra (pars compacta) terminate in the striatum by synapsing with cholinergic neurons. The latter are short interneurons confined to the striatum, and they synapse with GABA'ergic neurons. The GABA'ergic neurons, in turn, terminate in the substantia nigra (pars reticularis) by synapsing with dopaminergic neurons. In this scheme dopaminergic neurons are inhibitory, and cholinergic neurons are facilitatory. Acetylcholine stimulates dopamine release, whereas dopamine, as a feedback mechanism, inhibits the release of acetylcholine. (GABA itself inhibits dopamine neurons. Acetylcholine blocks GABA'ergic neurons in order to facilitate dopamine release.)

Complexities of the Dopamine-Acetylcholine Interaction

The preceding hypothesis—namely, that striatal acetylcholine stimulates the release of dopamine, which, in turn, inhibits the release of acetylcholine—does not explain all the clinical facts. For example, dopaminergic drugs exert much stronger effects than comparable doses of anticholinergic drugs, both in humans and in animals. Connections between dopaminergic neurons and noncholinergic neurons (especially GABA'ergic) without cholinergic interneurons may be partly responsible for this fact (Tarsy, 1977). In Parkinson's disease, anticholinergic drugs are less effective than L-dopa at any stage of the disease, but especially so during later stages. One reason for this phenomenon may be that anticholinergic agents restore the dopamine-acetylcholine balance at a markedly subphysiological level of dopamine activity, whereas L-dopa restores the balance at a near-normal level of dopamine activity (Hornykiewicz, 1971). Another suggested explanation for the relatively lesser efficacy of anticholinergic drugs in comparison with L-dopa may be a development of tolerance to the anticholinergic actions (Tarsy, 1977). It is possible that tolerance develops more rapidly to anticholinergic than to dopaminergic effects. Alternatively, anticholinergic drug effects may simply be weaker, indirect, and dependent on the presence of at least some dopaminergic function.

A balance between cholinergic and noradrenergic systems in the brain has also been described.

PATHOLOGY OF THE CHOLINERGIC SYSTEM

As noted previously, striatal cholinergic deficits have been demonstrated in the brains of patients with Huntington's disease. It is worth adding that, although Parkinson's disease is presumed to be associated with central cholinergic hypoactivity, the levels of striatal choline acetyltransferase in the brains of patients with this disease are normal.

There is some pharmacologic evidence to implicate cholinergic pathology in affective disorders. Cholinomimetic drugs sometimes improve manic symptoms and aggravate depression. Cholinergic hypofunction is suspected in patients with mania, and cholinergic hyperactivity in patients with depression. There is, however, little direct evidence of a primary disturbance of cholinergic mechanisms in affective disorders. Experimental support for involvement of the cholinergic system in schizophrenia is lacking.

ACETYLCHOLINE AND TARDIVE DYSKINESIA

The hypothesis of striatal cholinergic deficit in tardive dyskinesia (Gerlach et al., 1974; Gianutsos & Lal, 1976) has originated from two basic assumptions: first, that there is a reciprocal relationship between dopamine and acetylcholine in basal ganglia, and second, that there is an apparent nigrostriatal dopaminergic hyperactivity in tardive dyskinesia. The evidence for and limitations of both these assumptions have already been reviewed. The hypothesis of cholinergic hypofunction in tardive dyskinesia itself suggests several testable predictions, which we now examine.

1. There should be evidence of cholinergic deficit in patients with tardive dyskinesia. Few attempts have been made to study cholinergic activity directly in patients with tardive dyskinesia. One reason for this is the lack of suitable methods for judging central cholinergic function in man. Nagao *et al.* (1979) measured cyclic 3', 5'-guanosine monophosphate (cGMP) in the CSF of 12 patients with dyskinesia and 15 controls. They postulated that CSF levels of cGMP might indicate central cholinergic activity, as suggested by Ebstein, Biederman, Rimon, *et al.* (1976). Nagao *et al.* found no difference between patients with and without dyskinesia in CSF-cGMP concentrations. Obviously, more work along similar lines is necessary for studying cholinergic function in tardive dyskinesia.

   2. *Symptoms of tardive dyskinesia should improve with cholinergic drugs.* The results of treating tardive dyskinesia with cholinergic agents are discussed in Chapter 10. Suffice it to say here that the available cholinergic drugs have not been found to demonstrate consistent or specific anti-dyskinetic effects. There is, however, a need for developing more potent cholinomimetic drugs.

   3. *Anticholinergic drugs should produce dyskinesias and should predispose to and aggravate neuroleptic-induced tardive dyskinesia.* Anticholinergic drug-induced oral dyskinesias and choreoathetosis have been reported only rarely (see Chapter 8). Although Klawans (1973) suggested that anticholinergic agents might predispose to neuroleptic-induced tardive dyskinesia, evidence to support this assertion has been weak (see Chapter 4).

   Thus the available data do not support a theory of a primary disturbance in cholinergic activity as being the principal pathophysiological mechanism in tardive dyskinesia. It is possible, however, that some cholinergic dysfunction secondary to a disturbance in catecholaminergic activity may be present in certain subgroups of patients with tardive dyskinesia.

SUMMARY

The existence of an interaction between dopaminergic and cholinergic systems in the basal ganglia is generally undisputed. The nature and extent of such an interaction, and its role in the pathophysiology of various diseases, are, however, uncertain. The concept of a simple seesaw type of relationship between the two neurotransmitters has probably been overstated. The available data indicate that acetylcholine facilitates the release of dopamine, which, as a feedback mechanism, inhibits cholinergic neurons in the striatum. The GABA'ergic neurons are also presumed to be involved in this interaction. In general, anticholinergic drugs have weaker effects on movement disorders than dopaminergic agents. There is as yet no strong evidence to support the theory of a primary cholinergic deficit in tardive dyskinesia. It is probably fair to conclude that any striatal hypoactivity of the cholinergic system in tardive dyskinesia is likely to be mild and secondary to catecholamine pathology.

5-HYDROXYTRYPTAMINE (SEROTONIN)

$$HO-\text{[indole ring]}-CH_2\text{-}CH_2\text{-}NH_2$$

PHYSIOLOGY

The dietary precursor of serotonin is an essential amino acid, L-tryptophan. Serotonin is synthesized as follows:

L-Tryptophan
↓ (Tryptophan hydroxylase)
L-5-Hydroxytryptophan
↓ (Aromatic amino acid decarboxylase)
5-Hydroxytryptamine + CO_2

Serotonin is catabolized by MAO. The end product of serotonin catabolism is 5-HIAA. CSF–5-HIAA levels are often used as an index of central serotonergic function.

The cell bodies of serotonergic neurons are localized in the raphe nuclei in the lower midbrain and upper pons. Their axons terminate in various areas of the brain, the majority going to the hypothalamus. Table 5-1 summarizes the localization of serotonergic cell groups (Dahlström & Fuxe, 1964, 1965; Voogd & Huijzen, 1979).

Catecholamine–Serotonin Balance

Prange, Sisk, and Wilson (1973) and Hornykiewicz (1976) have commented on a catecholamine–serotonin balance in the basal ganglia. Dopamine and norepinephrine facilitate locomotor activity, whereas serotonin tends to suppress it. Changes in catecholamine functioning can often be compensated for by suitable alterations in serotonergic activity.

PATHOLOGY

There are few major neuropsychiatric disorders in which a pathology of the central serotonin system is considered to be primarily responsible. Secondary changes in serotonergic mechanisms are, however, believed to occur in a number of diseases. Thus a 50% decrease in the concentration of nigrostriatal serotonin in patients with Parkinson's disease probably represents an attempt to restore indolamine–catecholamine balance disturbed by a severe deficit of catecholamine levels (Hornykiewicz, 1976). Significantly subnormal concentrations of CSF-5-HIAA have been found in Parkinson's disease, senile dementia, presenile dementia, and neuroleptic-induced parkinsonism (Chase et al., 1970; Gottfries et al., 1971). Some hypotheses of the biochemistry of schizophrenia and major affective disorders involve disturbances of serotonin metabolism, too. Serotonergic pathology has also been linked to certain sleep and autonomic disorders and to migraine.

SEROTONIN AND TARDIVE DYSKINESIA

Prange, Sisk, and Wilson (1973) hypothesized that a deficit of serotonin activity in the basal ganglia might contribute to the pathogenesis of tardive dyskinesia. Although these investigators (Prange, Wilson, Morris, et al., 1973), in a single-blind trial, found L-tryptophan to be useful in four patients with tardive dyskinesia, a double-blind study in three patients showed that the drug was no better than a placebo. Jus, Jus, Gautier, et al. (1974) also had negative results with D, L-tryptophan.

We (Jeste, De Lisi, Zalcman, et al., 1981) found no significant difference in the plasma 5-hydroxytryptamine concentrations (measured by a liquid chromatographic assay) between young male patients with tardive dyskinesia and controls. CSF-5-HIAA studies have yielded conflicting findings. Chase et al. (1970) reported low levels of CSF-5-HIAA in adult patients with tardive dyskinesia, and Winsberg et al. (1977) obtained similar results in children with neuroleptic-withdrawal-emergent dyskinesia. On the other hand, Curzon (1973), Nagao et al. (1979), and Pind and Faurbye (1970) found no significant differences between the CSF concentrations of 5-HIAA of dyskinetic patients and those of controls. Even in the studies by Chase et al. (1970) and Winsberg et al. (1977), the differences between patients with dyskinesia and controls were less striking for 5-HIAA levels than for HVA levels in the CSF.

The available data suggest that a contribution of the serotonergic system to the pathophysiology of tardive dyskinesia is either minor or secondary to disturbances in other systems.

GABA (L-γ-AMINOBUTYRIC ACID)

$$CH_2-CH_2-CH_2-COOH$$
$$|$$
$$NH_2$$

PHYSIOLOGY

L-γ-Aminobutyric acid (GABA) is an amino acid. Although it was first synthesized about a century ago, knowledge of its role as a neurotransmitter in the human brain has been recent and is still quite incomplete.

GABA is formed from L-glutamic acid through the action of the enzyme L-glutamic acid decarboxylase (GAD). The activity of GAD is restricted mostly to the central nervous system, although some activity is also found in the kidneys and possibly in the fibroblasts. GABA is metabolized by GABA-glutamate transaminase (GABA-T) to succinic semialdehyde. The metabolism of GABA is intimately related to the Krebs cycle and thus to carbohydrate metabolism (Cooper *et al.,* 1978).

GABA is found in many areas of the brain and spinal cord, although its highest concentrations are present in the substantia nigra, globus pallidus, and hypothalamus. GABA exerts powerful inhibitory effects when applied to neurons and is believed to act as a neurotransmitter.

GABA–Dopamine Link

Studies by Bunney and Aghajanian (1976a), Hornykiewicz (1976), and others suggest the existence of a GABA–dopamine link in the basal ganglia (Figure 6-2). The GABA'ergic system seems to exert an inhibitory control over the activity of dopaminergic neurons. It is postulated that limbic system GABA serves to reduce locomotor activity, counteracting dopaminergic influence.

PATHOLOGY

A severe decrease in the levels of GABA and in the activity of GAD in the basal ganglia, probably resulting from neuronal loss, is the principal known biochemical abnormality in Huntington's disease (Bird, 1978; Hornykiewicz, 1976). GABA'ergic deficits in the basal ganglia are also found in Alzheimer's disease and Parkinson's disease; in the latter condition, the GABA'ergic activity is probably reduced as a compensatory attempt to restore the GABA–dopamine balance in the wake of a severe dopamine deficiency. Pharmacologic data in humans and animals support the hypothesis of decreased GABA turnover in certain types of seizure disorders.

GABA'ERGIC MECHANISMS IN TARDIVE DYSKINESIA

The apparent antagonism between nigrostriatal dopamine and GABA in their effects on locomotion suggests that, if tardive dyskinesia is associated with dopaminergic hyperactivity, it may also be associated with GABA'ergic deficit. Standefer and Dill (1977) found that intrastriatal injections of the GABA antagonists picrotoxin and bicuculline produced myoclonus in rats; concomitant administration of GABA prevented these abnormal movements. There is, however, little evidence to indicate that neuroleptic-induced tardive dyskinesia in humans is associated with GABA'ergic hypoactivity. Although chlorpromazine and many other neuroleptics are known to reduce the reuptake of GABA into the presynaptic neurons (Cooper et al., 1978), the contribution of such an effect to the pathogenesis of tardive dyskinesia is unclear. McGeer and McGeer (1979) studied the activity of GAD in 50 regions from the brains of 11 chronic schizophrenic patients with a history of prolonged neuroleptic treatment. (The number of patients with tardive dyskinesia was not specified.) The investigators found no significant differences between the schizophrenics and 28 normal controls in the activity of GAD in most regions of the brain.

Chase and Tamminga (1979) reported that four patients with tardive dyskinesia had significantly lower CSF concentrations of GABA (139 ± 70 pmol/ml) than 21 controls (544 ± 63 pmol/ml). The clinical relevance of this finding is uncertain. It is worth noting that the four dyskinetic patients were drug free at the time of the study. Recently, Zimmer, Teelken, Meier, et al. (1981) found that CSF concentrations of GABA were significantly *higher* in 13 chronically ill neuroleptic-treated inpatients (450 ±

120 pmol/ml) than in 17 controls (350 ± 90 pmol/ml). Interestingly, neuroleptic withdrawal for 4 weeks resulted in a significant drop, to near control values, in the CSF-GABA levels of the schizophrenic patients. A number of investigators have tried drugs with presumptively GABA'ergic effects in the treatment of patients with tardive dyskinesia (see Chapter 10). The results are not conclusive of specific antidyskinetic effects of such drugs.

SUMMARY

A reduction in nigrostriatal GABA activity in tardive dyskinesia is possible, but unproven. Large-scale postmortem biochemical studies of brains from tardive dyskinesia patients, aimed at studying the GABA system (e.g., assays of GAD), are lacking. Hence the severity and the extent of any pathology of the GABA system in tardive dyskinesia are not known. On the basis of the available pharmacologic data, it seems unlikely that a disturbance of the GABA'ergic processes might be playing a central role in the pathogenesis of tardive dyskinesia.

ENKEPHALINS

Several groups of investigators, including Pert and Snyder (1973), discovered specific opiate receptors in mammalian brain. This discovery led to a search for endogeneous opiates. Hughes, Smith, Kosterlitz, et al. (1975) were the first to isolate two opiates in the brain. These two pentapeptide enkephalins were called "methionine-enkephalin" and "leucine-enkephalin." The highest concentrations of these enkephalins are found in the caudate and globus pallidus; also, the enkephalin receptors are highly localized in the caudate (Kuhar, Pert, & Snyder, 1973). A number of structurally related endorphins have been discovered in different parts of the body. The functional significance of the endorphins is not yet clear. It is thought that the two enkephalins, methionine-enkephalin and leucine-enkephalin, which have a very short half-life in vivo, act as neurotransmitters. Strategies for exploring possible dysfunctions of endorphin systems in different disorders include measuring endorphins in blood, urine, and CSF and studying the effects of pharmacologic challenges with agonists and antagonists. Berger (1981) has reviewed the literature on studies of endorphin function in schizophrenia. Both an excess and a deficiency of endorphin activity in schizophrenia have been postulated. There is some evidence, although it is rather weak, to support both the hypotheses.

On the basis of the reportedly high concentrations of enkephalins and their receptors in the striatum, Diamond and Borison (1978) postulated a potential role for the enkephalins in extrapyramidal function. The investigators studied the effects of drugs such as naloxone and reserpine on rats with unilaterial 6-hydroxydopamine-induced lesions in the substantia nigra. Diamond and Borison concluded that presynaptic enkephalin interneurons facilitate, and postsynaptic enkaphalin interneurons inhibit, nigrostriatal dopaminergic activation. The authors suggested that these antagonistic effects of presynaptic and postsynaptic enkephalin neurons may be a "fine-tuning" mechanism for nigrostriatal dopaminergic activity. In another experiment on an animal model of tardive dyskinesia, Diamond and Borison (1979) found that methionine-enkephalin blocked stereotypy induced by apomorphine and amphetamine in haloperidol-pretreated rats. In contrast, the opiate antagonist naloxone potentiated such stereotypy. The researchers proposed that a potentiation of central enkephalin mechanisms may be an effective treatment for tardive dyskinesia.

In contrast to this suggestion, Carlsson (1980) reported that prolonged treatment with an opiate, methadone, increased the susceptibility of monkeys to neuroleptic-induced dyskinesia (see Chapter 9).

We found only one clinical study on the effects of opiate agonist and antagonist drugs on tardive dyskinesia. Bjørndal, Casey, and Gerlach (1980) tried three drugs in eight dyskinetic patients: FK33-824 (a synthetic analogue of methionine-enkephalin), morphine, and naloxone (an opiate receptor antagonist). There was no overall significant effect of any of these agents, except for suppression of dyskinesia upon administration of FK33-824 to two patients receiving neuroleptics in high doses.

In view of the preliminary nature of the work done until now, it is too early to comment on a possible contribution of the enkephalin system to the pathophysiology of tardive dyskinesia.

ESTROGENS

A number of investigators have found a higher prevalence of tardive dyskinesia in women than in men (see Chapter 2). This observation has led to speculations regarding the role of estrogens in the pathogenesis of tardive dyskinesia. The available data on this point have, however, been somewhat conflicting.

One group of researchers (Bedard, Langelier, & Villeneuve, 1977; Villeneuve, Langelier, & Bedard, 1978) suggested that estrogens may protect against dyskinesia. Increased prevalence of tardive dyskinesia among postmenopausal women appeared to favor their hypothesis. The investigators observed an improvement in L-dopa-induced dykinesia in one female patient and in neuroleptic-induced tardive dyskinesia in another woman during periods of raised circulating estrogen activity. They postulated an antidopaminergic effect of estrogens in the extrapyramidal system. Two other reports were cited as offering indirect evidence for this hypothesis: Gratton's (1960) observation of an apparent sensitization to neuroleptic-induced parkinsonism, in both genders, by administering estrogens, and an unpublished finding of Raymond (cited by Bedard *et al.*, 1977) that 17-estradiol reversed the effects of dopaminergic drugs on prolactin release. Recently, Villeneuve, Cazejust, and Cote (1980) reported some improvement in tardive dyskinesia among male patients treated with conjugated estrogens in an open trial. Also favoring the hypothesis of antidopaminergic activity of estrogens are animal experiments (Naik, Kelkar, & Sheth, 1978) showing enhanced behavioral responses to amphetamine and β-phenylethylamine following oophorectomy.

In contrast to the preceding theory is the work suggesting that estrogens may have a dyskinesia-enhancing action. There have been clinical reports of dyskinesia presumably induced by estrogens (Koller, Weiner, Klawans, *et al.*, 1979). Choreiform movements have been reported as possible side effects of contraceptive tablets containing estrogens (*Physicians' Desk Reference*, 1982, p. 1775). Nausieda, Koller, Weiner, et al. (1979) found that stereotypy response to amphetamine and apomorphine was significantly reduced in female guinea pigs following oophorectomy. Subsequent chronic administration of estradiol again increased the responsiveness to the dopaminergic agents.

In another experiment, Gordon, Borison, and Diamond (1980) noted that long-term coadministration of estradiol and haloperidol increased dopamine receptor supersensitivity, whereas treatment with estradiol following haloperidol pretreatment tended to reduce such supersensitivity.

In sum, it appears that estrogens may have some dyskinesia-suppressing action, although their prolonged use may possibly aggravate underlying pathology (catecholaminergic hyperactivity) in tardive dyskinesia.

OTHER ENDOCRINE FUNCTIONS

Earlier, a reference was made to studies showing no significant difference in the serum or plasma prolactin and growth levels between patients with dyskinesia and controls.

Rosenbaum, Maruta, Jiang, *et al.* (1979) found that 13 of their 18 patients with dyskinesia had elevated urinary free cortisol levels. Also, there was an inverse relationship between urinary free cortisol and serum thyroid stimulating hormone concentrations. On the basis of a report (Carroll, Curtis, Davies, *et al.,* 1976) of high urinary free cortisol levels in primary affective disorders, but not in schizophrenia, Rosenbaum concluded that a subgroup of dyskinesia patients might have endocrine dysfunction similar to that seen in primary affective disorders. However, the patients with dyskinesia in this study fulfilled most of the research diagnostic criteria for depression rather than for schizophrenia. Hence it is difficult to associate the findings with tardive dyskinesia per se.

Clinical and animal studies with α-melanocyte stimulating hormone (MSH) and MSH release inhibiting factor (MIF-1) are described in Chapter 10. Briefly, these agents did not appear to have noticeable effects on tardive dyskinesia.

In sum, there is little evidence so far to suggest significant endocrine dysfunction in tardive dyskinesia.

NEUROLEPTIC METABOLISM

Despite widespread use of neuroleptics, measurement of blood levels of these drugs is still not done on a regular clinical basis. Although sensitive chemical assays for measuring certain neuroleptics, such as chlorpromazine, and their metabolites are available (see Rivera-Calimlim *et al.,* 1978), such methods are usually expensive, cumbersome, and time consuming. Also, they do not distinguish between pharmacologically active and inactive metabolites of drugs (Cohen, Herschel, Miller, *et al.,* 1980).

Recently, Creese and Snyder (1977) developed a radioreceptor assay in which neuroleptic activity is determined by tritiated spiroperidol displacement. The advantage of this technique is that it measures total dopamine receptor blocking activity rather than concentration of a particular neuroleptic or its metabolites. It has been shown that there is a strong correlation between dopamine receptor blockade and therapeutic potency of neuroleptics (Creese & Snyder, 1977). Several groups of investigators have reported significant correlations between serum concentrations of neuroleptics measured with a radioreceptor assay and dosage, as well as psychopathology scores (e.g., Calil, Avery, Hollister, et al., 1979; Rosenblatt, Pary, Bigelow, et al., 1980). In a study of haloperidol tissue levels in rats, Cohen et al. (1980) found excellent correspondence among results obtained with the radioreceptor assay, radioimmunoassay, and the gas chromatography–mass spectrometry method. The researchers also reported high correlations between serum and brain levels of haloperidol in individual animals. On the other hand, there are some puzzling data which suggest caution in interpreting results with the radioreceptor assay. For example, it is unclear why thioridazine produces several times higher blood levels with this assay than other neuroleptics used in comparable doses (Calil et al., 1979).

As noted in Chapter 4, there are frequently no significant differences between dyskinetic and nondyskinetic patients in the amount of neuroleptic intake. This observation raises the possibility of differential metabolism of the drugs in the two groups. It is conceivable that some patients who metabolize the neuroleptics inefficiently may develop high blood and tissue levels of the drugs, predisposing them to tardive dyskinesia. Our studies support such a possibility in some, but not all, of the patients with tardive dyskinesia. We (Jeste, Rosenblatt, Wagner, et al., 1979; Jeste, Linnoila, Wagner, et al., in press) measured serum neuroleptic levels in eight dyskinetic women over the age of 50 years who were receiving thioridazine or mesoridazine and in eight controls who were also being treated with the same drugs. The two groups were matched for gender and primary psychiatric diagnosis and for mean age, height, weight, and length of neuroleptic treatment. Five patients from each group were also matched for the daily dose of neuroleptic. With a radioreceptor assay, the mean ratio of serum level to daily dose of neuroleptics was 6.3 in patients with tardive dyskinesia and 1.4 in controls. A similar significant difference was found using a liquid chromatographic assay of Skinner, Gochnauer, and Linnoila (1981). The difference was significant whether we compared all 16 patients from the two groups or only the ten dose-matched patients. Interestingly, the metabolite of thioridazine that was found in highest concentrations in dyskinetic patients was sulforidazine. Sulforidazine has been shown to have the maximum affinity, among thioridazine metabolites, for α-noradrenergic and dopaminergic receptors (Cohen et al., 1979).

Hence our results offer additional support to the postulated contribution of the catecholaminergic, including noradrenergic, system to the pathophysiology of tardive dyskinesia. We did not find significant differences between dyskinesia and control subjects in the mean α-1-acid-glycoprotein concentrations in the serum. The latter measurement is believed to reflect inflammatory activity. Hence the high serum neuroleptic levels in the dyskinetic patients did not seem to be a result of an inflammatory process (Jeste, Linnoila, Wagner, *et al., in press*). A 1-year follow-up showed that the ratio of serum level to daily dose of neuroleptics was stable in five patients who continued to receive neuroleptics. (Neuroleptics had been withdrawn in the other 11 patients by their primary physicians.) We must add that our results do not necessarily imply a cause-and-effect relationship between high serum neuroleptic levels and tardive dyskinesia in our patients.

In another study of serum neuroleptic levels in tardive dyskinesia, we compared six young male inpatients with tardive dyskinesia and six matched controls. These 12 subjects were being treated with different types of neuroleptics, including haloperidol, chlorpromazine, thiothixene, and fluphenazine. Using a radioreceptor assay, we found no significant difference in the serum neuroleptic levels between dyskinetic patients and controls (Jeste, De Lisi, Zalcman, *et al.,* 1981). This result suggests that the finding of high serum levels of neuroleptics may be restricted to a subgroup of dyskinetic patients.

Studies of pharmacokinetics in large numbers of patients with tardive dyskinesia and matched controls are warranted in order to explore further a possible association between inefficient metabolism of neuroleptics and development of tardive dyskinesia.

OVERVIEW OF BIOCHEMICAL HYPOTHESES

A GENERAL CRITIQUE

A number of points need to be made before considering a composite biochemical hypothesis of tardive dyskinesia.

What Are These Hypotheses Supposed to Explain?

Biochemical hypotheses do not necessarily explain causes of a disorder; they try to clarify some of the mechanisms involved in the pathophysiology of that disorder. For instance, it would be wrong to say that catecholaminergic hyperactivity causes tardive dyskinesia. The proper statement would be that neuroleptics produce tardive dyskinesia in susceptible individuals through the mechanism of catecholaminergic hyperactivity.

Problems in Conducting Biochemical Studies

Probably the greatest problem in this area is a lack of adequate technology. Considerable biochemical advances have been made during the past several decades. Yet, we still do not have reliable methods for measuring the activity of various neurotransmitters *in vivo*. The available technology is inadequate for studying pathophysiological mechanisms in the brains of living patients.

Second, lack of specific drugs hampers pharmacologic testing of a hypothesis. For example, drugs that act selectively on presynaptic dopaminergic receptors, irrespective of dosage, are not yet available.

Third, clinical experiments are subject to many sources of error. Selection of patients (with proper diagnosis and stated severity of illness) and well-matched controls, methods for collecting CSF or blood, and assay techniques all involve known and unknown variables, which may have a crucial influence on the results of the study.

Fourth, clinical studies are fraught with practical, ethical, and medicolegal problems. Thus undertaking prospective, long-term studies in which matched groups of patients receive different treatments (e.g., one group gets only neuroleptics, a second group receives neuroleptics and antiparkinsonian drugs, a third group gets only antiparkinsonian drugs, etc.) would be unacceptable, since the patients would need to be treated according to the research design rather than the individual patients' needs at various times.

Problems in Interpreting Biochemical Studies

The problems just cited with regard to conducting studies also make their interpretation difficult. Although the limitations of reports with "positive" findings (including the fact that such reports tend to be published much more often than those with "negative" findings) are often stressed, the shortcomings of "negative" reports, too, should be considered. Because the unavailability of adequate techniques may make it difficult to test a particular hypothesis properly, negative findings with the available methods should not result in premature dismissal of a hypothesis.

A given disorder such as tardive dyskinesia may have different subtypes on the basis of clinical, pharmacologic, or biochemical parameters. Some of these subtypes may overlap in certain respects.

It is necessary to separate facts from theory. For instance, an investigator may postulate that tardive dyskinesia results from a deficiency of a neurotransmitter, N, and then claim to have proved his hypothesis by showing that patients with tardive dyskinesia improve when treated with an N-agonist drug. Even assuming that the clinical study was flawless, the demonstrated efficacy of an N-agonist drug does not necessarily reflect on the mechanisms underlying tardive dyskinesia. It is possible that the drug may have acted nonspecifically (e.g., as a sedative) or in other ways unrelated to the investigator's hypothesis. A finding that is presumed to be consistent with the investigator's original hypothesis does not necessarily testify to the correctness of the hypothesis; alternative explanations must be considered.

There is sometimes a danger of self-fulfilling prophecies. As an example, the screening tests for neuroleptics may include tests for dopamine-blocking effects. It would then not be surprising if the neuroleptic action were found to correlate strongly with dopamine receptor blockade.

The use of animal models to prove a hypothesis about a particular disorder is particularly hazardous. The advantages and limitations of animal models are discussed in Chapter 9.

Problems in Formulating Biochemical Theories

A theory serves the useful function of forming order from a mass of fragmented data. It may also provide a number of testable hypotheses. On the other hand, a rigid theory may result in foreclosure and consequent inattention to data that do not fit the theory. Taking a theory or a model too literally may hamper further progress.

Anticipating internal mechanisms mostly on the basis of pharmacologic responses and other clinical data may sometimes yield inaccurate theories. Thus two decades ago one might have suggested a cholinergic excess as the primary pathogenic mechanism in Parkinson's disease on the basis of therapeutic response to anticholinergic drugs. Recent work indicates, however, that the primary pathology in this disease may be a loss of dopamine neurons and that acetylcholine levels in the postmortem brains of patients with Parkinson's disease tend to be normal.

The oft-repeated admonition to scientists that association does not necessarily mean causation, is never outdated.

The desire for parsimonious hypotheses may result in oversimplifications. An example is the seesaw theory of dopamine–acetylcholine interaction, which has recently been found to be somewhat simplistic. Theories that assume disturbances in the function of only one neurotransmitter in only one area of the brain may be overlooking other chemical changes, whether primary or secondary. Similarly, the terminology of a theory may seem to explain a phenomenon without really doing so.

One unsolved problem in biochemical theories is partly a philosophical one. Do the biochemical changes in diseases represent the body's attempts at normalization, or are they evidence of a failure of compensatory mechanisms, or both?

COMPOSITE BIOCHEMICAL HYPOTHESIS

All the problems involved in biochemical studies discussed here make it difficult and even premature to construct "the" biochemical theory of tardive dyskinesia. If and when such a theory emerges, it would be expected to explain the following clinical facts:

1. Persistent tardive dyskinesia is commonly associated only with the use of neuroleptics.
2. Neuroleptics are the most effective known suppressors of the symptoms of tardive dyskinesia.
3. There is as yet no satisfactory evidence that the commonly used neuroleptics differ in their ability to produce or suppress tardive dyskinesia.
4. Constitutional susceptibility is a necessary factor in the etiology of tardive dyskinesia.
5. Aging predisposes to the development of dyskinesia.
6. Tardive dyskinesia is not primarily related to psychiatric disorders such as schizophrenia.
7. Symptoms of tardive dyskinesia are reversible in some patients and persistent in others.

Regarding biochemical data in patients with tardive dyskinesia, there are few established facts. The available studies, however, may permit us to make the following conclusions:

1. There is pharmacologic evidence (mostly indirect) to suggest nigro-striatal catecholaminergic hyperactivity in tardive dyskinesia.

2. Long-term administration of neuroleptics to animals produces postsynaptic dopamine receptor supersensitivity in the basal ganglia, as judged by biochemical and behavioral studies.
3. There is an interaction between dopamine and other neutotransmitters (especially norepinephrine, acetylcholine, serotonin, and GABA) in the basal ganglia.
4. The contributions of noradrenergic system and presynaptic mechanisms to the pathogenesis of tardive dyskinesia have received insufficient attention.
5. The role of acetylcholine, GABA, and serotonin in the pathophysiology of tardive dyskinesia is probably secondary to catecholamine disturbances, at least in the majority of dyskinetic patients.
6. There is little evidence of major endocrine dysfunction in dyskinetic patients.
7. The possibility that altered metabolism of neuroleptics may play a role in the pathogenesis of tardive dyskinesia in at least some patients needs to be studied carefully.

In view of the clinical and biochemical data considered here, a tentative hypothesis can be proposed. Tardive dyskinesia is associated with nigrostriatal catecholaminergic (dopamine + norepinephrine) hyperactivity. Postsynaptic dopamine receptor supersensitivity is probably a normal accompaniment of prolonged treatment with neuroleptics. Although such supersensitivity may be the likely explanation for withdrawal-emergent dyskinesias, it may not be a sufficient mechanism for the production of tardive dyskinesia. Presynaptic catecholaminergic hyperactivity is probably necessary for tardive dyskinesia to occur. Constitutional predisposition may be in the form of such presynaptic hyperactivity (perhaps lower MAO or structural damage). Although the available neuropathological techniques have failed to reveal structural abnormalities in the nigrostriatal systems in patients with tardive dyskinesia, it is very likely that subtle damage to the neurons is present. Such damage may also explain the persistence of dyskinesia in some patients and the increased prevalence of persistent tardive dyskinesia in the elderly. The possibility that long-term use of neuroleptics produces either derangement of enzyme functions or subtle neuronal damage cannot be ruled out. We believe that tardive dyskinesia represents a breakdown in the body's homeostatic mechanisms and should therefore be considered an indication of decompensation in the basal ganglia. Other neurotransmitter systems, such as acetylcholine and GABA, may be a part of this derangement of the regulatory processes.

There is a need for intensified research on neurochemical abnormalities in tardive dyskinesia. Presynaptic dopaminergic mechanisms and the noradrenergic system in the basal ganglia seem at present to be the best candidates for this purpose. The possible contribution of different types of dopamine receptors (e.g., D_1 and D_2) also requires study. The possibility of abnormal peripheral metabolism of neuroleptics as a contributing factor to tardive dyskinesia in subgroups of patients deserves further scrutiny. On the clinical side, development of tests to predict high as well as low risk of tardive dyskinesia may be beneficial.

CHAPTER VI

Neurophysiology and Neuropathology

NEUROPHYSIOLOGICAL BASIS

The terms "extrapyramidal system," "basal ganglia," and "nigrostriatal system" are often used loosely and sometimes interchangeably. A clearer understanding of the anatomy and physiology of these structures would be helpful for studying the pathophysiological basis of tardive dyskinesia. Of the three structures, the extrapyramidal system is the most encompassing, whereas the nigrostriatal system is a narrow and specific component of it.

EXTRAPYRAMIDAL SYSTEM

Kinnier Wilson is generally credited with introducing the concept of the extrapyramidal system (Adams & Victor, 1977). For phylogenetic reasons, Wilson called it the "older motor system," which, in contrast to the newer pyramidal motor system, was thought to include all nonpyramidal structures that were primarily concerned with motor function. In recent times, however, the extrapyramidal system has been given the role of a functional, rather than an anatomic, unit.[1] The extrapyramidal system is mainly responsible for static, postural activities, whereas the pyramidal system is principally involved in voluntary movements. Normal execution of

---

[1]Voogd and Huijzen (1979) assert that the pyramidal and extrapyramidal systems are so closely interrelated that the notion that these two systems are even functionally independent needs to be abandoned.

voluntary movements is not possible without the activity of the extra-pyramidal system in maintaining tone and posture. Some authorities, such as Adams and Victor (1977), divide the extrapyramidal system into two parts: basal ganglia and cerebellum. Others do not consider the cerebellum to be a part of the extrapyramidal system.

The term "basal ganglia" is used to refer to some or all of the major subcortical gray masses at the base of the cerebral hemispheres (Figure 6-1). Most neuroanatomists and neurophysiologists agree on the inclusion of the corpus striatum (comprised of caudate nucleus, putamen, and globus pallidus), substantia nigra, claustrum, and subthalamic nucleus of Luys as parts of the basal ganglia. There is a variable amount of disagreement over the inclusion of other possible constituents, such as amygdaloid nuclei, red nucleus, substantia innominata of Reichert, pars incerta, fields H_1 and H_2 of Forel, thalamus, and brain stem reticular formation (Adams & Victor, 1977; Vick, 1976). Of all these structures, the nigrostriatal system (substantia nigra and corpus striatum) has received the most attention in recent neuropsychiatric literature dealing with extrapyramidal system disorders.

EMBRYOLOGY

The brain develops from three primary vesicles: prosencephalon, or forebrain; mesencephalon, or midbrain; and rhombencephalon, or hindbrain. The prosencephalon itself differentiates into two parts: telencephalon, which gives rise to the two cerebral hemispheres, and diencephalon, from which arise the thalamic, hypothalamic, and epithalamic nuclei, and other structures enclosing the third ventricle. The corpus striatum and pars reticularis of substantia nigra are derived from telencephalon, the subthalamic nucleus of Luys is derived from diencephalon, and most of the midbrain (including pars compacta of substantia nigra, red nucleus, and midbrain reticular formation) is derived from mesencephalon. The corpus striatum is divisible into two parts: neostriatum, consisting of caudate nucleus and putamen, and paleostriatum, which is composed of globus pallidus. Phylogenetically, globus pallidus is the oldest component of the striatum. It is also interesting to note that, although the neurons of substantia nigra are present in the fish brain, they are not pigmented. The pigment (neuromelanin) of the substantia nigra increases with evolution, and its highest concentrations are found in the most highly evolved mam-

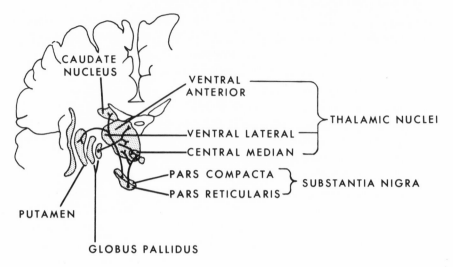

Figure 6-1. Basal ganglia. Shaded areas represent some of the principal components of the basal ganglia.

mals (Forrest, 1974). Ontogenetically, too, the substantia nigra in humans becomes increasingly pigmented during childhood and adolescence. The function of neuromelanin is as yet unknown.

ANATOMY OF THE NIGROSTRIATAL SYSTEM

Corpus striatum, the largest subcortical cell mass, consists of caudate and lentiform nuclei, the latter being subdivided into putamen and globus pallidus. Striatum owes its name to a grossly striped appearance because of the white fibers of internal capsule located between the gray caudate and putamen, the medullary laminae separating putamen and globus pallidus, and inner and outer pallidal segments. Caudate and putamen, which constitute neostriatum, share embryologic, cytologic, and functional similarities (Carpenter, 1976). Histologically, both are homogeneous structures with many small neurons, among which large cells are scattered (Voogd & Huijzen, 1979). Neostriatum receives afferent fibers from diverse sources—telencephalon (cerebral cortex), diencephalon (intralaminar thalamic nuclei), and mesencephalon (substantia nigra). Paleostriatum comprises globus pallidus, which, as its name suggests, appears pale because of numerous myelinated fibers. Globus pallidus contains large, fusiform cells. It receives afferent projections from the neostriatum and subthalamic nucleus of Luys. The major efferent pathways from the striatum arise in the medial pallidal segment; they exit by way of ansa lenticularis and fasciculus lenticularis and terminate in thalamus. From there, they project to the frontal motor area. These efferent bundles are topographically organized. Recent neuroanatomical work suggests that the ventrolateral nucleus of thalamus is a vital link in the efferent fiber system from the basal ganglia (and cerebellum) to the motor cortex. The remaining striatal efferents, originating in the lateral pallidal segment, terminate in the subthalamic nucleus of Luys.

Substantia nigra, which extends the length of the midbrain, consists of two portions: pars compacta and pars reticularis. The pars compacta (the A_9 area) is rich in large, polygonal pigmented cells containing dopamine. The pars reticularis is poor in cells, but is richer than the pars compacta in its content of the GABA-synthesizing enzyme, GAD. The striatum and the substantia nigra are reciprocally and topographically linked (Carpenter, 1976). Nigral efferents originating in the pars reticularis travel to the thalamus; their function is not well understood. Nigrostriatal fibers, which arise in the pars compacta, convey dopamine to the striatum.

Nauta and Mehler (1969) note two characteristics of the connections of the nigrostriatal system that are not shared by any other area of the brain, with the sole exception of the cerebellum. First, the striatum receives direct afferents from all major subdivisions of the neocortex (in a topographically oriented fashion). Second, the striatal efferents to the thalamus terminate in the ventrolateral and ventroanterior nuclei, which seem to constitute "the major thalamic gateway to the precentral cortex."

PHYSIOLOGY OF THE NIGROSTRIATAL SYSTEM

According to Denny-Brown and Yanagisawa (1976), the nigrostriatal system is comparable to a clearinghouse, which collects samples of ongoing cortical activity projected to it and then, on a competitive basis, can facilitate any one and suppress all others. This system also stands out because it is rich in the content of a number of neurotransmitters, especially dopamine, norepinephrine, acetylcholine, substance P, GABA, and enkephalins (Hong, Yang, Fratti, *et al.*, 1977). Figure 6-2 shows the postulated interaction among dopaminergic, GABA'ergic, and cholinergic neurons in the nigrostriatal system. Research during the past 25 years has shown that the limbic system and corpus striatum are linked to each other both directly and indirectly. These two forebrain structures are not mutually isolated, as was thought initially, but influence the activity of each other to a considerable extent (Nauta & Domesick, 1978).

The functional role of neuromelanin pigments found in the substantia nigra (as well as other nuclei such as the interpeduncular nucleus, the locus ceruleus, and the dorsal motor nucleus of the vagus) is unclear. According to Mann, Yates, and Barton (1977), neuromelanin pigments are probably waste products of cell metabolism and reflect neuronal activity in the catecholamine system. The relationship between possible neuroleptic effects on these pigments and the induction of extrapyramidal side effects is not well understood.

Figure 6-2. Interaction of dopamine, GABA, and acetylcholine neurons. (See text in Chapters 5 and 6.)

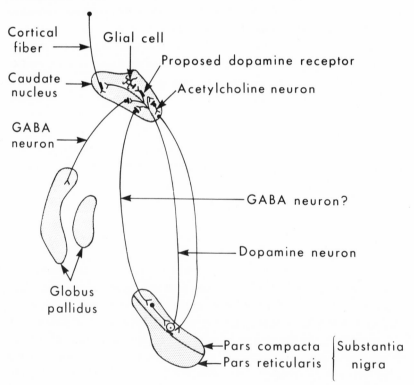

The principal functions of this area are concerned with postural adjustments, associated movements, and motoric integration. Its lesions result in impairment of voluntary movements and disinhibition of involuntary activity.

PATHOLOGY OF THE BASAL GANGLIA

Adams and Victor (1977) and others have outlined clinicopathological correlations between certain syndromes and principal locations of morbid anatomy in the basal ganglia. So far, the most convincing evidence for such correlations has been found in Parkinson's and Huntington's diseases. The neuropathology of tardive dyskinesia is unclear, although the nigrostriatal system is usually believed to be involved. Table 6-1 summarizes the major sites of lesion in related extrapyramidal system disorders. It is postulated that damage to the basal ganglia results in removal of inhibitions over cortically induced involuntary movements, so that abnormal movements, such as those of chorea, are manifested.

Klawans and Rubovits (1974) have attempted to explain localization of symptoms of tardive dyskinesia on a possible neuropathological basic. According to them, the areas of the caudate related to the complex, fine movements of the face and hands may be affected by long-term neuroleptic administration more than other parts of the caudate, and hence the typical orofacial dyskinesia and limb chorea in patients with tardive dyskinesia. This is an interesting, but speculative, hypothesis. There is as yet no direct evidence that the caudate is involved in the pathophysiology of tardive dyskinesia. However, the Klawans–Rubovits theory that localized neuronal lesions are responsible for symptom localization in tardive dyskinesia is attractive and deserves further exploration.

SUMMARY

Corpus striatum and substantia nigra are principal components of the extrapyramidal system. They are rich in their content of neurotransmitters, such as dopamine, norepinephrine, acetylcholine, and GABA. Also, these structures have direct and topographically oriented fiber connections with all the major subdivisions of the neocortex. It has been demonstrated that the caudate and putamen are atrophied in patients with Huntington's

Table 6-1. Primary Extrapyramidal Sites of Lesion in Certain Disorders

Disorder	Extrapyramidal site of lesion
Huntington's disease with chorea	Caudate and putamen
Parkinson's disease	Substantia nigra (and locus ceruleus)
Hemiballismus and hemichorea	Contralateral subthalamic nucleus of Luys and prerubral area
Athetosis and dystonia	Putamen
Tardive dyskinesia	Nigrostriatal system (?)

disease, whereas the substantia nigra and locus ceruleus show degeneration in patients with Parkinson's disease. Direct evidence linking lesions of the nigrostriatal system to tardive dyskinesia is still lacking.

NEUROPATHOLOGICAL STUDIES

Stereotyped motor manifestations, a positive relationship with old age, and a tendency to be persistent in many patients are clinical characteristics that suggest that tardive dyskinesia may be associated with brain damage. Demonstration of structural damage in substantia nigra and striatum in Parkinson's disease and Huntington's disease, respectively, further increases the possiblility that lesions in the same region may be associated with persistent tardive dyskinesia, another extrapyramidal system disorder. Moreover, the presence or absence of neuronal damage may explain why tardive dyskinesia is irreversible in some patients, but not in others.

Investigators have used different strategies to study a possible relationship between tardive dyskinesia and brain dysfunction. These include clinical evaluations, neurological investigations (e.g., skull X ray, electroencephalography, CT scan, neuropsychological testing), and postmortem examinations of brains from patients who had tardive dyskinesia. The findings of these studies have not been consistent. A number of investigators have not found a positive correlation between evidence of brain damage and tardive dyskinesia. This probably reflects an inadequacy of the available techniques to detect small structural damage in the nigrostriatal area.

A number of investigators have reported neuropathological findings in humans as well as in animals who had received long-term neuroleptic treatment (see Baldessarini *et al.*, 1980; Jellinger, 1977; Tarsy & Baldessarini, 1974). The relevance of these studies to tardive dyskinesia is uncertain, since the disorder is not synonymous with long-term neuroleptic treatment. (As stated earlier, only a proportion of patients so treated develop tardive dyskinesia.) Furthermore, such neuropathological studies have not revealed satisfactorily specific lesions that might be attributable to direct actions of neuroleptics on neural tissues. In this chapter, only studies of patients with tardive dyskinesia are considered.

CLINICAL DIAGNOSIS OF BRAIN DAMAGE

Early reports (e.g., Hunter *et al.*, 1964) indicated that tardive dyskinesia was seen most frequently in older and brain-damaged subjects. Since then, it has often been assumed that patients with organic mental syndromes are more likely to develop tardive dyskinesia than those without brain damage. Table 6-2 lists studies that examined the relationship between tardive dyskinesia and a clinically diagnosed brain syndrome. The criteria for

Table 6-2. Association between Clinical Diagnosis of Organic Mental Disorder and Tardive Dyskinesia

Investigators	Relationship between dyskinesia and "organicity"
Faurbye, Rasch, and Petersen (1964)	Absent
Pryce and Edwards (1966)	Absent
Crane and Paulson (1967)	Present
Siede and Muller (1967)	Absent
Degkwitz and Wenzel (1967)	Absent
Greenblatt, Stotsky, and DiMascio (1968)	Absent
Heinrich, Wagener, and Bender (1968)	Absent
Edwards (1970)	Present
Brandon, McClelland, and Protheroe (1971)	Absent
Crane (1974)	Absent
Bell and Smith (1978)	Absent
Simpson, Varga, Lee, *et al.* (1978)	Absent
Jeste, Potkin, Sinha, *et al.* (1979)	Absent
Jeste (unpublished data)	Absent

detecting brain damage varied among studies. The majority of investigators diagnosed brain damage on the basis of clinical examination and past history. Simpson, Varga, Lee, *et al.* (1978) used a long checklist of factors suggestive of "organicity"—for example, lobotomy, epilepsy, mental retardation, and alcoholism. Pryce and Edwards (1966) and Edwards (1970) judged brain damage to be present when there was strong evidence of any of these: clinically diagnosed organic mental syndrome, leukotomy, any of the signs of "organicity" listed by Shapiro, *et al.* (1956)—such as focal cerebral attacks, abnormal electroencephalogram (EEG)—and inability to learn the meaning of six out of ten new words in six trials in the Modified Word-Learning Test of Walton, White, and Black (1959).

Only 2 of the 14 studies summarized in Table 6-2 found a positive relationship between tardive dyskinesia and "organicity." The sensitivity of the measures for detecting brain damage and the method for comparing dyskinesia patients with controls are important variables. Thus Edwards (1970), Pryce and Edwards (1966), and Simpson, Varga, Lee, *et. al.* (1978), used relatively more objective measures for diagnosing brain damage as compared to many other investigators. Using age-matched controls, Pryce and Edwards (1966) found no significant difference between the dyskinesia group and the control group in the proportion of patients with "organicity"; there was a rather high prevalence of brain damage in both groups. On the other hand, Edwards (1970) selected controls matched not only for age, but also for total phenothiazine intake, and reported a significantly higher prevalence of "organicity" in dyskinesia patients as compared to controls.

Table 6-3 summarizes studies that specified the prevalence of tardive dyskinesia in schizophrenia, other "functional" disorders, and organic mental syndrome. There was no significant difference in the overall weighted mean prevalence of dyskinesia in the three diagnostic groups. This result confirms the finding of most researchers (see Chapter 4) that patients with clinically diagnosed brain damage are not significantly more prone to develop tardive dyskinesia than patients without obvious brain damage.

Some investigators examined the relationship between type of tardive dyskinesia and brain damage. We (Jeste, Potkin, Sinha, *et. al.,* 1979) did not find EEG abnormalities that could discriminate between reversible and persistent tardive dyskinesia. In a study of outpatients, Chouinard, Annable, Ross-Chouinard, *et. al.* (1979) reported that, among patients with tardive dyskinesia, those with brain damage tended to have more severe dyskinesias.

Table 6-3. Tardive Dyskinesia and Primary Psychiatric Diagnoses

Investigators	Schizophrenia		Other "functional" disorders		Organic mental syndrome		Total	
	n^a	% TD[b]	n	% TD	n	% TD	n	% TD
Faurbye, Rasch, and Petersen (1964)	216	34.7	92	18.5	109	15.6	417	26
Crane and Paulson (1967)	96	8.3	5	20	81	22.2	182	14.8
Brandon, McClelland, and Protheroe (1971)	453	20.8	146	21.2	311	28.3	910	23.4
Simpson, Varga, Lee, et al. (1978)	2124	11.5	365	9	830	9.9	3319	10.8
Jeste, Potkin, Sinha et al. (1979)	28	32.1	29	31	31	9.7	88	23.9
Jeste (unpublished data)	75	32	3	0	17	35.3	95	31.6
TOTAL	2992	15.2	640	14.2	1379	15.5	5011	15.2

[a] n = total number of patients.

[b] % TD = percentage of patients with tardive dyskinesia.

Several other possibilities need to be explored systematically. For example, patients with brain damage may develop dyskinesia with relatively small amounts of neuroleptics or a short duration of neuroleptic treatment, or organic impairment may increase susceptibility to tardive dyskinesia only among certain subgroups of patients. It should be stressed that the detection of brain damage with a mental status examination is usually related to cortical dysfunction. A brief clinical examination is unlikely to uncover subtle forms of subcortical damage, unless gross weakness or cognitive deficits are present. (It is conceivable that specific kinds of cortical damage may increase the risk of tardive dyskinesia.) On the other hand, severe tardive dyskinesia may lead to a false impression of cortical dysfunction, especially on tasks involving motor performance.

NEUROLOGICAL INVESTIGATIONS

Table 6-4 summarizes 12 studies of neurological investigations in patients with tardive dyskinesia. Six of these 12 studies found an association between dyskinesia and a specific neurological abnormality.

Radiology

Faurbye et. al. (1964) performed skull X ray and pneumoencephalograms in seven elderly schizophrenic patients with tardive dyskinesia. They found atrophic changes that were not different from those "commonly seen in schizophrenics of the same age group." Gelenberg (1976) referred to a personal communication by Duvoisin, who had noted caudate atrophy in the pneumoencephalogram of a woman with severe dyskinesia. Pandurangi, Devi, and Channabasavanna (1980) found caudate atrophy in three of their five patients with tardive dyskinesia in whom pneumoencephalography was done. Interestingly, these three patients also proved refractory to treatment, suggesting that they had persistent tardive dyskinesia. Studies of CT scans in dyskinetic patients are considered separately.

Electroencephalography

Gardos, Cole, and La Brie (1977b) reported that an abnormal EEG discriminated between tardive dyskinesia and control groups. Ten of their 50 subjects (23 with dyskinesia and 27 controls) had an abnormal EEG,

Table 6-4. Neurological Tests for Brain Damage in Tardive Dyskinesia

Investigators	Test	Relationship between dyskinesia and brain damage
Faurbye, Rasch, and Petersen (1964)	Radiological	Absent
Pryce and Edwards (1966)	Neuropsychological	Absent
Edwards (1970)	Neuropsychological	Present
Gelenberg (1976)	CT scans	Absent
Crayton, Smith, Klass, *et al.* (1977)	H reflex	Present
Gardos, Cole, and La Brie (1977b)	EEG	Present
Simpson, Varga, Lee, *et al.* (1978)	EEG	Absent
Jeste, Potkin, Sinha, *et al.* (1979)	EEG	Absent
Wegner, Struve, Kantor, *et al.* (1979)	EEG	Present
Famuyiwa, Eccleston, Donaldson, *et al.* (1979)	Neuropsychological and CT scans	Present
Jeste, Wagner, Weinberger, *et al.* (1980); Jeste, Weinberger, Zalcman, *et al.* (1980)	CT scans	Absent
Pandurangi, Devi, and Channabasavanna (1980)	Pneumoencephalography	Present in patients with persistent tardive dyskinesia

although the investigators did not define "abnormal EEG." In contrast, Jeste, Potkin, Sinha, *et. al.* (1979) and Simpson, Varga, Lee, *et. al.* (1978) found, in terms of the EEG abnormalities present, no significant difference between patients with and without dyskinesia. Studies of B-mitten pattern in the EEGs of dyskinetic patients are discussed later.

Electromyography

Faurbye *et al.* (1964) noted spontaneous electromyographic activity in dyskinetic patients; also, the regular rhythm characteristic of Parkinson's disease was missing in the patients with facial dyskinesia. The researchers found that the muscle activity in tardive dyskinesia was similar to that in athetosis.

Neuropsychological Tests

Clinical neuropsychology deals with behavioral expressions of brain dysfunctions. Neuropsychological tests are designed to diagnose the presence, severity, and, if possible, nature and location of brain damage. These tests differ in their reliability and validity. It is usually more difficult to detect mild subcortical dysfunction than comparable cortical dysfunction. In recent years neuropsychological test batteries, such as the Halstead–Reitan battery, are being increasingly employed to aid in localization of brain damage.

There are only a few reports on neuropsychological test performance in patients with tardive dyskinesia. Pryce and Edwards (1966) compared 21 elderly female patients with dyskinesia and 21 controls matched for age, gender, primary psychiatric diagnosis, and length of current admission. As one of the measures of brain dysfunction, the investigators administered the Modified Word-Learning Test of Walton et al. (1959). Inability to learn the meaning of six out of ten new words in six trials was presumed to indicate brain dysfunction. There was no difference between the performance of the experimental group and that of the control group, with both groups having a rather high prevalence (83%) of "organicity." Edwards (1970) repeated this study, employing controls matched not only for age, but also for phenothiazine intake. He then found a significant difference between the dyskinesia and control groups. Of the patients with dyskinesia who could be tested, 73% had impairment on the test, as opposed to 32% of the controls. Famuyiwa et al. (1979) reported that their dyskinesia patients performed significantly worse than controls on Inglis's Paired Associate Learning Test, but the two groups did not differ in the scores on the Withers–Hinton Clinical Test of the Sensorium.

Ivnik (1979) administered the Halstead–Reitan test battery to a 58-year-old man with dyskinesia, both before and after neuroleptics were discontinued. The patient showed improvement clinically as well as on the test battery after the withdrawal of neuroleptics.

Neuropsychological test batteries are theoretically superior to single tests; the former are, however, often difficult to administer and interpret in a population of chronically hospitalized, elderly psychiatric patients. Patients' motivation, intelligence, primary psychiatric diagnosis, and current treatment are among the major variables that may affect performance on neuropsychological tests. The problem of localizing brain damage in tardive dyskinesia is compounded by the fact that the commonly employed tests are not very useful for judging brain stem dysfunction. Continued research is warranted on neuropsychological test performance in patients with dyskinesia.

B-Mitten EEG Pattern

Struve and his associates have reported an association between B-mitten pattern in EEG and certain psychiatric disorders. This pattern consists of a sharp wave followed by a higher voltage slow wave, and the whole complex resembles the thumb and hand of a mitten. It occurs bilaterally and synchronously over frontal and frontal-central areas during stages 3 and 4 of sleep. It is best seen in monopolar recordings. The B-mitten pattern is age related, occurring mostly between 15 and 50 years of age. First described by Gibbs, Gibbs, Tasher, et al. (1960), the mittens are thought to be subcortical in origin. They are rare in normal controls and are primarily associated with psychiatric dysfunction. Struve and Klein (1976) suggested a relationship between mittens and affective dysregulation (especially the dysphoric type) in various diagnostic categories.

In an EEG study of patients with and without tardive dyskinesia, Wegner, Struve, Kantor, et al. (1979) observed B-mitten pattern in 20 of 21 dyskinesia patients and in only 7 of 21 matched controls. The investigators reported that they found no evidence that neuroleptic treatment or the dyskinesia itself produced the mittens. They suggested that the mitten pattern might indicate susceptibility to tardive dyskinesia, especially in younger adults (since mittens were rare in dyskinetic patients over the age of 40). Further work is necessary to explore the possibility that the subcortical mitten dysrhythmia may be an electroencephalographic expression of a disorder of the midbrain (containing substantia nigra) and that such a disorder increases susceptibility to neuroleptic-induced tardive dyskinesia.

H-Reflex Studies

Peripheral neuronal dysfunction has been shown to be present in several movement disorders. A common approach to assessing the excitability of the spinal α-motoneuron pool is the study of the H reflex. The H reflex is an electrically evoked spinal monosynaptic reflex. It is elicited by stimulation of sensory fibers (mainly IA fibers from muscle spindle receptors); the reflexly evoked muscle action potential is then recorded with an electro-myographic apparatus. Usually, an electrode is placed in the popliteal fossa over the posterior tibial nerve, and square wave pulses are adminis-tered. Electromyographic recording is made by means of surface elec-trodes placed over the belly and distal tendon of the soleus muscle. Abnor-malities of the H reflex have been observed in a number of disorders, in-cluding Parkinson's disease (McLeod & Walsh, 1972) and schizophrenia (Crayton, Meltzer, & Goode, 1977). It has been suggested that a part of the normal H reflex curve may be under dopaminergic influence (Crayton, Smith, Klass, et al., 1977).

Crayton, Smith, Klass, et al. (1977) studied H reflex curves in 31 schizophrenic patients with tardive dyskinesia and compared them with curves in schizophrenic patients without dyskinesia and with those in nor-mal controls. The investigators found an absence of H reflex in nine pa-tients with dyskinesia, but in none of the subjects without dyskinesia. The absence of H reflex in dyskinesia patients was not related to the dyskinetic movements themselves. Also, there was no clinical evidence of peripheral neuropathy in these patients. The researchers therefore suggested that an excessive inhibition of the reflex by spinal or supraspinal mechanisms might be responsible for the absent H reflex.

A surprising finding in this study was that patients with severe dyskin-esia had higher values for Hx (peak of the H reflex curve) as compared to patients with mild dyskinesia or no dyskinesia. It is believed that the height of Hx is inversely related to the dopaminergic tone. Patients with Parkin-son's disease have high values for Hx, and these values tend to return toward normal on treatment with L-dopa. On the basis of the hypothesis of nigrostriatal dopaminergic hyperactivity in tardive dyskinesia, one would expect an association between low values for Hx and moderate to severe tardive dyskinesia. Since the results were just the opposite of this expecta-tion, Crayton, Smith, Klass, et al. (1977) suggested that other neuro-transmitters, such as acetylcholine or GABA, might also be implicated in the pathophysiology of tardive dyskinesia.

It is not yet possible to assess the significance of the preceding find-ings for the pathophysiology of tardive dyskinesia. These results, how-ever, deserve further evaluation, particularly in light of the recent demon-stration of a nigrospinal dopaminergic pathway (Commissiong et al., 1979) and the role of dopamine and norepinephrine (present in the ventral horn of the spinal cord) in the regulation of γ- and α-motoneurons.

Computed Tomography

One of the most notable advances in neuroradiology was the introduction of CT scans in 1972. Hounsfield and Cormack shared the Nobel prize in medicine and physiology in 1979 for their development of CT scans (also called "computerized axial tomography," or CAT scans). This technique involves very low amounts of radiation and has, for the first time, enabled a noninvasive visualization of the brain for detecting structural abnormalities in large numbers of patients. The introduction of CT scans has resulted in their being substituted for pneumoencephalography as a common diagnostic procedure for a variety of neurological disorders, such as Huntington's disease.

Gelenberg (1976) reported an absence of significant abnormalities in CT scans of eight patients with tardive dyskinesia. The subjects' ages ranged from 17 to 56 years. All the patients carried the primary diagnosis of chronic undifferentiated or paranoid schizophrenia. The severity of dyskinesia was mild to moderate. With an average of three cuts per subject, the CT scans were read in a qualitative, rather than a quantitative, manner. Famuyiwa et al. (1979) concluded that their patients with dyskinesia had a significantly higher prevalence of CT scan abnormalities than controls. An analysis of their data shows, however, that the two groups did not differ in mean scores on any of the four variables studied. The only observed difference was based on the use of an arbitrary cutoff point for defining the normal ventricular index. Nine of 10 dyskinesia patients and 14 of 26 controls had an "abnormal" ventricular index, although the means for the two groups were not significantly different.

Jeste, Wagner, Weinberger, et al. (1980) studied CT scans of 12 elderly female inpatients with moderate to severe tardive dyskinesia and of 12 controls matched for gender, age (mean 69.5 years), primary diagnosis (schizophrenia in 10 and organic mental syndrome in 2 patients), and length of neuroleptic therapy (mean 19.6 years). We obtained an average of 12 cuts (range 8 to 14) per subject. The scans were read "blind" by two physicians, including a neuroradiologist. A quantitative analysis was done on the following measures: bifrontal/bicaudate ratio to assess caudate atrophy, planimetric assessment of lateral ventricle/brain ratio, focal abnormalities, and measures for cortical atrophy and cerebellar atrophy. The CT scans of the patients were also compared to those of 42 patients with Huntington's disease done earlier with the same scanner. We found no caudate atrophy in CT scans of our patients (with or without dyskinesia) as compared to patients with Huntington's disease and no significant differences between dyskinesia patients and controls in their CT scan abnormalties.

A subsequent study of CT scans in male schizophrenic patients under 50 years of age confirmed the absence of significant differences between CT scan abnormalities of dyskinesia patients and those of patients without dyskinesia (Jeste, Weinberger, Zalcman, et al., 1980). We considered the possibility that chronic neuroleptic treatment itself might have produced CT scan abnormalities in both groups. However, a separate study in our laboratory (Weinberger, Torrey, Neophytides, et al. 1979) found that hospitalization and neuroleptic treatment were not correlated with the CT scan abnormalities seen in a subgroup of chronic schizophrenic patients.

It is necessary to add that the available techniques for analyzing CT scans are inadequate for detecting fine structural abnormalities in certain areas such as the brain stem. Hence the negative results with CT scans of patients with tardive dyskinesia do not rule out the possibility of neuronal damage in substantia nigra in these patients.

POSTMORTEM STUDIES OF BRAINS

Postmortem neuropathological and neurochemical studies have proved to be useful in understanding the chemical pathology underlying disorders such as Huntington's and Parkinson's diseases. Unfortunately, there have been few such sophisticated and well-controlled studies of the brains of patients with tardive dyskinesia. Table 6-5 summarizes the published reports on postmortem examination of the brains of dyskinesia patients.

Problems with Postmortem Studies in Tardive Dyskinesia

A number of factors make a simple interpretation of postmortem neuropathological studies difficult. These factors are as follows:

1. There are general methodological issues, such as the time elapsed between death and removal of the brain, storage of the brain, and use of sophisticated quantitative techniques to analyze multiple morphological and neurochemical changes.

Table 6-5. Postmortem Studies of Brains

Investigators	Number of subjects	Patient characteristics	Findings	Comments
Grunthal and Walther-Buhl (1960)	1P[a]	Treated with perphenazine.	Damage of inferior olive.	Patient had persistent "dystonic hyperkinesia."
Hunter, Blackwood, Smith, et al. (1968)	3P	Women, aged 25, 70, and 77 years. Neuroleptic therapy for more than 2 years.	No specific or significant lesions on neuropathological and neurochemical study.	All patients had persistent tardive dyskinesia.
Gross and Kaltenbach (1969)	3P	Two men (aged 42, 55) and one woman (aged 40).	Lesions of caudate in all three patients and of sub-stantia nigra in one patient.	Two patients were chronic alcoholics; the third probably had Huntington's disease.
Dynes (1970)	1P	Man, aged 76. Chronic alcoholic.	Generalized atrophy, including substantia nigra, globus palli-dus, and hippocampus.	Korsakoff's psychosis was sus-pected clinically.
Christensen, Moller, and Faurbye (1970)	28P 28C[b]	21 had tardive dyskinesia. Diagnosis was schizophrenia or organic brain syndrome. All dyskinetic patients were women (mean age 74). Con-trols were mostly men (mean age 69).	Degeneration in substantia nigra in 27 of 28 dyskinetic patients and in 7 of 28 controls. Gliosis in brain stem in 25 of 28 dyskinetic pa-tients and in 4 of 28 controls.	Similar changes in patients with tardive dyskinesia and in those with spontaneous dys-kinesia. In the former group, mean age at onset of neuro-leptic administration was 69.
Jamielity, Kosc, and Lukaszewicz (1976)	1P	Man, aged 54.	Atrophic changes, mainly in substantia nigra.	
Jellinger (1977)	9P 14C	Three women, six men. Mean age 53.3 (range 40 to 70).	Swelling of large neurons and glial satellitosis in caudate in five patients and one control.	No correlation between inten-sity of neuropathology and of clinical syndrome.
Ule and Struwe (1978)	1P	Woman, aged 66.	Degenerative changes in nigro-striatal area.	

[a]P = patients with tardive dyskinesia.

[b]C = controls.

2. With two exceptions (Christensen, Moller, & Faurbye, 1970; Jellinger, 1977), the studies in Table 6-5 have been done on three or fewer patients and have not employed controls. Of the ten brains from dyskinetic patients examined in these six studies, three brains had no specific or significant lesions; three had atrophic changes in caudate, two in other parts of striatum; four had degenerative changes in substantia nigra and one in the olivary nucleus. (Some brains had multiple lesions.) In several of the brains with lesions in specified parts, there was also generalized atrophy, as might be expected, since most of the patients were either middle-aged or elderly. Thus there were no specific and consistent neuropathological lesions associated with tardive dyskinesia *per se*.

3. It is difficult to isolate the effect of variables such as age, physical illnesses, alcoholism, and dementia on the neuropathology seen.

4. The antemortem clinical diagnosis of tardive dyskinesia is also sometimes questionable. For instance, a patient of Gross and Kaltenbach (1969) had a clinical history highly suggestive of Huntington's disease. On postmortem examination, he had pronounced caudate atrophy. Kaufman (1977) has presented neuropathological findings in three patients who were diagnosed as having tardive dyskinesia. The author found, on a thorough review of the history, that there was little basis for diagnosing tardive dyskinesia in one patient while the other two had developed neurological manifestations before neuroleptic treatment was begun. Both the clinical features and the postmortem findings were consistent with diagnoses of Huntington's disease, Alzheimer's disease, and normal pressure hydrocephalus in the three patients.

5. The study by Christensen *et al.* (1970) included the largest number of patients and controls (28 in each group). However, the experimental and control groups were not well matched on factors such as gender and age. The mean age at which neuroleptic treatment had been begun in the patients with tardive dyskinesia was unusually late—namely, 69 years. Moreover, there was no indication that the lesions found in the brains of patients with tardive dyskinesia (degenerative changes in substantia nigra and gliosis in brain stem) were significantly different from those in patients with spontaneous dyskinesia.

6. Jellinger (1977) reported that five of his nine patients with dyskinesia and only 1 of the 14 controls had neuronal damage in the

caudate. The damage was not related to length of neuroleptic treatment, nor was there a positive correlation between the intensity of the neuropathological changes and the clinical dyskinesia.

On the positive side, the presence of lesions in the nigrostriatal region in many of the patients with tardive dyskinesia (Table 6-5) is in accordance with the hypothesized pathology in basal ganglia in this syndrome. However, it is not clear whether the lesions observed were specific to tardive dyskinesia. Forrest, Forrest, and Roizin (1963) and Roizin, True, and Knight (1959) described pathological changes in the basal ganglia in patients (nondyskinetic?) chronically treated with neuroleptics.

Careful and methodologically sophisticated postmortem studies of the brains of dyskinesia patients and of well-matched controls are necessary for a better understanding of the pathophysiology of tardive dyskinesia. These should include analyses of the chemical constituents and different types of receptors in substantia nigra, caudate, and other basal ganglia. It is also necessary to explore the possibility that different subtypes of tardive dyskinesia may be associated with somewhat different kinds of neuropathology.

SUGGESTIONS FOR FURTHER NEUROPATHOLOGICAL STUDIES

There is a need to compare sufficient numbers of patients with tardive dyskinesia and well-matched controls on various clinical and laboratory measures of neuropathology. At least two groups of controls, with and without a history of prolonged neuroleptic treatment, should be used. Prospective long-term studies of patients both on and off medication are warranted. Attempts should be made to correlate possible neurological dysfunction with other behavioral measures, such as severity of tardive dyskinesia and psychopathology. It will also be valuable to compare, in prospective investigations, patients having persistent tardive dyskinesia with those having reversible tardive dyskinesia.

In patients with reversible tardive dyskinesia, a comparison of test results during the two clinical states—with and without dyskinesia—may help determine whether any neurological dysfunction found is secondary to the clinical state of dyskinesia. (If the dysfunction persists when the patient is nondyskinetic, it is not secondary to the presence of dyskinesia per se.) Employing newer techniques, such as positron emission tomography, or PET scans, would be useful for detecting certain functional aberrations in different brain areas in patients with tardive dyskinesia.

SUMMARY

It is widely suspected that tardive dyskinesia, especially the persistent form, is likely to be associated with structural brain abnormalities. However, the majority of the studies done so far have failed to substantiate this assumption. With future advances in the techniques of neuropathological investigations, a possible organic substrate of persistent tardive dyskinesia may be detected.

CHAPTER VII

Dyskinesias in Children
and Adolescents

HISTORY

Tardive dyskinesia was initially thought to be restricted to elderly, brain-damaged patients. Subsequent reports of dyskinesia in young adults dispelled this impression. Yet, it was not until 15 years after tardive dyskinesia was first reported in adults that neuroleptic-induced dyskinesia in children was first described. This time lag is difficult to explain since many psychotic children and adolescents receive long-term neuroleptic treatment, and the prevalence of tardive dyskinesia in this age group (Table 7-1) has been reported to be 8% to 20%. There is still a dearth of literature on tardive dyskinesia in children and adolescents.

PREVALENCE STUDIES

Table 7-1 summarizes five prevalence studies. Three of these studies described tardive dyskinesia (Frank & Djavadi, 1980; McAndrew, Case, & Treffert, 1972; Paulson, Rizvi, & Crane, 1975); the others reported the prevalence of withdrawal-emergent dyksinesia (Engelhardt *et al.*, 1975; Winsberg *et al.*, 1977).

McAndrew *et al.* (1972) examined 86 boys and 39 girls who had been hospitalized and had received neuroleptics. The children ranged in age from 4 to 16 years (median 13.6 years). Fifty-two patients were psychotic, while the others suffered from behavior problems or personality dis-

171

Table 7-1. Prevalence of Dyskinesia among Neuroleptic-Treated Children and Adolescents

Investigators	Age (years)	n^a	$\%^b$	Type of dyskinesia	Localization	Variables related to dyskinesia
McAndrew, Case, and Treffert (1972)	4–16 (median 13.6)	125	8	Withdrawal-emergent reversible tardive	Upper limbs, face, lower limbs	Length and amount of neuroleptic intake, but not brain damage
Engelhardt, Polizos, and Waizer (1975)	5–16 (mean 9.6)	47	48	Withdrawal-emergent	Trunk, head, limbs	Treatment with certain neuroleptics, mainly fluphenazine and butaperazine
Paulson, Rizvi, and Crane (1975)	11–16	103	20.4	Persistent tardive	Limbs, tongue, trunk	—
Winsberg, Hurwic, and Perel (1977)	?c	6	50	Withdrawal-emergent	?	Lower CSF-HVA and 5-HIAA; normal cAMP
Frank and Djavadi (1980)	?	120	18.3	Tardive	Limbs, face	Not related to use of specific neuroleptics, drug holidays, or polypharmacy

$^a n$ = number of patients treated with neuroleptics.

$^b \%$ = percentage of patients with dyskinesia.

^{c} ? = not stated.

orders. The investigators diagnosed tardive dyskinesia in ten children, including seven with childhood schizophrenia and three with behavior problems. In all cases the symptoms appeared in 3 to 10 days after withdrawal of neuroleptics and subsided in 3 to 10 months.

Paulson *et al.* (1975) found that 103 children (aged 11 to 16), out of 2145 residents of a state facility for the mentally retarded, had received prolonged neuroleptic treatment. Twenty-one of these patients (i.e., about 20%), including 15 girls and 6 boys, were diagnosed as having mild to moderate tardive dyskinesia. The symptoms probably appeared while the children were being treated with neuroleptics. Administration of neuroleptics was continued because of psychiatric problems. A 4-year follow-up of 15 patients showed that the dyskinesia was worse in 4 and unchanged or less severe in 11 patients.

Polizos, Engelhardt, and Hoffman (1973) and Polizos, Engelhardt, Hoffman, *et al.* (1973) noticed a high prevalence of involuntary movements associated with neuroleptic withdrawal in 34 children. The same group of researchers (Engelhardt *et al.*, 1975) later expanded their series to a total of 47 children, all schizophrenic and ranging in age from 5 to 14 years (mean 9.6 years). There were 141 instances of abrupt drug withdrawal in the 47 patients. (A number of children had more than one period of neuroleptic withdrawal in the course of drug studies.) Forty-eight percent of the patients developed dyskinesia within 1 to 29 days (mean 12 days) of neuroleptic withdrawal. The symptoms disappeared spontaneously within 15 days in one-third of the children. The remaining children were given a neuroleptic within 1 week of developing dyskinesia, for clinical reasons; the symptoms remitted within 2 weeks of reinstituting pharmacotherapy.

Winsberg *et al.* (1977) studied six psychotic children who had been on neuroleptics for 3 to 12 months. Three of these children developed dyskinesia within 4 weeks of drug withdrawal.

Frank and Djavadi (1980) diagnosed tardive dyskinesia in 22 of 120 adolescents (i.e., 18.3% prevalence) who had been psychiatric inpatients for a long time. Autistic and mentally retarded children seemed to be particularly susceptible to tardive dyskinesia (18 of 33 with dyskinesia).

Thus the reported prevalence of tardive dyskinesia in children and adolescents ranges between 8% and 20%. The prevalence of withdrawal-emergent dyskinesia in this age group seems to be much higher (about 50%) than in adults. It is likely that in some cases the withdrawal-emergent dyskinesia may herald the onset of tardive dyskinesia, although in a majority of instances it may remit spontaneously.

CASE REPORTS

Browning and Ferry (1976) reported choreiform movements of the head, neck, and upper extremities in a severely disturbed 10-year-old boy treated with prochlorperazine for 3 years. The dyskinesia first appeared within a few weeks of drug withdrawal and was still present 4 months later.

McLean and Casey (1978) presented the case of a 12-year-old boy who developed buccolingual masticatory dyskinesia, choreoathetosis, and dystonias following 2 years of treatment with moderate doses of neuroleptics. The abnormal movements worsened on withdrawing neuroleptics, but improved with deanol.

Caine, Margolin, Brown, et al. (1978) described a 15-year-old boy with Gilles de la Tourette's syndrome who developed tardive dyskinesia following haloperidol treatment for 4 years. The dyskinesia was characterized by abnormal movements of the extremities and trunk, which persisted despite withdrawal of medication for a month. At that time haloperidol was reinstituted because of aggravation of the Tourette's syndrome and the appearance of psychotic symptoms. The neuroleptic administration reduced the severity of the dyskinesia.

Mizrahi, Holtzman, and Tharp (1980) also reported the onset of tardive dyskinesia in a 7-year-old boy with Gilles de la Tourette's syndrome who had been treated with haloperidol for 5 months. The patient's dyskinesia was localized to the neck, head, face, and tongue. Tongue protrusion was so severe that the frenulum was excoriated from repeated contact with the lower incisors. A dental shield was fitted over the incisors to prevent further damage. Haloperidol was discontinued, and ethosuximide was begun. Two months later, the dyskinesia had completely disappeared.

Petty and Spar (1980) described a 10-year-old girl who developed choreoathetoid movements affecting the face, mouth, extremities, and trunk following prolonged treatment with neuroleptics. The dyskinesia was still present 3 months after withdrawal of neuroleptics.

Gualtieri, Barnhill, McGimsey, et al. (1980) reviewed the literature on this subject and also presented a case report of tardive dyskinesia in an adolescent.

MANIFESTATIONS

The frequent assertion that orofacial dyskinesia is rare in children and adolescents is not borne out by the published reports. It is, however, true that, in younger patients with dyskinesia, orofacial symptoms are usually not present in isolation and that involvement of the limbs and trunk tends to be a more prominent feature. It is likely that buccolingual masticatory manifestations are more common in older children and adolescents than in younger ones. In a study of 14 children with withdrawal dyskinesia (mean age 9.6 years), Polizos, Engelhardt, Hoffman, *et al.* (1973) found that only one patient had oral symptoms. In contrast, McAndrew *et al.* (1972) noted a facial tic in six of their ten patients (mean age of population 13.6 years) with tardive dyskinesia. McLean and Casey (1978), Moline (1975), Paulson *et al.* (1975), and Tarsy, Granacher, and Bralower (1977) described orofacial involvement in their patients ranging in age from 11 to 19.

In most of the reported cases of neuroleptic-related dyskinesia in childhood, the children had choreiform movements of the upper limbs. Lower limbs and trunk were also affected in a sizable proportion of young dyskinetic patients. One interesting feature was the frequent concomitant presence of other extrapyramidal symptoms, such as akathisia (McAndrew *et al.*, 1972), ataxia (Engelhardt *et al.*, 1975), and dystonias (McLean & Casey, 1978).

As in adults, the dyskinesia in children shows at least temporary aggravation on withdrawal of neuroleptics and suppression with reinstitution of the medication. The symptoms are absent during sleep. Antiparkinsonian drugs are of no benefit in the treatment of childhood dyskinesia.

VARIABLES RELATED TO DYSKINESIA

McAndrew *et al.* (1972) reported a positive correlation between tardive dyskinesia and length of neuroleptic treatment, total drug intake, and daily dose prior to neuroleptic withdrawal. The dyskinetic patients had been treated with neuroleptics for a mean of 32.5 months. The mean total drug intake was equivalent to 403 g of chlorpromazine, and the median daily termination dose was equivalent to 400 mg of chlorpromazine. The investigators, however, found no relationship between dyskinesia and brain damage as rated on a scale that encompassed clinical, neurological, historical, laboratory, and psychological test findings.

Engelhardt *et al.* (1975) observed that the incidence of withdrawal-emergent dyskinesia was related to the type of neuroleptic.[1] Fluphenazine

---

[1]Further analysis of the data of Engelhardt *et al.* shows, however, that the incidence of withdrawal-emergent dyskinesia might be at least partly related to the total amount of neuroleptic administered. Thus fluphenazine (which was associated with a 79% incidence of withdrawal-emergent dyskinesia) had been given in mean amounts equivalent to 533 g of chlorpromazine, whereas chlorpromazine (with a 31% incidence of withdrawal-emergent dyskinesia) had been administered in mean amounts of 46 g.

withdrawal had the highest propensity for inducing withdrawal dyskinesia, whereas chlorprothixene withdrawal did not produce dyskinesia in any child. Among the remaining drugs, butaperazine, haloperidol, thiothixene, and mesoridazine were more often associated with withdrawal dyskinesia than chlorpromazine, thioridazine, and trifluoperazine. The investigators reported that the occurrence of withdrawal dyskinesia was not related to age, length of treatment, total dosage, prewithdrawal dosage, history of extrapyramidal side effects during treatment, or the chemical class of the neuroleptic. The authors also concluded that gradual withdrawal of neuroleptics did not significantly reduce the incidence of dyskinesia.

Frank and Djavadi (1980) noted that development of tardive dyskinesia did not appear to be related to the use of any particular neuroleptics, polypharmacy versus single compounds, medication changes, or drug holidays. In the only published biochemical study of childhood dyskinesia, Winsberg et al. (1977) reported that children without withdrawal dyskinesias had three times higher mean concentrations of CSF-HVA as compared to children with dyskinesia. The two groups did not differ in CSF levels of cAMP. The researchers suggested that presynaptic disturbances may be associated with withdrawal dyskinesias.

TREATMENT

Neuroleptic withdrawal seems to be the best treatment. Although neuroleptics are the most effective agents for suppressing dyskinesia, their long-term continued use in dyskinetic patients might be potentially hazardous. Paulson et al. (1975) found that continued administration of neuroleptics for a 4-year period to children with tardive dyskinesia had variable effects on the severity of dyskinesia. The symptom severity at the 4-year follow-up was described as unchanged in six patients, worse in four, and less in five cases. Antiparkinsonian and other medications have little effect on childhood dyskinesias. Frank and Djavadi (1980) reported that four of their five adolescents with severe tardive dyskinesia had remission of dyskinesia following discontinuation of neuroleptics.

SUMMARY

Although the literature on tardive dyskinesia in children is scanty, the following tentative conclusions can be drawn from the available information:

1. Tardive dyskinesia occurs in 8% to 20% of children and adolescents receiving prolonged neuroleptic treatment. Although persistent dyskinesia is probably less common in children than in adults, it is certainly not rare in the younger age group.

2. Phenomenologically, tardive dyskinesias in children and adults are similar, except for the predominance of limb involvement over orofacial dyskinesia in children.

3. Neuroleptic withdrawal is associated with short-term dyskinesias in a large proportion (40% to 50%) of children. These dyskinesias remit either spontaneously or as a result of reinstituting neuroleptics.

4. Long-term use of neuroleptics in children is justified only if there is evidence that, for individual patients, discontinuing medication would result in the development of neuropsychiatric symptoms of an unacceptable severity.

5. There is no satisfactory treatment for childhood dyskinesias apart from discontinuation of neuroleptics.

CHAPTER VIII

Dyskinesias with Nonneuroleptic Drugs

Dyskinesias have been reported as side effects of short-term or long-term treatment with a number of different drugs. A consideration of such dyskinesias may be helpful to get a proper perspective of neuroleptic-induced tardive dyskinesia. Dyskinesias produced by L-dopa resemble the neuroleptic-induced tardive dyskinesia most closely; hence they are discussed here at some length. Dyskinesias caused by most other drugs are generally acute, self-limited, and, sometimes, toxic effects. It is indeed remarkable that neuroleptics are the only drugs that induce persistent tardive dyskinesia in large numbers of patients.

L-DOPA

Introduction of high-dosage L-dopa therapy for patients with Parkinson's disease almost revolutionized the treatment of that disease. Yet, as with neuroleptics, dyskinesias induced by L-dopa have proved to be a serious concern. There are a number of similarities between the abnormal involuntary movements produced by L-dopa and those produced by neuroleptics. Indeed, L-dopa-induced dyskinesias are often taken as a clinical prototype of neuroleptic-induced tardive dyskinesias; this has led some investigators to believe that the pathophysiology of the movement disorders caused by these two types of drugs is similar. There are, however, many differences between the dyskinesias resulting from the use of L-dopa and those due to use of neuroleptics. Barbeau, Mars, Gillo-Joffrey, *et al.* (1970), Klawans (1973), Weiner and Bergen (1977), and Yahr (1970) have ably reviewed the data on L-dopa-induced dyskinesias.

HISTORY

Cotzias, Van Woert, and Schettes (1967) and Cotzias, Papavasiliou, and Gellene (1969) were the first to report on the value of long-term, high-dosage L-dopa treatment in patients with Parkinson's disease. Even in their initial communications on this subject, they referred to the occurrence of dyskinesias caused by L-dopa. There has been no reluctance to accept the entity of L-dopa-induced dyskinesias, nor has there been a dramatic overall increase in the prevalence of this complication over the last 15 years.[1]

PREVALENCE

The reported prevalence of L-dopa-induced dyskinesias has ranged from 40% to 80%. It is interesting to note that the 80% prevalence was reported as early as 1969 by Barbeau. According to McDowell (1970), if every patient with Parkinson's disease had a progressive increase in the dose of L-dopa beyond the point of maximal improvement, we would see a 100% prevalence of dyskinesias.

MANIFESTATIONS

Barbeau et al. (1970) have proposed a descriptive classification of the abnormal movements produced by L-dopa. The classification is based on the localization of the signs. The four principal classes are cephalic, trunk, upper extremity, and lower extremity dyskinesias. These include a total of 47 different kinds of involuntary movements. Barbeau et al. assert that such abnormal movements are rarely observed in spontaneous extrapyramidal disorders; the only conditions with similar phenomena are von Economo's encephalitis and neuroleptic-induced tardive dyskinesias. L-Dopa-induced involuntary movements are often intermittent and sometimes unilateral.

[1]There has been a slight shift of focus in the literature on L-dopa-induced dyskinesias. Whereas the initial studies dealt mostly with dyskinesias caused by high-dose therapy relatively early in the treatment course, more recently there has been an interest in dyskinesias seen in patients maintained on lower doses of L-dopa for longer periods of time (Tarsy, 1981). Whether the latter type of dyskinesias are more akin to neuroleptic-induced tardive dyskinesias is unclear.

TREATMENT-RELATED VARIABLES IN ETIOLOGY

Dosage of L-dopa therapy is the single most important determinant of the prevalence of dyskinesias produced by this drug. Dyskinesias are more likely to occur in patients treated with relatively high doses of the drug.

Duration of treatment is less crucial than dosage. Although the majority of patients who develop L-dopa-induced dyskinesias do so within 3 to 12 months of the onset of treatment, a gradual increase in the prevalence continues over a 5-year period.

Another variable in the etiology of dyskinesias is the type of drug used. Among related drugs, L-dopa is the one most commonly used in Parkinson's disease and the one most frequently associated with dyskinesias. Other similar drugs, such as D, L-dopa, carbidopa + L-dopa combination, bromocriptine, and amantadine also produce dyskinesias. Cotzias, Papavasiliou, Fehling, *et al.* (1970) reported induction of dyskinesia with apomorphine in a patient with Parkinson's disease.

A final variable is concomitant treatment. The effect of anticholinergic agents on L-dopa-induced dyskinesias is uncertain. Yahr (1970) found no change in the intensity of this movement disorder when anticholinergic drugs were added. Weiner and Bergen (1977), however, reported improvement in L-dopa-induced dyskinesias in one-third of their patients when the doses of concomitant anticholinergic medication were reduced; this is consistent with Birket-Smith's (1974) observation that anticholinergic drugs increased L-dopa-induced dyskinesias.

PATIENT-RELATED VARIABLES

Primary neurological illness for which L-dopa was prescribed in a particular patient is an important determinant of the prevalence of dyskinesias. L-Dopa-induced dyskinesias are most likely to occur in patients with Parkinson's disease. They have also been seen, although rarely, in patients with dystonia musculorum deformans that has been treated similarly. Administration of L-dopa in high doses to patients with other (nonextrapyramidal) neurological disorders or to persons without apparent structural brain damage has not been known to result in dyskinesias; however, the number of such persons who have received long-term high-dosage L-dopa therapy has been quite small. Animal experiments show that facial dyskinesias can be produced in normal monkeys by chronic treatment with L-dopa, provided that extremely high amounts of the drug are given.

Generally, L-dopa produces dyskinesias in those patients who have had considerable improvement in parkinsonian symptoms as a result of the treatment. This does not necessarily suggest an inverse relationship between the symptoms of Parkinson's disease and dyskinesia. The two coexist in some patients, indicating that therapeutic effects and dyskinesia induction by L-dopa may occur through somewhat different mechanisms.

Lateralization of L-dopa-induced limb dyskinesias in patients with hemiparkinsonism or in patients operated upon stereotaxically is uncertain. The dyskinesias are more prone to involve, first, the affected side in patients with hemiparkinsonism and are less likely to occur initially on the operated side in patients treated with thalamotomy. Yet, with passage of time, both sides eventually may be affected by the abnormal movements. The orofacial dyskinesias produced by L-dopa are not related to the severity of Parkinson's disease.

Duration of Parkinson's disease may also affect the incidence of L-dopa-induced dyskinesias; the longer the duration of illness, the greater the chances of developing dyskinesias with L-dopa. Such a relationship is, however, not always apparent.

Aging is a relatively less important predisposing factor for L-dopa-induced dyskinesias than it is for neuroleptic-induced tardive dyskinesia.

Regarding the factor of constitutional susceptibility, some patients manifest dyskinesias with relatively small total amounts of L-dopa, whereas other patients do not have dyskinesias even after years of high-dosage treatment. The average daily dose of the drug in patients with and without dyskinesias may be similar. This suggests that biochemical, neuropathological, or other types of individual characteristics may predispose certain patients to develop abnormal movements with L-dopa therapy. The exact nature of such predisposing constitutional factors is not known.

PATHOGENESIS

The mechanism of production of dyskinesias with L-dopa is not clear. It is generally thought that supersensitivity of postsynaptic dopamine receptors in the nigrostriatal system is responsible for these dyskinesias. Elicitation of dyskinesias in patients with Parkinson's disease by a dopamine receptor agonist such as apomorphine is consistent with this hypothesis (Cotzias *et al.*, 1970). However, it is not clear whether the postulated supersensitivity results primarily from denervation or from prolonged treatment with L-dopa. One theory states that progressive loss of dopaminergic neurons in the nigrostriatal system, which is presumed to be the central lesion in Parkinson's disease, leads to denervation supersensitivity of postsynaptic receptors. Administration of L-dopa to parkinsonian patients results in an uncontrolled delivery of dopamine onto the supersensitive dopamine receptors in the extrapyramidal system, the result being dyskinesias (Carlsson, 1970). Absence of L-dopa-induced dyskinesias in neurologically normal persons supports this hypothesis. On the other hand, rarity of spontaneous dyskinesias early in the course of Parkinson's disease argues against denervation supersensitivity. (In early stages of Parkinson's disease, some dopamine is still being released and might be expected to stimulate the supersensitive receptors; Tarsy & Baldessarini, 1977.)

Work by Klawans and Margolin (1975) suggests that chronic dopaminergic stimulation may contribute to the development of dopmine receptor supersensitivity. The investigators found that chronic administration of amphetamine to normal guinea pigs resulted in increased responsiveness to amphetamine as well as to apomorphine. The clinically observed positive correlation between duration of high-dosage L-dopa therapy and incidence of dyskinesias also conforms with the hypothesis that chronic dopaminergic stimulation leads to dopamine receptor supersensitivity.

As stated earlier, parkinsonian symptoms and L-dopa-induced dyskinesias coexist in some patients. Klawans (1973) and Weiner and Bergen (1977) explain this observation on the basis of a two-receptor hypothesis. They postulate that different types of dopamine receptors are involved in the pathogenesis of parkinsonian symptoms and dyskinesias.

Carlsson (1970) believes that certain mechanisms other than dopamine receptor supersensitivity may also underlie L-dopa-induced movement disorders. These may be related to minor metabolites of dopamine or to other monoamines, especially serotonin. Cholinergic hypofunctioning in the striatum has been implicated, too. Strong evidence to confirm these hypotheses is lacking.

CLINICAL COURSE

Continued treatment with L-dopa usually leads to an increase in the severity of dyskinesias and to the spread of symptoms to other areas of the body. On the other hand, dosage reduction or withdrawal of the drug almost always results in remission of the involuntary movements. To our knowledge, persistent dyskinesias induced by L-dopa (i.e., those that persist long after the drug is discontinued) have not been reported.

ON-OFF PHENOMENA

Some patients who have been on L-dopa for more than a year manifest sudden and dramatic changes in symptomatology, called the "on–off phenomenon." Periods of dyskinesia and hypermotility ("on" periods) alternate with periods of parkinsonian immobility ("off" periods). The pathophysiology of this penomenon is unknown. Sometimes there is an association between elevated plasma L-dopa levels and "on" periods, and between low plasma L-dopa levels and "off" periods.

TREATMENT

The only satisfactory treatment for L-dopa-induced dyskinesias is to lower the dose of the drug. This may, however, result in a worsening of the parkinsonian symptoms. The clinician needs to strike a balance between the dose of L-dopa that is too high and produces dyskinesia and the dose that is so low as to be ineffective in the treatment of Parkinson's disease. In some cases the patient may have to accept mild dyskinesia as a price to be paid to obtain relief from parkinsonian akinesia and rigidity. A number of other drugs have been tried in the treatment of L-dopa-induced dyskinesias, but they have generally proved to be of limited value.

COMPARISON WITH NEUROLEPTIC-INDUCED TARDIVE DYSKINESIA

Despite the phenomenological similarities between the abnormal involuntary movements produced by long-term treatment with L-dopa and those produced by treatment with neuroleptics, there are a number of differences between the two types of dyskinesias. Gerlach (1977) compared a group of 16 psychotic patients having neuroleptic-induced tardive dyskinesia with a group of 16 Parkinson's disease patients having L-dopa-induced dyskinesia. He found that neuroleptic-caused movements were more likely to involve the oral region, whereas L-dopa therapy often produced hyperkinesias in the neck and extremities. With age, L-dopa-induced dyskinesias also tended to affect the mouth and face. In a recent study, however, we found that buccolingual masticatory dyskinesias were significantly more likely to occur in neuroleptic-treated patients than in age-matched L-dopa-treated patients (Karson, Jeste, & Wyatt, unpublished data).

Table 8-1 compares the main characteristics of dyskinesias resulting from long-term administration of neuroleptics and of L-dopa. The principal distinguishing features of the L-dopa-induced dyskinesias are that they usually result from high-dosage therapy, may occur relatively early in the treatment course, and are rarely, if ever, permanent.

OTHER CATECHOLAMINERGIC DRUGS

AMPHETAMINE[2]

Oral and other stereotypies have been known to occur in amphetamine addicts. Ashcroft, Eccleston, and Waddell (1965) described a physical sign that was "widely recognized" among the "amphetamine fraternity." It consisted of continuous chewing or teeth-grinding movements and rubbing the tongue along the inside of the lower lip, often resulting in traumatic ulcers on the tongue and lip.

Dyskinesias also occur in patients treated with therapeutic doses of amphetamine; Mattson and Calverley (1968) were probably the first to report such cases. The authors described four patients, ranging in age from 3 to 51 years, who were treated with dextroamphetamine sulfate for conditions such as hyperactivity and narcolepsy. The subjects developed different types of dyskinesias, including lip smacking, grimacing, twitching of eyelids, twisting of head and neck, and choreoathetoid movements of extremities, as a result of *d*-amphetamine intake. The dyskinesias appeared to be an idiosyncratic reaction to the therapeutic doses of the drug, since no other signs of amphetamine toxicity were present. Discontinuing the drug always led to disappearance of the abnormal movements. Since three of these patients had evidence of brain damage, Mattson and Calverley thought that *d*-amphetamine probably unmasked a subclinical extrapyramidal disorder in them. Amphetamine-induced dyskinesias are, however, not restricted to brain-damaged patients. Eveloff (1968) described

[2]There is a large amount of literature on amphetamine dyskinesias in Sweden, where they are included as a part of the "punding" syndrome.

Table 8-1. Comparison of Tardive Dyskinesias Induced by L-Dopa and Neuroleptics

Variable	L-Dopa	Neuroleptics
Prevalence		
Overall prevalence	40% to 80%	5% to 40%
Progressive rise in prevalence since first reports	Not seen	Seen
Manifestations		
Oral manifestations	Common	More common
Limb dyskinesias	Common	Less common
Intermittent dyskinesias	Frequent	Uncommon
Unilateral dyskinesias	Frequent	Rare
Drug-withdrawal dyskinesias	Rare	Frequent
Etiologic factors		
Daily high doses	Important	Less important
Length of treatment	Less important	More important
Effect of concomitant anticholinergic treatment	Uncertain	Little
Primary illness	Parkinsons's disease	Unimportant
Need for predisposing brain damage	Present	Not apparent
Relationship to therapeutic effects of the drug	Sometimes	Absent
Predisposing constitutional factors	Probable	Probable
Aging as predisposition	Less important	Important
Pathophysiology		
Dopamine receptor supersensitivity	Probable	Presumed
Role of the other neurotransmitters	Possible	Possible
Course		
Relationship between duration and severity of dyskinesia	Positive	Variable
On–off phenomena	Sometimes	Not reported
Persistence on drug withdrawal	Not reported	In 67% of patients
Treatment		
Dose reduction	Effective	Sometimes effective
Dose increase	Dyskinesia worsens	Dyskinesia may be masked
Effect of other drugs	Variable	Variable

involuntary lateral movements of the jaw as an acute side effect of *d*-amphetamine in an 18-year-old neurologically normal girl.

d-Amphetamine has been shown to aggravate neuroleptic-induced tardive dyskinesia (Chapter 10).

APOMORPHINE

Cotzias *et al.* (1970) described a case of apomorphine-induced dyskinesia in a patient with Parkinson's disease; the patient had previously developed dyskinesia with L-dopa.

METHYLPHENIDATE

This is an amphetamine-like central nervous system stimulant. Mattson and Calverley (1968) reported acute dyskinesias involving the head and neck and choreoathetoid movements of the extremities in a 3-year-old girl who was given 5 mg of methylphenidate hydrochloride. The movements disappeared on stopping the drug, but later reappeared when the patient was given d-amphetamine. Golden (1974) described a patient in whom Gilles de la Tourette's syndrome made its appearance following methylphenidate administration. Denckla, Bemporad, and MacKay (1975) reported that, among children receiving methylphenidate, tics developed *de novo* in 14 and became worse in 6 children who had preexisting tics. The tics involved muscles of the face, eyelids, jaw, head, neck, limbs, and trunk. The primary clinical diagnosis was minimal brain dysfunction in 19 cases, and Gilles de la Tourette's syndrome in 1. The appearance or aggravation of tics with methylphenidate in these patients showed no consistent relationship with duration or dose of the drug. In all cases except one, the tics improved on stopping methylphenidate.

FENFLURAMINE

This drug is sometimes used in the treatment of obesity. Although it is similar to amphetamine in several of its pharmacologic actions, it is presumed to cause more sedation than central nervous system stimulation, unlike amphetamine. Brandon (1969) described a case of fenfluramine-induced acute oral dyskinesia. The patient, an 18-year-old man, manifested teeth-grinding and facial dyskinesias on ingesting the drug. According to Shoulson and Chase (1974), fenfluramine stimulates postsynaptic serotonergic receptors and has no consistent dopaminergic activity.

AMANTADINE

This drug is often used in patients with Parkinson's disease. It potentiates catecholaminergic activity. It is less potent than L-dopa in its therapeutic activity, but is also thought to have fewer side effects than L-dopa. Pearce (1970) first reported a case of lingual–facial dyskinesia produced by amantadine. The patient was a 68-year-old woman with Parkinson's disease. Amantadine treatment resulted in an improvement in parkinsonian symptoms, but also caused dyskinesia.

Amantadine has been used unsuccessfully in patients with neuroleptic-induced tardive dyskinesia (see Chapter 10).

MAO INHIBITORS

Stancer (1979) described two patients (aged 62 and 38 years, respectively) with primary affective disorder who developed involuntary chewing movements after combined tranylcypromine-lithium therapy for more than a year. In both cases the movements persisted after tranylcypromine was discontinued and lithium was given alone. It is unclear whether the dyskinesias in Stancer's patients were caused by tranylcypromine or lithium or both.

SUMMARY

Dyskinesias similar to those induced by neuroleptics and L-dopa have been reported with a number of catecholaminergic agents. Abnormal movements caused by amphetamine, methylphenidate, fenfluramine, and amantadine are almost always reversible. Whether MAO inhibitors produce persistent dyskinesias in a few patients is uncertain.

NONNEUROLEPTIC CATECHOLAMINE ANTAGONISTS

METOCLOPRAMIDE

This is a benzamide, presumed to be a selective D_2 receptor antagonist (see Chapter 5). Metoclopramide is used clinically in the treatment of upper gastrointestinal symptoms such as heartburn, nausea, and vomiting.

Melmed and Bank (1975) reported two cases of acute facial dyskinesia along with dystonias following metoclopramide ingestion. Ethylbenztropine produced rapid symptom relief in both patients (aged 18 and 34 years, respectively). Walsh (1975) described two similar cases. Tardive dyskinesia following long-term administration of metoclopramide was first reported by Lavy, Melamed, and Penchas (1978). The patient, a 48-year-old man, received the drug for 6 years. Ten days after he abruptly stopped it, he developed buccolingual masticatory dyskinesia consisting of sucking, chewing, grimacing, and tongue protrusions. Readministration of metoclopramide resulted in an almost complete disappearance of the movements. When the drug was withdrawn again, the dyskinesias recurred; they subsided when metoclopramide was given again. Kataria, Traub, and Marsden (1978) also described metoclopramide-induced tardive dyskinesia.

DROPERIDOL

This butyrophenone is used as a sedative in preanesthetic medication. Patton (1975) reported the occurrence of acute orofacial dyskinesias and dystonias with grimacing, tongue protrusion, and perioral spasms in a 41-year-old man following droperidol administration. The symptoms cleared within 1 minute of intravenous injection of diphenhydramine.

NONNEUROLEPTIC PHENOTHIAZINES

Among the phenothiazines likely to produce tardive dyskinesia, the following nonneuroleptic agents were included by the American College of Neuropsychopharmacology–FDA Task Force (1973); promethazine, thiethylperazine, and propiomazine. Long-term clinical experience with these agents is, however, rather limited.

METHYLDOPA

Yamadori and Albert (1972) described a 59-year-old hypertensive man who developed choreoathetoid movements of the extremities, trunk, and face following treatment with methyldopa for 25 days. The involuntary movements ceased within a day of discontinuing the drug.

ANTICHOLINERGIC AGENTS

The relationship of anticholinergic drugs to tardive dyskinesia is discussed in Chapter 4 under "Antiparkinsonian Drugs."

MISCELLANEOUS DRUGS

TRICYCLIC ANTIDEPRESSANTS

Sedivec, Valenova, and Paceltova (1970) reported five cases of tricyclic-induced tardive dyskinesia (orofacial). All the patients were women over 50 years of age with evidence of brain damage (cerebral arteriosclerosis in three patients, "more advanced brain damage due to senility" in one, and carbon monoxide intoxication in one). It is not mentioned whether the patients had also been treated with neuroleptics. In most cases dyskinesia persisted for a number of months after withdrawal of tricyclics (imipramine, amitriptyline, or nortriptyline).

Fann, Sullivan, and Richman (1976) presented two cases of tricyclic-induced dyskinesia (orofacial dyskinesia in one patient and choreoathetosis in the other). The patients, aged 37 and 44, had also received neuroleptics. Dyskinesia dissappeared within 2 weeks of discontinuing the tricyclics in both subjects. Although the investigators suggested that the anticholinergic activity of the drugs might be responsible for the dyskinesias, the noradrenergic action also deserves consideration (see Chapter 5).

Two other cases of oral dyskinesia attributed to tricyclic antidepressants have been reported by Deckret, Maany, Ramsey, et al. (1977) and Woogen, Graham, and Angrist (1981).

ANTIHISTAMINE DRUGS

Thach, Chase, and Bosma (1975) described two women, aged 55 and 65, who developed blepharospasm and dyskinesia involving the mouth, tongue, face, and, in one case, hands, following prolonged oral intake (for a number of years) of antihistaminic decongestants. The antihistamine drugs taken by these patients included brompheniramine, chlorpheniramine, and phenindamine. One patient improved on stopping the medication, but the other one did not. Both patients improved with a trial of haloperidol. The investigators found substantially low CSF-HVA accumulations during probenecid loading in the two patients. This suggested a similarity in the pathophysiological mechanisms (involving central dopamine pathways) underlying tardive dyskinesias induced by chronic treatment with neuroleptic and antihistamine drugs.

Thach et al. (1975) cited a case report by Worz. The latter described a 60-year-old woman with oral dyskinesia resulting from prolonged use of mebhydroline, a nonphenothiazine antihistamine. Davis (1976) reported the case of a 57-year-old man who developed left-sided orofacial dyskinesia, including blepharospasm, following ingestion of antihistamine decongestants for about 20 years. The dyskinesia remitted within 6 weeks of stopping the offending agents.

ANTICONVULSANTS

Abnormal involuntary movements are sometimes seen as a sign of acute or chronic intoxication with various anticonvulsants. Orofacial and limb dyskinesias similar to neuroleptic-induced tardive dyskinesias are, however, associated only with the use of diphenylhydantoin or phenytoin. Two exceptions are case reports by Kirschberg (1975) and Joyce and Gunderson (1980). Kirschberg's patient, a 15-year-old epileptic girl, developed tongue protrusion, lip smacking, and limb dyskinesias when ethosuximide was added to her phenobartitone–phenytoin regimen. Intravenous administration of diphenhydramine hydrochloride produced dramatic improvment in the dyskinesias. The patient of Joyce and Gunderson (1980) was a 51-year-old man who developed acute orofacial dyskinesia following an overdose of carbamazepine. Discontinuation of the drug resulted in rapid relief of symptoms.

Ahmad, Laidlaw, Houghton, *et al.* (1975), Chadwick, Reynolds, and Marsden (1976), and Dravet, Bernardina, Mesdjian, *et al.* (1980) have reviewed the literature on anticonvulsant-induced dyskinesias. Cerebral pathology, patient's age, type or duration of epilepsy, and duration of treatment do not seem to make any major contribution to the etiology of dyskinesias caused by these drugs. The serum concentrations of phenytoin are found to be in the toxic range in many of the affected patients. The dyskinesias are generally rapidly reversible by discontinuing or reducing the dose of phenytoin or, occasionally, by administering intravenous diazepam. Chadwick *et al.* (1976) hypothesized that phenytoin probably shares some biochemical actions, such as dopamine-blocking effect, with the neuroleptics.

DeVeaugh-Geiss (1978) reported the case of a 55-year-old man in whom haloperidol-induced tardive dyskinesia was aggravated by phenytoin in spite of subtherapeutic serum phenytoin level. Since a large number of patients receive neuroleptics and phenytoin concomitantly, this case report is of clinical interest.

It is again noteworthy that, considering the frequency of long-term administration of phenytoin to patients with brain damage, persistent tardive dyskinesia produced by this drug has, to the best of our knowledge, not been reported.

BENZODIAZEPINES

Kaplan and Murkofsky (1978) first reported a case of oral–buccal dyskinesia associated with low-dose benzodiazepine treatment. The patient, a 63-year-old man, had never been treated with neuroleptics. The dyskinesia disappeared within 72 hours of discontinuing diazepam and flurazepam.

Rosenbaum and De La Fuente (1979) described five patients with benzodiazepine-induced dyskinesias and another patient whose neuroleptic-induced tardive dyskinesia was aggravated by the use of a benzodiazepine. All the patients were over 50 years of age; five were women. All had orofacial dyskinesias. The symptoms remitted on withdrawal of the responsible drugs in two cases; the remaining patients were treated with a combination of tricyclic antidepressants and lithium. The benzodiazepines involved were diazepam, clorazepate, and lorazepam.

ANTIMALARIAL DRUGS (4-AMINOQUINOLINES)

Akindele and Odejide (1976) described four cases of involuntary movements induced by amodiaquine. Later, Umez-Eronini and Eronini (1977) reported five similar cases, except that the involuntary movements had been caused by chloroquine. According to Majumdar (1977), other 4-aminoquinolines, such as cycloquine and hydroxychloroquine, may also produce the same reaction. He believed that the side effect was a result of the action of the drugs on dopamine receptors in the nigrostriatal system.

The abnormal movements caused by the antimalarial agents differ from the neuroleptic-induced tardive dyskinesias in several respects. The former represent an acute, idiosyncratic reaction to the drugs, reported mostly in children and young adults. The symptoms include protrusion of the tongue, muscle spasms (producing torticollis, etc.), tremors of the hands, and excessive salivation. They remit spontaneously on withdrawal of the antimalarial and also respond quickly to anticholinergic, antihistamine, or sedative drugs. Thus the involuntary movements caused by the 4-aminoquinolines are comparable to the acute extrapyramidal reaction (dystonias) induced by neuroleptics and not to the tardive dyskinesias.

LITHIUM

Any association between lithium and tardive dyskinesia is unclear. We have not found published reports of cases in which tardive dyskinesia could be attributed to lithium treatment alone. Several authors have, however, described patients in whom lithium seemed to contribute to the development, reinduction, or aggravation of tardive dyskinesia.

Crews and Carpenter (1977) reported a case of lithium-induced aggravation of tardive dyskinesia. A 46-year-old woman had developed tardive dyskinesia following prolonged neuroleptic therapy. On starting lithium, the severity of dyskinesia appeared to correlate with serum lithium levels, toxic levels being associated with increased severity. Beitman (1978) described a 56-year-old woman whose tardive dyskinesia cleared shortly after stopping neuroleptics. Two years later she was put on lithium, with no neuroleptics. After 2 years of lithium treatment, she had a recurrence of facial dyskinesia similar to that which she had experienced earlier. Administration of trihexyphenidyl produced only a temporary improvement. We have already referred to Stancer's (1979) report of tardive dyskinesia with tranylcypromine and lithium in two patients.

Lithium has also been tried in the treatment of neuroleptic-induced tardive dyskinesia, but the results have usually been unsatisfactory (see Chapter 10).

Thus there is no consistent relationship between lithium and tardive dyskinesia. In spite of the large number of patients who have had long-term treatment with lithium, few cases have been reported in which lithium alone produced tardive dyskinesia. In individual patients, however, lithium may aggravate or improve neuroleptic-induced dyskinesia.

ESTROGENS

Estrogens have been reported to induce choreiform dyskinesias in a few patients (Koller *et al.*, 1979). Yet, some investigators believe that estrogens may protect against the development of tardive dyskinesia (see Chapter 5). Thus the association between estrogens and dyskinesia is quite unclear.

SUMMARY

Dyskinesias resulting from brief or prolonged treatment have been reported with a number of drugs other than neuroleptics. These drugs may be classified into three main groups:

1. Catecholaminergic agents—L-dopa, amphetamine, methylphenidate, amantadine, fenfluramine, tranylcypromine, tricyclic antidepressants, and apomorphine.
2. Dopamine antagonists—metoclopramide, droperidol, methyldopa (and promethazine).
3. Drugs with other or uncertain mechanisms of action—anticholinergic agents, antihistamine drugs, anticonvulsants (especially phenytoin), benzodiazepines, antimalarial agents (4-aminoquinolines), lithium, and estrogens.

With the exception of L-dopa and d-amphetamine, the number of cases of dyskinesias produced by other drugs has been relatively small. A cause-and-effect relationship between those drugs and dyskinesias is therefore not yet established on an epidemiologic basis. Moreover, dyskinesias presumptively elicited by those agents have been of different varieties. In many patients the movement disorder was apparently an acute, idiosyncratic reaction to a drug (e.g., 4-aminoquinoline) and rapidly subsided either on withdrawing that drug or on administering agents with sedative, antihistaminic, or anticholinergic action. In a few cases the dyskinesia became manifest only after prolonged treatment with a drug (e.g., tricyclic antidepressant) and was thus tardive dyskinesia. Even in these patients, persistence of symptoms after drug withdrawal has been rare.

Thus two notable facts emerge from a consideration of non-neuroleptic-induced dyskinesias. First, the only drugs that have been commonly associated with such dyskinesias have been catecholaminergic agents. The most important of these, L-dopa, induces dyskinesias after long-term, high-dosage therapy almost exclusively in patients with structural damage in the extrapyramidal region. Second, persistent tardive dyskinesias with nonneuroleptic agents have been extremely rare. Hence the induction, by neuroleptics, of persistent dyskinesias in a large number of patients without apparent structural brain damage is a unique phenomenon.

CHAPTER IX

Animal Models

INTRODUCTION

Animal models are commonly employed in both psychopathology and psychopharmacology. They are used in the hope of gaining a better understanding of the mechanisms underlying mental illnesses and of ways to prevent and manage those disorders (e.g., preclinical screening of new drugs to predict their usefulness in psychiatric patients). An example of an animal model that may be helpful in studying the neurochemistry of schizophrenia is amphetamine-induced or phenylethylamine-induced stereotypy (Borison & Diamond, 1978; Wyatt, Gillin, Stoff, *et al.,* 1977). The paradigm of conditioned avoidance response has long been used to screen drugs for neuroleptic properties. Animal models have also been proposed for depression, aggression, alcoholism, drug-induced hallucinations, and other conditions (see Stoff, Gillin, & Wyatt, 1978).

NEED

In-depth longitudinal and cross-sectional studies of large numbers of patients with psychiatric illnesses and matched controls are difficult because of ethical, medicolegal, and practical problems, not to mention methodological issues such as certain unavoidable differences between patient and control groups. Experimental surgical procedures (such as brain lesions) or neurophathological studies of brain tissue after controlled administration of a drug for varying lengths of time can be done only in animals.

Baldessarini and Fischer (1975) state that a model is an experimental compromise—that is, it consists of a simple experimental system that represents a more complex and less readily accessible system. Thus a rat with amphetamine-induced stereotypy is presumed to represent a patient with schizophrenia. An ideal or "model" model should have the same etiology, symptomatology, mediating mechanisms, and treatment responses as the human condition it is supposed to represent (Murphy, 1976). Few animal models in psychiatry or neurology satisfy all of these criteria. Most animal models, at best, only partly mimic selected aspects of a complex human syndrome.

RATIONALE

During the course of evolution, the size and complexity of the brain as well as the structure and function of its individual areas underwent enormous changes. Yet, certain phylogenetically older regions, such as the nigrostriatal system, are remarkably similar in lower animals and humans, especially in terms of neurochemistry, and so justify use of specific animal models for certain human conditions (Matthysse & Haber, 1975).

LIMITATIONS

Simplicity is both a merit and a drawback of animal models. Long-term prospective studies of patients to be treated with different neuroleptics according to a rigid research schedule may be impractical, whereas studying large numbers of matched groups of rats to be treated similarly is quite feasible. Yet, a question arises about the comparability of data obtained from 300-g normal rats "treated" with daily intraperitoneal injections of a neuroleptic for several weeks and data from chronic schizophrenic patients who received oral neuroleptics, usually along with other drugs, for a number of years. Ignoring the various psychobiosocial variables that contribute to the human condition may lead to simplistic interpretations of results obtained from animal studies.

A major problem with some animal models, rightly stressed by Kornetsky (1977), is that of relevance of the model to the human syndrome it is believed to represent. There may be a good model, but of the wrong thing. As discussed later, one example of this problem may be the animal model of tardive dyskinesia based on neuroleptic-induced striatal postsynaptic dopamine receptor supersensitivity. There is little doubt that neuroleptic administration causes such supersensitivity. The unresolved issue, however, is whether this supersensitivity is responsible for persistent tardive dyskinesia. Until that question is answered, it is somewhat premature to make conclusions about tardive dyskinesia based solely on experiments with the supersensitivity model.

To conclude, animal models have an undisputed place in psychiatric research. However, it is necessary to bear in mind their limitations so as to avoid overinterpreting the data. According to Harlow (cited by Kornetsky, 1977), "One has to be crazy to use animal models for studying human psychopathology, but one is also crazy not to use animal models since they offer some valuable insights."

ISOMORPHISM CRITERIA

To judge the relevance of an animal model to a clinical syndrome, it is useful to define certain essential features of the syndrome that the animal model is expected to share. In considering animal models of schizophrenia, Matthysse and Haber (1975) introduced the concept of isomorphism derived from systems theory. Isomorphism between two systems (in this case a clinical syndrome and its animal model) requires that every formal or specific characteristic of one system should have a precise counterpart in the other, even if the objects involved in the two systems are not the same. (For example, aggravation by catecholamine agonists and improvement with neuroleptics are two of the formal characteristics of human schizophrenia that should be shared by a proposed animal model.) Since it is unreasonable to expect that an animal model would have all the characteristics of the human syndrome, it is important to specify the essential features of the clinical disorder that a good animal model should share. Thus the phenomenology and localization of drug-induced stereotypy, which are at least partly species-dependent, may not be considered a crucial component of the tardive dyskinesia syndrome for the purposes of validating an animal model.

Two other terms that are frequently used in referring to the relevance of an animal model to the human condition are "homology" and "analogy." Homologous animal models are those that correspond in etiology to specific human disorders (Kornetsky, 1977). Few animal models in neurology or psychiatry are homologous, if only because the etiology of the human disorders themselves is frequently not known. Analogous animal models are those that are faithful to some features of the clinical syndrome

(Stoff *et al.*, 1978). For instance, oral stereotypy induced by various drugs in rodents may be conceived of as an analogous model of oral dyskinesia in man; yet, the two conditions may differ considerably in terms of etiology, pathophysiology, and pharmacologic responses. (The term "analogy" is generally employed to refer to the content of behavior and is therefore narrower in its implications than "isomorphism.")

Following is our list of isomorphism criteria against which the various available animal models of tardive dyskinesia may be evaluated:

1. Induction by prolonged or repeated, but not by acute, neuroleptic treatment.
2. Higher incidence or greater effects in older than in younger animals.
3. Spontaneous onset either during the course of prolonged neuroleptic administration or following withdrawal of neuroleptics.
4. Persistence of the abnormal behavior (which is postulated to be the analog of human tardive dyskinesia) in at least a proportion of animals long after neuroleptics have been discontinued.
5. Temporary suppression of the abnormal behavior by acute neuroleptic administration and worsening on neuroleptic withdrawal.
6. Nonresponse to, or aggravation by, anticholinergic drugs.

In the remainder of the chapter, we will assess the validity of the individual animal models against these criteria. There are few models that have been tested and shown to satisfy all of these criteria. Of the various models, the one based on neuroleptic-induced striatal postsynaptic dopamine receptor supersensitivity has been the most popular. It is, however, less satisfactory than the other major model—namely, neuroleptic-induced dyskinesias in monkeys. A number of miscellaneous animal models, such as naturally occurring dyskinesia-like disorders and amphetamine-induced stereotypy, have also been employed, but their validity as models of tardive dyskinesia is largely unproven.

NEUROLEPTIC-INDUCED STRIATAL POSTSYNAPTIC DOPAMINE RECEPTOR SUPERSENSITIVITY

The most widely studied animal model for tardive dyskinesia has been postsynaptic dopamine receptor supersensitivity in the striatum following chronic neuroleptic treatment. Such supersensitivity can be inferred from behavioral (increased responsiveness to dopaminergic drugs such as amphetamine and apomorphine) or biochemical (increased number of striatal dopamine receptor binding sites) experiments. Rodents (rats and mice) have been the animals most frequently employed for this purpose. (Eibergen & Carlson, 1976, used rhesus monkeys.)

BACKGROUND

There were few systematic attempts to formulate a hypothesis of the pathophysiology or to construct a suitable animal model for neuroleptic-induced tardive dyskinesia until about 1970. When increasing reports of similar dyskinesias produced by L-dopa in patients with Parkinson's disease began appearing in the literature during the late 1960s, they seemed also to offer a clue to the mechanisms underlying dyskinesias due to neuroleptics. Carlsson (1970) and Klawans, Ilahi, and Shenker (1970) proposed that dyskinesias caused by L-dopa and neuroleptics were secondary to denervation supersensitivity of striatal postsynaptic dopamine receptors. Carlsson (1970) suggested that loss of dopaminergic neurons in the nigrostriatal area led to supersensitivity in Parkinson's disease and that this supersensitivity contributed to the clinical efficacy of L-dopa treatment in Parkinson's disease. Long-term neuroleptic treatment produces similar supersensitivity as a consequence of prolonged blockade of postsynaptic dopamine receptors—a form of "disuse supersensitivity" (Sharpless, 1969).

Work by Carlsson and Lindqvist and others (see Bunney & Aghajanian, 1976b) has shown that acute administration of neuroleptics leads to an increased release of dopamine and an increased firing of dopamine neurons. These changes are thought to be a result of a feedback mechanism, suggesting neuroleptic-induced blockade of dopamine receptors. The ability of most, but not all, of the neuroleptics to block dopamine receptors has been found to correlate well with their antipsychotic efficacy. It is assumed that blockade of postsynaptic dopamine receptors in the mesolimbic and mesocortical areas is responsible for the antipsychotic property of neuroleptics (although there is some controversy about this) and that a similar blockade in the nigrostriatal system is responsible for parkinsonism. Prolonged blockade of striatal dopaminergic receptors may lead to dopaminergic supersensitivity in that region of the brain, so that, according to this hypothesis (see Chapter 5), even small amounts of dopamine released there might produce dopaminergic hyperactivity clinically manifesting as tardive dyskinesia.

Experimental evidence for neuroleptic-induced striatal dopamine receptor supersensitivity came during the 1970s.[1] Klawans and Rubovits (1972), Tarsy and Baldessarini (1973, 1974), and a number of other researchers reported that chronic administration of dopamine-receptor-blocking neuroleptics (as well as other antidopaminergic drugs such as α-methyl-p-tyrosine [AMPT] and reserpine, but not other central nervous system depressants), followed by drug withdrawal, resulted in a lowering of the threshold for stereotypy produced by dopaminergic agents such as amphetamine and apomorphine. Burt, Creese, and Snyder (1977) and other investigators presented biochemical evidence of an increased number of striatal dopamine receptors after long-term use of neuroleptics. There is thus little doubt that chronic administration of neuroleptics produces striatal dopamine receptor supersensitivity; the main question is about the relevance of this phenomenon to tardive dyskinesia.

VALIDITY

Following is a discussion of the applicability of each of the isomorphism criteria to this putative model of tardive dyskinesia (summarized in Table 9-1).

1. Induction by chronic, but not acute, neuroleptic treatment. Christensen, Fjalland, and Nielsen (1976) showed that even a single injection of a neuroleptic produced dopamine receptor supersensitivity. The investigators reported that a single dose of a neuroleptic led to dopamine receptor blockade, which was replaced within 2 days by receptor supersensitivity; such supersensitivity (as judged by increased response to apomorphine and methylphenidate) lasted for several days to a week.

2. Higher incidence or greater effects in older animals. Smith and Leelavathi (1980) found that older rats treated with neuroleptics had greater responses to both apomorphine and amphetamine as compared to younger rats treated similarly. In contrast, Tanner and Domino (1977)

---

[1]It was, however, a Russian scientist, Schelkunov (1967), who first described increased response to dopaminergic drugs in animals pretreated with neuroleptics for long periods. He considered the likelihood that this effect might be due to presynaptic actions of neuroleptics resulting in increased synthesis and turnover of catecholamines.

Table 9-1. Application of Isomorphism Criteria to Two Principal Animal Models
of Tardive Dyskinesia

	Animal model[a]	
Criterion	Postsynaptic dopamine receptor supersensitivity	Dyskinesias in monkeys
Induction by chronic, but not acute, neuro-leptic treatment	−	+
Higher incidence or greater effects in older animals	+ or ?	Not tested
Spontaneous onset during or following neuro-leptic treatment	+	+
Persistence long after neuroleptic withdrawal	− or ?	+
Suppression by acute neuroleptic administration	+	+
Nonresponse to, or aggravation by, anticholin-ergic treatment	±	+

[a] + indicates presence and − indicates absence of that requirement in the animal model; ?
suggests uncertain status.

reported an increased effect only with amphetamine, not with apomorphine, in older gerbils. Furthermore, Smith and Leelavathi (1980) observed that chronic neuroleptic administration also produced significant
presynaptic biochemical changes, such as an increased uptake of catecholamines in cortical synaptosomes. It is therefore not at all certain that the
increased responsiveness of older neuroleptic-treated animals to catecholaminergic drugs is mostly due to postsynaptic receptor supersensitivity.

3. *Spontaneous onset during or following neuroleptic treatment.* Behavioral demonstration of dopaminergic receptor supersensitivity requires challenge with a dopaminergic agent such as apomorphine days
after the neuroleptic administration has been discontinued. If a dopaminergic drug is given during the course of neuroleptic treatment, there is a
diminished reponse to that drug. (One exception to this is a report by
Clow, Jenner, Theodorou, *et al.,* 1979, that rats had an exaggerated response to apomorphine at the end of 6 months of continuous trifluoperazine treatment.) Thus the behavioral manifestation of neuroleptic-induced
supersensitivity is neither spontaneous nor usually seen during the course
of neuroleptic administration. (In contrast, clinical tardive dyskinesia
often occurs while the patients are still on neuroleptics and in the absence
of precipitating dopaminergic drug challenges.)

Biochemical demonstration of increased dopamine receptor binding suggesting receptor supersensitivity does not need administration of a dopaminergic agent. It is not clear, however, whether the observed receptor supersensitivity entirely explains the enhanced responsiveness to dopaminergic drugs. Whereas 3-week administration of a neuroleptic, such as haloperidol, produces only a 20% to 25% increase in the number of binding sites for striatal dopamine receptors (Burt et al., 1977; Kobayashi, Fields, Kruska, et al., 1977), similar neuroleptic treatment causes an 80% enhancement of behavioral response to dopamine agonists (Gnegy, Uzunov, & Costa, 1977). Furthermore, dopamine receptor supersensitivity following chronic neuroleptic treatment is of a much smaller magnitude than that resulting from injections of 6-hydroxydopamine into the nigrostriatal system (Burt et al., 1977).

Interesting work by Engel et al. (1976) suggests the role of presynaptic mechanisms in the effects of chronic neuroleptic treatment. The Swedish researchers found that long-term administration of penfluridol to mice or rats was followed by a marked locomotor stimulation coincident with a significant increase in the activation of tyrosine hydroxylase in the striatum. The authors concluded that an increased synthesis of striatal dopamine might be involved in the pathogenesis of spontaneous hyperactivity following chronic neuroleptic use.

Clow, Theodorou, Jenner, et al. (1980) and Smith and Leelavathi (1980) have reported the occurrence of spontaneous oral stereotypy in chronic neuroleptic-treated rats. Such stereotypy tends to be reversible on drug withdrawal (Clow et al., 1980b). Glassman and Glassman (1980) studied the effects of long-term administration of neuroleptics to brain-damaged rats. The investigators found that rats with ablated frontal sensorimotor cortex showed more vacuous chewing movement following a 6-week treatment with a neuroleptic than did occipitally damaged rats or normal controls that had been treated in the same way. The effect was still apparent 1 month after neuroleptic withdrawal. Neurochemical mechanisms responsible for this phenomenon are not known. It is possible, however, that stereotypy induced by chronic neuroleptic treatment in rats (as in monkeys) may be a more valid model for tardive dyskinesia, at least the reversible type, than pharmacologic or biochemical demonstration of postsynaptic dopamine receptor supersensitivity.

4. Persistence long after neuroleptic withdrawal. Both the behavioral and biochemical manifestations of dopaminergic supersensitivity induced by neuroleptics in animals usually disappear within a few days or weeks of stopping the drugs.

Recently, Clow, Theodorou, Jenner, *et al.* (1980a, 1980b) reported the results of a 12-month study of continuous administration of trifluoperazine and thioridazine to rats. The researchers found that the various behavioral and biochemical changes produced by the 1-year treatment with neuroleptics, including spontaneous mouthing movements, increased response to apomorphine, and increased number of binding sites for striatal dopamine receptors, were reversible and disappeared within weeks of neuroleptic discontinuation. The only biochemical alteration that was still present 6 months after drug withdrawal[2] was an enhanced stimulation of striatal adenylate cyclase by dopamine. Since the significance and the behavioral correlates of this latter phenomenon are not known, its possible relationship with tardive dyskinesia cannot yet be judged.

5. *Response to neuroleptic challenge and withdrawal.* This isomorphism criterion is fully satisfied by the supersensitivity model. Acute administration of a neuroleptic diminishes behavioral response to dopamine agonists, whereas the dopaminergic response is at its maximum several days after neuroleptic discontinuation.

6. *Response to anticholinergic agents.* Different investigators have reported conflicting results with concomitant use of anticholinergic drugs and neuroleptics. Smith and Davis (1975) found that long-term administration of haloperidol and benztropine mesylate to rats produced significantly less response to apomorphine than did administration of haloperidol alone. On the other hand, Borison, Havdala, and Diamond (1979) observed that haloperidol and benztropine in combination induced greater responsiveness to apomorphine in rats as compared to haloperidol alone. Christensen and Nielsen (1979) and Tarsy and Baldessarini (1974) reported that addition of atropine to a neuroleptic regimen did not affect dopaminergic supersensitivity to a noticeable degree. The possible effect of anticholinergic treatment on neuroleptic blood levels was not measured in any of these studies.

SUMMARY

It is thus apparent that the supersensitivity model does not satisfactorily meet several of the isomorphism criteria for tardive dyskinesia. The relevance of the supersensitivity model to tardive dyskinesia is uncertain.

[2]The average life span of a rat is 3 years (compared with 70 years for a human). Hence 1 year of neuroleptic administration followed by drug withdrawal for 6 months in a rat is equivalent to neuroleptic treatment for 23 years followed by withdrawal for 11.5 years in a human.

As suggested by Tarsy and Baldessarini (1977), postsynaptic dopamine receptor supersensitivity may help explain neuroleptic-withdrawal-emergent dyskinesia. It seems that dopaminergic supersensitivity is a normal and universal response to neuroleptic administration. This response is related to the length and amount of prior neuroleptic treatment, but is probably a reversible phenomenon that disappears within a few days or weeks of termination of drug treatment.

Future research should try to explore differences among strains of animals that develop greater supersensitivity and those that develop less supersensitivity. We (Jeste, Stoff, Potkin, *et al.,* 1979) found that the amount of behavioral supersensitivity might be related to the animals' baseline response to amphetamine. Further studies along similar lines, but using inbred strains of animals, may be useful for improving the understanding of pharmacogenetics. Also, the effects of chronic neuroleptic administration on spontaneous locomotion and spontaneous oral stereotypy need careful investigation.

DRUG-INDUCED DYSKINESIAS IN MONKEYS

It is generally expected that monkeys would provide animal models that closely simulate the human syndromes. This is indeed the case with drug-induced dyskinesias. Principally, three types of drugs have been used to produce experimental dyskinesias in monkeys: L-dopa and other catecholaminergic agents, narcotics such as methadone, and neuroleptics such as haloperidol and chlorpromazine. The resultant dyskinesias can be classified into three categories: acute reversible, tardive reversible, and tardive persistent.

L-DOPA AND OTHER CATECHOLAMINERGIC AGENTS

Neurologists have long been interested in L-dopa-induced dyskinesias in monkeys as an animal model of similar dyskinesias produced by L-dopa in patients with Parkinson's disease. Paulson (1973) reported that acute parenteral, but not chronic oral, administration of L-dopa to normal rhesus monkeys resulted in the appearance of dyskinesias. Acute intraperitoneal injection of 2 to 3 g of L-dopa produced severe abnormal movements, whereas oral administration of more than 2 g of L-dopa daily for more than 6 months failed to elicit any movement disorders. Mones (1973) and Sassin,

Taub, and Weitzman (1972) also found that parenteral (intraperitoneal or intravenous) administration of L-dopa or apomorphine led to acute reversible dyskinesias in normal monkeys. In another set of interesting studies, Ng, Gelhard, Chase, et al. (1973) and Sax, Butters, Tomlinson, et al. (1973) observed that lesions of the caudate, either surgical or 6-hydroxy-dopamine-induced, reduced the threshold for dyskinesias in monkeys produced by L-dopa and apomorphine.

Validity

The studies enumerated here parallel two findings in humans—namely, induction of acute, but not chronic, dyskinesias by L-dopa in normal persons and reduced threshold for dyskinesias in patients with nigrostriatal damage. Phenomenologically, too, there are many similarities between human and simian dyskinesias caused by L-dopa. The validity of this animal model for neuroleptic-induced tardive dyskinesias is, however, questionable or untested.

NARCOTICS

Carlson (1980) and Eibergen and Carlson (1976) have conducted a number of experiments on the effects of long-term administration of methadone and morphine in monkeys (as well as in guinea pigs). Although prolonged narcotic treatment per se did not induce dyskinesias, it markedly reduced the threshold for oral dyskinesias elicited by methamphetamine or apomorphine. This phenomenon was observed even after the animals had been withdrawn from the narcotic for as long as 26 months. Methadone induced greater sensitivity to methamphetamine than did morphine; furthermore, methadone was more effective in this respect when given parenterally rather than orally. Stress also lowered the threshold for the effects of methamphetamine following chronic narcotic pretreatment. Acute administration of chlorpromazine, spiroperidol, or clozapine blocked or abolished methamphetamine-induced dyskinesias, whereas phenobarbitone and diazepam had no such effect.

Validity

The main drawback of this animal model for studying tardive dyskinesia is that the narcotic-treated monkeys did not develop dyskinesia unless they were challenged with a drug such as methamphetamine. As pointed out by

Carlson (1980), the main value of this animal model may be suggesting a testable hypothesis that methadone-maintenance patients are at an increased risk of developing oral dyskinesia with catecholaminergic drugs.

NEUROLEPTICS

A number of investigators have succeeded in producing dyskinesias in monkeys by giving prolonged neuroleptic treatment. There have been some differences in the results obtained by different researchers. Yet, dyskinesias in monkeys induced by long-term neuroleptic administration constitute the most satisfactory animal model of tardive dyskinesia that is available today.

Deneau and Crane (1969) reported that several of their 17 rhesus monkeys given chlorpromazine, 30 mg/kg daily, by a nasogastric tube for more than 6 months developed abnormal involuntary movements. These movements were a combination of dyskinesias (especially of the tongue) and dystonias and lasted for less than 24 hours after each dose of the drug.

Paulson (1972) confirmed the findings of Deneau and Crane in rhesus monkeys treated with chlorpromazine for at least 3 months. Interestingly, similar use of haloperidol in ten rhesus monkeys failed to elicit abnormal movements.

Weiss, Santelli, and Lusink (1977) reported, however, that administration of haloperidol, .5 to 1 mg/kg, orally (in a fruit drink) 5 days a week for several months induced severe movement disorders in cebus and squirrel monkeys. The movement disorders consisted of brief and sometimes violent hyperkinetic episodes, bizarre postures, and buccolingual movements. Such reactions occurred 1 to 6 hours after drug intake and usually lasted for only a few minutes. The tendency for an abnormal reaction to a challenging dose of haloperidol was, however, present as long as 508 days after chronic haloperidol administration had been discontinued. Weiss and Santelli (1978) later found that weekly oral doses of haloperidol, .25 to .5 mg/kg, were probably more potent than 5-days-a-week administration of similar amounts in causing the abnormal responsiveness to acute haloperidol intake. The investigators concluded that intermittent administration of haloperidol was effective in inducing movement disorders in nonhuman primates.

Messiha (1980) reported that monkeys that received 10 to 180 mg of chlorpromazine daily for more than 1 year developed buccolingual dyskinesias, whereas those treated with 100 to 120 mg/day for 4 months did not. Biochemical studies showed that the animals with dyskinesia had significantly greater urinary excretion of dopamine and norepinephrine as compared to drug-free controls. In the CSF, too, the dyskinetic monkeys had higher concentrations of the catecholamine metabolites DOPAC and HVA and of the serotonin metabolite 5-HIAA when compared with controls, although the difference missed statistical significance for DOPAC and HVA. Messiha's data support presynaptic, rather than postsynaptic, hyperactivity of catecholamine systems in neuroleptic-induced dyskinesias.

The most convincing demonstration of neuroleptic-induced persistent tardive dyskinesia in monkeys has been reported by Barany, Ingvast, and Gunne (1979) and Gunne and Barany (1979). Four of 11 cebus monkeys who received .05 to 1 mg/kg of haloperidol daily by mouth for 3 to 35 months developed buccolingual and/or choreiform limb and trunkal dyskinesias. The abnormal movements generally became more severe with continued neuroleptic administration. In two monkeys the signs were still present 3 months after haloperidol was discontinued. Interestingly, the dyskinesia in one of these two animals had been reversible after 5 months of haloperidol treatment, but became persistent following a further 12 months of treatment. Acute administration of a neuroleptic suppressed the dyskinesia temporarily, whereas drug withdrawal resulted in a shortlasting aggravation of symptoms. Although "tardive dyskinesia" occurred in only 4 of the 11 monkeys treated with neuroleptics, acute dystonia and parkinsonism were observed in all the animals. Anticholinergics relieved dystonia and parkinsonism. In another experiment Gunne and Barany (1979) used the rebound worsening of preexisting dyskinesia following neuroleptic withdrawal as a test of the liability of a particular neuroleptic to produce tardive dyskinesia. The researchers concluded, from their results, that haloperidol, chlorpromazine, and fluphenazine were much more likely to induce tardive dyskinesia than clozapine and thioridazine.

Validity

The chronic neuroleptic-induced dyskinesias in monkeys, particularly those reported by Gunne and Barany, meet most of the isomorphism criteria for human tardive dyskinesia, including persistence of symptoms months after the drugs have been stopped (Table 9-1). Much more work is necessary, however. Studies of biochemistry and neuropathology in the dyskinetic monkeys versus controls, comparison of various treatment practices for their propensity to produce or prevent tardive dyskinesia, and long-term studies of the effects of different drugs (GABA'ergic agents, norepinephrine antagonists, etc.) on the treatment of dyskinesia would be of considerable theoretical and practical importance. At the same time, drawing conclusions based on acute drug challenge studies should be tempered with caution. For example, there are no hard clinical data to suggest that thioridazine is less likely to cause tardive dyskinesia than chlorpromazine or that deanol is useful in treating tardive dyskinesia, thus questioning the conclusions derived by Gunne and Barany (1979) and Barany and Gunne (1979), respectively, from their work with monkeys.

MISCELLANEOUS ANIMAL MODELS

A number of proposed animal models of tardive dyskinesia are described in this section. They either do not satisfy, or have not been tested for, most of the isomorphism criteria.

NATURALLY OCCURRING DYSKINESIA-LIKE DISORDERS IN ANIMALS

Background

A number of spontaneously occurring (hereditary or acquired) movement disorders have been described in various animal species. Koestner (1973) has presented an excellent review of the literature on this subject. Broadly, the disorders can be classified into three groups:

1. Genetically transmitted conditions—These include the so-called dancing mice (subgrouped as "waltzer," "shaker," "jerker," etc.), dancing rats, dancing guinea pigs, acrobat rabbits, and Scottish terrier dogs with hyperkinetic episodes precipitated by exercise. Of all these animals, the best known is the Japanese dancing mouse, or the "waltzer," described since the year 80 B.C. The animals exhibit stereotyped circling movements, shaking of the head, and deafness. These traits are believed to be transmitted by means of autosomal recessive genes, although gene mutations may also play a role in the production of the abnormal movements. There are some reports of striatal atrophy in the dancing mice.

2. Noninherited delay in myelination—Affected young pigs and lambs have congenital tremors that gradually improve with progressive myelination.

3. Acquired disorders—Ingestion of yellow star thistle, which grows in dry and weedy pastures, has been known to produce acute focal necrosis in the globus pallidus and substantia nigra in horses. Clinically it manifests as difficulty in eating and drinking, continuous chewing movements, tongue protrusion, muscular rigidity, and drowsiness.

A condition that is particularly relevant to a discussion of spontaneous and tardive dyskinesia in humans is the oral stereotypy observed in farm animals, probably as a response to an inadequate environment or boredom (Sharman, 1978). It consists of repetitive chewing or licking movements, sometimes called the "licking disease." It is seen in cows, pigs, sheep, horses, and other farm animals. Metoclopramide has been shown to induce oral stereotypies in pigs, and these have been found to be associated with increased dopamine metabolites, HVA, and DOPAC in the brain. Sharman (1978) has suggested that the oral stereotypies in farm animals result from an increased release of dopamine in specific areas of the brain.

Validity

The movement disorders in animals mentioned here occur spontaneously and are not neuroleptic-induced. Applicability of other isomorphism criteria for tardive dyskinesia has been mostly untested. Phenomenologically, the abnormal movements in rodents and other lower animals are distinct from human tardive dyskinesia. Despite these shortcomings, a study of the naturally occurring movement disorders in animals may be useful for understanding certain genetic, biochemical, and neuropathological aspects of iatrogenic dyskinesias.

ELECTROPHYSIOLOGICAL CHANGES IN BRAIN FOLLOWING CHRONIC NEUROLEPTIC TREATMENT

Background

Glassman (1976) has proposed a systems theory of tardive dyskinesia. According to him, there are three "echelons," or levels, of brain function that are relevant to tardive dyskinesia and schizophrenia: the lowest echelon is the brain stem, the middle one is the basal ganglia, and the highest is the frontal cortex. Whereas schizophrenia results from a disturbance of function of the highest echelon, tardive dyskinesia is caused by neuroleptic-induced disorganization of the middle-echelon function, leading to a release of the lowest echelon from higher control. To test this hypotheesis, Glassman, Glassman, and Frew (1977) have been studying electrophysiological changes in various areas of the brains of cats receiving chronic neuroleptic treatment. Electrodes are implanted at multiple cortical and subcortical loci, and EEG and evoked potentials are recorded over periods of months or years before, during, and after long-term courses of neuroleptic administration. The investigators have observed stereotyped licking and certain other movements associated with neuroleptic use. The electrophysiological findings are not consistent.

Validity

The published data are too scanty to judge the validity of this animal model.

OTHER EFFECTS OF CHRONIC NEUROLEPTIC ADMINISTRATION

In addition to striatal dopamine receptor supersensitivity, a number of other changes result from chronic neuroleptic use in animals. We have already referred to presynaptic biochemical alterations (Engel et al., 1976; Smith & Leelavathi, 1980), spontaneous hyperactivity (Engel et al., 1976), and oral stereotypy (Clow et al., 1980b; Smith & Leelavathi, 1980).

Burki (1979) described a biochemical test for predicting the liability of a drug to produce tardive dyskinesia. Striatal HVA content was measured in rats pretreated for 6 days with the test drug and challenged on the 7th day with 3 mg/kg haloperidol orally. According to Burki, pretreatment with only the "classical neuroleptics" known to induce tardive dyskinesia desensitizes the striatal dopamine system to the effect of acute haloperidol on day 7. Clozapine, amphetamine, atropine, and morphine did not have such desensitizing action. Until considerably more work is done, validity of such a test to predict occurrence of tardive dyskinesia should be taken as unproven.

ACUTE AMPHETAMINE-INDUCED STEREOTYPY

Background

Amphetamine produces stereotyped behavior in a number of animal species. Experimental evidence suggests that this effect of amphetamine is mediated through catecholaminergic mechanisms. Attempts to separate dopaminergic from noradrenergic influences and mesolimbic from striatal sites of action in amphetamine-induced stereotypy and locomotor hyperactivity have not always led to consistent results. Rubovits and Klawans (1972) proposed that stereotypy produced by amphetamine may serve as an animal model of tardive dyskinesia, for the following reasons:

1. Both amphetamine-induced stereotypy and tardive dyskinesia involve abnormal involuntary movements that are repetitive and usually localized in the orofacial region.
2. The same biochemical mechanism (striatal dopaminergic hyperactivity) probably underlies both the phenomena. Decreasing the dopaminergic activity reduces both types of abnormal movements.
3. Anticholinergic drugs reduce the threshold for amphetamine-induced stereotypy and worsen tardive dyskinesia.

Validity

This animal model is based on presumed striatal dopaminergic hyperactivity in tardive dyskinesia. Since this mechanism does not explain all of tardive dyskinesia, or even all of amphetamine-induced stereotypy, the basic assumption is open to question. Of the six isomorphism criteria described earlier, only two are satisfied by this model—namely, temporary suppression by neuroleptics and worsening by anticholinergic agents.

SUPERSENSITIVITY INDUCED BY CHRONIC ADMINISTRATION OF AMPHETAMINE

Background

The effects of chronic amphetamine administration have been of interest both to neurologists (as an animal model for L-dopa-induced dyskinesias) and to psychiatrists (as an animal model for schizophrenia). Klawans and Margolin (1975) reported that long-term treatment of guinea pigs with amphetamine resulted in enhanced responsiveness to amphetamine as well as to apomorphine. Ellison, Eison, Huberman, *et al.* (1978) found that continuous long-term administration of amphetamine, through silicone pellets implanted subcutaneously in rats, had a selective toxic effect on striatal dopamine neurons. Reduced activity of tyrosine hydroxylase was found in the caudate 110 days after the pellet was removed.

Validity

Chronic amphetamine-induced dopaminergic supersensitivity (as well as spontaneous oral stereotypy) is a suitable analogue of dyskinesias induced by catecholamine agonists. Its relationship to neuroleptic-induced tardive dyskinesia is unclear.

6-HYDROXYDOPAMINE-INDUCED DENERVATION SUPERSENSITIVITY

Background

Ungerstedt (1971) demonstrated that stereotaxic injection of 6-hydroxydopamine, a specific toxin against catecholamine neurons, produced degeneration of the nigrostriatal dopamine system. Such denervation was followed, after some days, by an apparent development of receptor supersensitivity. Ungerstedt, Avemo, Avemo, *et al.* (1973) suggested that unilateral 6-hydroxydopamine-induced lesions of the substantia nigra might be used to indicate potential antiparkinsonian activity of drugs. Systemic administration of dopaminergic agents in these animals results in a rotational behavior. Agents such as L-dopa, which have predominantly presynaptic action, produce contralateral circling, whereas those such as apomorphine, which act postsynaptically, cause ipsilateral circling. Since the rotational model is thus helpful for detecting dopaminergic or antiparkinsonian activity of drugs, it may also be expected to indicate dyskinesia-inducing action of the drugs. (Agents that reduce parkinsonian symptoms tend to induce or worsen dyskinesia.)

Validity

This model is more applicable to dyskinesias induced by catecholaminergic drugs, such as L-dopa, in Parkinson's disease rather than to neuroleptic-induced tardive dyskinesias. As noted in Chapter 5, the contribution of denervation supersensitivity to the causation of tardive dyskinesia is uncertain.

OTHER ANIMAL MODELS

Coyle and Schwarcz (1976) proposed kainic-acid-induced striatal lesions as an animal model of Huntington's disease. Stereotaxic injection of small amounts of kainic acid, a structural analogue of glutamate, selectively damages cell bodies in the striatum. This results in an increased effect of amphetamine, but not of apomorphine, in inducing stereotypy.

Robin, Pelfreyman, and Schechter (1979) reported the occurrence of dyskinesia in rats with intrastriatal injections of GABA-transaminase (GABA-T) inhibitors. Such dyskinesia was blocked by injections of GABA and muscimol.

The relevance of these and other similar models to neuroleptic-induced tardive dyskinesia remains to be studied.

SUMMARY

A number of animal models of tardive dyskinesia have been proposed. Two of these deserve serious consideration: neuroleptic-induced striatal postsynaptic dopamine receptor supersensitivity and neuroleptic-induced dyskinesias in monkeys. The supersensitivity model, although cheaper and easier, fails to meet some of the isomorphism criteria satisfactorily. Although neuroleptic treatment has been known to produce receptor supersensitivity, there is as yet no good evidence to show that such supersensitivity is responsible for persistent tardive dyskinesia.

Neuroleptic-induced dyskinesias in monkeys constitute a much better model of human tardive dyskinesia. Further research on this and similar models should seek answers to various unresolved questions regarding tardive dyskinesia: Do specific types of brain damage predispose to persistent dyskinesia? Is liability (biochemical or neuropathologic) to tardive dyskinesia genetically transmitted? Do different neuroleptics differ in their ability to cause dyskinesia? Do certain treatment practices (e.g., short and long drug-free periods) reduce or increase chances of producing persistent dyskinesia? Are treatments with noradrenergic-blocking or GABA'ergic drugs useful in specific biochemical subtypes of dyskinesia?

CHAPTER X

Treatment of Tardive Dyskinesia: Review of the Literature

INTRODUCTION

Lennox (1960) has stated that almost every drug that could pass the pharynx has been tried in the treatment of epilepsy. Although the situation with tardive dyskinesia has not quite reached that extent, the number of pharmacologic and other treatments used in this disorder during the past decade has been large.

Until the end of 1969, the reported treatments for tardive dyskinesia included administration or withdrawal of neuroleptics, use of antiparkinsonian agents, and use of some nondrug treatments, such as dental prosthesis. Of these, only neuroleptic withdrawal was employed to any major extent. Most of the early studies were nonblind. During the last few years, there have been a number of controlled, double-blind studies using a wide range of drugs. Apart from challenging the therapeutic nihilism that had surrounded the concept of irreversible tardive dyskinesia, these studies have also attempted to gain a better understanding of the neurochemistry of the disorder. Unfortunately, however, they have so far failed to unearth "the" treatment for tardive dyskinesia.

It is interesting to note that many investigators tried treatments for dyskinesia based on some rationale about the mechanism of action of those treatments. Although the neuropathology underlying tardive dyskinesia, and the mode of action of the treatments have so far eluded our understanding, the therapeutic maneuvers have had an impact on our knowledge of the syndrome.

The principal treatments for tardive dyskinesia may be considered under these headings:

1. Neuroleptics
   Dopamine blocking—for example, phenothiazines, butyrophenones
   Dopamine depleting—for example, reserpine, tetrabenazine
2. Other dopamine antagonists—for example, methyldopa, AMPT
3. Cholinergic drugs—for example, deanol, choline
4. GABA'ergic drugs—for example, diazepam, sodium valproate
5. Dopaminergic drugs—for example, amantadine, L-dopa
6. Anticholinergic drugs—for example, trihexyphenidyl, biperiden
7. Miscellaneous drugs—for example, lithium, pyridoxine
8. Withdrawal of neuroleptics
9. Nondrug treatments—for example, dental prosthesis, biofeedback

At the current state of knowledge and ignorance about the mechanism of action of different drugs, any classification of treatments for dyskinesia has to be tentative. Furthermore, many drugs have multiple chemical actions, and it may sometimes be difficult to decide which of these actions, if any, is of primary importance in the relief of symptoms. In this chapter, we review in some detail the literature on each of the major modalities tried in patients with tardive dyskinesia. This is followed by a general consideration of the methodological issues involved in the treatment studies and an overview of the relative place of different treatments in the management of tardive dyskinesia. Clinical guidelines for prevention and management of tardive dyskinesia are discussed in the next chapter.

DATA ANALYSIS

We reviewed all studies on the treatment of tardive dyskinesia published through December 1980. These also included individual case reports of treatments that are not commonly employed in clinical practice (e.g., apomorphine or deanol). Wherever feasible, we reanalyzed data in the published studies so as to obtain a rate of improvement based on the number of patients who had 50% or greater reduction in their symptoms. We found that, in a number of instances, the rate of improvement computed in this manner was much smaller than that reported by the investigators who had included patients with minimal or mild improvement in the category of improved patients. We think that an improvement criterion of a minimum 50% reduction in symptoms is warranted for a condition such as tardive dyskinesia in which spontaneous fluctuations in symptom severity are all too frequent. Also, since a large majority of the studies were short-term and nondouble-blind, it was necessary to use a strict criterion of improvement.

We divided the various treatments according to their known principal mechanism of action. Such a classfication of treatments has to be tentative and may need to be modified as more information about the actions of these drugs becomes available. Some studies employed multiple treatment approaches; we considered them under each separate treatment category.

TREATMENT MODALITIES

NEUROLEPTICS

It is paradoxical that neuroleptics could be considered a treatment for tardive dyskinesia, and it is even more intriguing that they are the most effective agents for suppressing the symptoms of dyskinesia. The use of neuroleptics as a treatment for tardive dyskinesia is controversial and poses a challenge to clinicians as much as to researchers.

The first article on the treatment of dyskinesia with a neuroleptic appeared in 1961. Prompted by reports of the use of tetrabenazine, a dopamine-depleting neuroleptic, for the relief of symptoms in Huntington's chorea, Brandrup (1961) tried tetrabenazine in another movement disorder—namely, neuroleptic-induced persistent dyskinesia—and got successful results in all four of his patients. Interestingly, no major studies on the treatment of dyskinesia with neuroleptics were reported throughout the 1960s.[1] The only treatment that was tried in dyskinetic patients on a significant scale during that decade was neuroleptic withdrawal. A progressive increase in the number of patients with persistent dyskinesia, and a failure to find a suitable alternative to neuroleptics in the treatment of schizo-

---

[1]There were two single case reports on the use of perphenazine (Rosin & Exton-Smith, 1965) and haloperidol (Gilbert, 1969). In both nonblind studies, patients improved with the respective neuroleptics.

phrenia, resulted in new studies on the use of neuroleptics in dyskinetic patients during the 1970s. About 40 reports on the treatment of dyskinesia with neuroleptics have been published during the past decade.

Table 10-1 lists studies that used neuroleptics to treat tardive dyskinesia. Case reports on treatment of individual patients with commonly prescribed neuroleptics such as chlorpromazine, thioridazine, or haloperidol have been excluded for practical reasons. Also excluded are reports of single parenteral administration of neuroleptics for dyskinesia (e.g., Bateman, Dutta, McClelland, et al., 1979). Of the 50 studies summarized in Table 10-1, 40 gave results in terms of the numbers of patients improved and not improved. Of the total 325 patients treated with neuroleptics, 67.4% had significant improvement in their dyskinesia. Neuroleptics as a group proved to be more effective than any other major treatment for suppressing the symptoms of tardive dyskinesia. We now discuss various aspects of the use of neuroleptics in patients with dyskinesia.

Differential Efficacy of Specific Neuroleptics

Some investigators have reported specific antidyskinetic action for individual neuroleptics. Duvoisin (1972) suggested that reserpine was unique in that it was the only effective neuroleptic that was not also a cause of persistent dyskinesia. He proposed that a difference between the mechanism of action of reserpine (which depletes intraneuronal catecholamines) and that of other neuroleptics (most of which block the effect of dopamine on postsynaptic receptors) may be primarily responsible for the uniqueness of reserpine.

In a crossover trial of three neuroleptics, Gerlach and Simmelsgaard (1978) found that haloperidol had significantly greater antidyskinetic effects than thioridazine and clozapine. The investigators suggested that the antidyskinetic actions of these neuroleptics were related to their antidopaminergic properties.

Clozapine has often been touted as a "revolutionary" neuroleptic in that it (presumably) does not owe its antipsychotic action to dopamine blockade or dopamine depletion (Matz, Rick, Oh, et al., 1974). On the basis of experiments with rats, Sayers, Burki, Ruch, et al. (1975) concluded that clozapine was uniquely different from "classical" neuroleptics such as chlorpromazine and haloperidol. Biochemically, long-term treatment with other neuroleptics produced tolerance to the increase in striatal HVA, whereas clozapine failed to affect the HVA content. Sayers et al.

Table 10-1. Treatment with Neuroleptics

Investigators	Study design	Dose (mg/24 h)	Length of treatment	Improved	Not improved	Total
				Number of patients		
Haloperidol						
Kazamatsuri, Chien, and Cole (1972b)	Double-blind	2-16	4 weeks	7	2	9
Kazamatsuri, Chien, and Cole (1973)	Double-blind	8-16	18 weeks	2	3	5
Gerlach, Thorsen, and Fog (1975)	Double-blind	9	3 weeks	5	0	5
Frangos and Christodoulides (1975)	Single-blind	8-15	15 weeks	7	3	10
Gerlach and Simmelsgaard (1978)	Probably double-blind	1.5-6 (average 5.25)	8 weeks	NS[a]	NS	16
Nair, Yassa, Ruiz-navarro, et al. (1978)	Double-blind	5	3 weeks	NS	NS	10
Jus, Jus, and Fontaine (1979)	Open	.5-2	3 years	24	4	28
TOTAL				45 (79%)	12	57 +26[b]
Thiopropazate						
Roxburgh (1970)	Double-blind	36-60	3 weeks	2	0	2
Carruthers (1971)	Open	36-60	NS	1	0	1
Singer and Cheng (1971)	Double-blind	45	3 weeks	18	5	23
Kazamatsuri, Chien, and Cole (1972b)	Single-blind	10-80	4 weeks	4	5	9
Bullock (1972)	Open	30	1-2 weeks	4	0	4

(continued)

Table 10-1. (continued)

Investigators	Study design	Dose (mg/24 h)	Length of treatment	Number of patients		
				Improved	Not improved	Total
Thiopropazate (continued)						
Curran (1973)	Open	Up to 45	Several months	2	0	2
Lal and Ettigi (1974)	Double-blind	30	2 weeks	5	4	9
DeSilva and Huang (1975)	Open	NS	18 months	0	1	1
Ananth, Ban, and Lehmann (1977)	Single-blind	20–40	4 weeks	1	9	10
Smith and Kiloh (1979)	Blind ratings	Up to 30	6 months	7	3	10
TOTAL				44 (62%)	27	71
Tetrabenazine						
Brandrup (1961)	Open	75–300	6–15 weeks	4	0	4
MacCallum (1970)	Open	150–200	Many months	2	0	2
Godwin-Austen and Clark (1971)	Double-blind	50–100	1 week	4	2	6
Kazamatsuri, Chien, and Cole (1972a)	Probably double-blind	50–150	6 weeks	14	6	20
Kazamatsuri, Chien, and Cole (1973)	Probably double-blind	100–200	18 weeks	2	4	6
TOTAL				26 (68.4%)	12	38

	Reserpine					
Villeneuve and Boszormenyi (1970)	Open	1	4–8 weeks	12	20	32
Sato, Daly, and Peters (1971)	Open	.25–4	NS	5	0	5
Duvoisin (1972)	Open	NS	NS	"Several"	0	"Several"
Crane (1973d)	Open	Up to 4	4 weeks	3	3	6
Fahn (1978)	Open	Up to 6 (with AMPT)	NS	7	0	7
Jus, Jus, and Fontaine (1979)	Open (multiple treatments simultaneously)	.25–1	3 years	28	8	36
Huang, Wang, Hasegawa, et al. (1980)	Double-blind	.75–1.5	2 weeks	NS	NS	10
TOTAL				55 (64%)	31	86 (+ an unspecified number)[b]
	Other neuroleptics					
Rosin and Exton-Smith (1965)	Open	*Perphenzaine* NS	1 week	1	0	1
Singer and Cheng (1971)	Open	24	3 weeks	14	0	14
Simpson and Varga (1974)	Probably single-blind	*Clozapine* 500–800	12 weeks	2	0	2
Gerlach, Thorsen, and Fog (1975)	Double-blind	225	3 weeks	0	6	6
Carroll, Curtis, and Kokmen (1977)	Open	Up to 1000	18 days	0	1	1
Simpson, Lee, and Shrivastava (1978)	Open	20–900	18 weeks	NS	NS	12

(continued)

Table 10-1. (continued)

Investigators	Study design	Dose (mg/24 h)	Length of treatment	Number of patients		
				Improved	Not improved	Total
Other neuroleptics (continued)						
Clozapine (continued)						
Gerlach and Simmelsgaard (1978)	Probably double-blind	37.5–225 (average 62.5)	4 weeks	1	6	7
Caine, Polinsky, Kartzinel, et al. (1979)	Double-blind	Up to 425 mg	4–7 weeks	0	2	2
Cole, Gardos, Tarsy, et al. (1980)	Open	50–500	Weeks to months	9	18	27
Gerbino, Shopsin, and Collora (1980)	Open	15–1200 (average 650)	Weeks to months	23	0	23
Trifluoperazine						
Lal and Ettigi (1974)	Double-blind	15	2 weeks	6	3	9
Pimozide						
Calne, Claveria, Teychenne, et al. (1974)	Double-blind	NS	6 weeks	NS	NS	20
Claveria, Teychenne, Calne, et al. (1975)	Double-blind	6–28 (average 18.8)	6 weeks	14	4	18
Gibson (1978a)	Open	NS	3 years	NS	NS	NS

	Design	Drug/Dose	Duration			
Gibson (1978a)	Open	*Depot fluspirilene* NS	3 years	NS	NS	NS
Doongaji (1977)	Open	*Penfluperidol* 20–120 mg/wk	Several months	1	0	1
Gerlach and Simmelsgaard (1978)	Probably double-blind	*Thioridazine* 75–300 (average 267.5)	3 months	NS	NS	16
Bucci (1971)	Open (with MAO inhibitor)	*Chlorpromazine* 300	10 months	8	2	10
Jeste, Olgiati, and Ghali (1977)	Blind ratings (q.i.d. vs. o.d. administration)	100–200	2 weeks each	2 (with q.i.d.)	0	2
Turek, Kurland, Hanlon, et al. (1977)	Double-blind	*Various neuroleptics* Individualized	12–40 weeks	NS	NS	48
TOTAL — other neuroleptics				49 (67.1%)	24	73 +96[b]

[a] NS = not stated.

[b] For these patients the numbers improved and not improved were not known.

predicted that tardive dyskinesia was unlikely to develop after clozapine and that clozapine might abolish tardive dyskinesia induced by other neuroleptics.

Based on a model of neuroleptic antagonism of dopamine-induced dyskinesias in guinea pigs, Costall and Naylor (1975) reported that pimozide and oxiperomide possessed specific antidyskinetic properties not shared by other neuroleptics such as thioridazine, haloperidol, fluphenazine, clozapine, tetrabenazine, and others.

An overview of the studies listed in Table 10-2 does not support significant superiority of any of the commonly used neuroleptics over others in the treatment of tardive dyskinesia. The proportion of patients improved with such neuroleptics ranges from 62% (thiopropazate) to 79% (haloperidol); the figures for tetrabenazine and reserpine are 68% and 64%, respectively. The total number of patients treated with other neuroleptics has been too small to justify separate statistical analyses; combining results for these "other" neuroleptics yields an improvement rate of 84%. It is worth noting that clozapine was the least effective of the neuroleptics tried for suppressing tardive dyskinesia. Doepp and Buddeberg (1975) noted that in certain cases clozapine even aggravated preexisting tardive dyskinesia. Also, at least two animal studies found that long-term treatment with clozapine was followed by behavioral evidence of striatal dopaminergic supersensitivity (Smith & Davis, 1976; Gianutsos & Moore, 1977). Suspected hematological side effects such as granulocytopenia and agranulocytosis further reduce the clinical value of clozapine. In short, clozapine has not fullfilled the initial hopes of being not only different from other neuroleptics, but also safe and potent, at least with regard to tardive dyskinesia.

There is thus no strong clinical evidence that any of the common neuroleptics possesses significantly greater antidyskinetic efficacy than others. It is much more likely that specific neuroleptics may have differential effects in individual patients because of differences in drug metabolism rather than because of any specific pharmacologic actions of the neuroleptics (Hollister, 1979). This would be consistent with a report of Gardos (1974) that, for individual schizophrenic patients, antipsychotic drugs were not interchangeable. For certain patients, specific enuroleptics may be most effective (Gerlach & Simmelsgaard, 1978); for large groups of patients, however, no overall superiority of one or more neuroleptics over others has been demonstrated.

Table 10-2. Summary of Studies with Neuroleptics

Neuroleptic	Number of studies	Daily dose (mean ± SD) mg	mg CPZ eq[a]	Number of patients Total	Percentage improved
Haloperidol	7	7.6 ± 3.9	317 ± 163	83	79
Thiopropazate	10	35.9 ± 10.5	150 ± 44	71	62
Tetrabenazine	5	138 ± 48	344 ± 121	38	68
Reserpine	7	1.6 ± 0.9	160 ± 90	96	64
Clozapine	8	394 ± 230	499 ± 291	75	51
Other	13	—	356 ± 167	138	84
TOTAL[b]	50	—	304 ± 132	501	67

[a]Neuroleptic doses were converted to chlorpromazine equivalents according to conversion table given in Chapter 1 (Table 1-1).
[b]Includes some repeats with different neuroleptics.

Do the Neuroleptics Have a Specific Antidyskinetic Action?

This question can be answered on the basis of three criteria:

1. Comparable efficacy of drugs with a similar mechanism of action. As noted previously, there are no significant differences among the common neuroleptics in their ability to suppress tardive dyskinesia.
2. Superiority over placebo in double-blind studies. There are 19 double-blind studies on the treatment of tardive dyskinesia with neuroleptics. Most of them show that neuroleptics are significantly better than placebo. The overall rate of improvement with neuroleptics in double-blind studies is 63%; this is not significantly different from the 69% rate of improvement in open and single-blind studies (Table 10-10).
3. Relative independence of the antidyskinetic effect from nonspecific actions such as sedation. Although different neuroleptics vary in their sedative properties, they do not differ significantly in their antidyskinetic efficacy. A number of studies have found that neuroleptics administered in doses that did not cause sedation produced significant improvement in dyskinesia (e.g., Gerlach & Simmelsgaard, 1978). Notwithstanding some case reports to the contrary, the presence and severity of tardive dyskinesia do not seem

to be related to the presence and severity of parkinsonism or of schizophrenic symptoms (see Chapter 4). This suggests that the dyskinesia-suppressing action of neuroleptics may be independent of acute extrapyramidal as well as antipsychotic effects of these drugs.

All these considerations permit one to conclude that neuroleptics probably have a specific dyskinesia-suppressing effect.

Studies on Long-Term Use of Neuroleptics in Tardive Dyskinesia

Such studies are important for understanding both beneficial and harmful effects of long-term administration of neuroleptics in patients with tardive dyskinesia. There are no standard definitions of "long-term" and "short-term" studies. We defined long-term studies as those in which neuroleptics were administered for more than 8 weeks; the remaining studies were classified as short-term ones. Excluding the 16 studies in which either the length of treatment was not mentioned or the results were not given in terms of numbers of patients improved or unimproved, we found 13 long-term studies and 21 short-term ones. Of the 117 patients who were given neuroleptics for more than 8 weeks, 77% improved; of the 95 patients treated for shorter periods, 61% improved. Thus it appears that the overall antidyskinetic efficacy of neuroleptics does not decrease with continued administration. Although Kazamatsuri *et al.* (1972a) and Gibson (1978a) reported that some of their patients seemed to develop tolerance to the antidyskinetic effects of neuroleptics, most other investigators did not notice significant tolerance.

The improvement in dyskinesia produced by neuroleptics is essentially symptomatic. Therefore, discontinuing their use, even after prolonged administration, has usually resulted in at least a temporary recurrence of dyskinetic symptoms. (An exception to this is the study by Jus, Jus, & Fontaine, 1979, discussed later in this section, which employed a "desensitization" technique.) The symptoms are characteristically more severe for 1 or 2 weeks following neuroleptic withdrawal, but then tend to stabilize at their pretreatment intensity.

Other Aspects of the Use of Neuroleptics in Tardive Dyskinesia

Administration Schedule. Jeste *et al.* (1977) found that dividing the total daily dose of a neuroleptic into four equal doses (four-times-a-day administration) was significantly more effective in suppressing dyskinesia than once-a-day administration of the total dose. Our subsequent experience has confirmed this observation in some patients. Maintaining a fairly stable concentration of neuroleptics in serum (and probably brain) over a 24-hour period (by giving multiple daily doses; Itoh, Yagi, Ohtusuka, *et al.*, 1980) might be presumed to result in a fairly steady blockade of dopamine receptors and therefore a constant suppression or masking of dyskinetic symptoms.

Dosage. The daily dose of the neuroleptics used has varied among different studies. Table 10-2 shows that the mean doses of neuroleptics employed in the treatment of tardive dyskinesia have been relatively low. Doses used in studies of treatment for chronic schizophrenia have been more than twice as high (Wyatt, 1976) as those used for the control of tardive dyskinesia (304 ± 132 mg chlorpromazine equivalents). It is fair to assume that, in the studies enumerated in Table 10-2, psychotic symptoms were also controlled in schizophrenic patients. This raises the possibility that at least some patients with tardive dyskinesia may be hyperresponsive to neuroleptics. Such a possibility is also consistent with our finding of significantly higher serum neuroleptic levels in elderly schizophrenic patients with tardive dyskinesia as compared with matched controls (see Chapter 5).

Combined Use with Other Drugs. Nair, Yassa, Ruiz-navarro, *et al.* (1978) found that combined use of sodium valproate and haloperidol controlled symptoms of dyskinesia, whereas neither drug administered alone was so effective. The authors speculated that simultaneous inhibition of dopaminergic activity (by haloperidol) and increase in GABA'ergic activity (by sodium valproate) in the substantia nigra might be necessary to produce remission of dyskinetic symptoms. Linnoila and Viukari (1979) observed, however, that combined administration of sodium valproate and a "low-potency" neuroleptic (e.g., chlorpromazine) was more effective than simultaneous use of sodium valproate and a "high-potency" neuroleptic. Fahn (1978) reported success with combined reserpine and AMPT treatment. All of these studies need replication.

"Desensitization" Technique

Because some investigators believe that tardive dyskinesia results from a supersensitivity of dopamine receptors, Jus *et al.* (1979) postulated that a desensitization of those receptors by continued use of neuroleptics might provide a basis for definitive treatment of the disorder. They conducted a 4-year trial in which neuroleptics and antiparkinsonian agents were slowly, but progressively, reduced, and reserpine or haloperidol or both were administered in small, slowly increasing and then decreasing doses. Of the 62 patients treated, 49 improved significantly. In 26 patients the improvement persisted after reserpine and haloperidol were withdrawn until the end of the study (about a year later). Eighteen patients had a recurrence of dyskinetic symptoms following withdrawal of reserpine and haloperidol; reinstitution of those drugs in the same small doses produced improvement again.

The overall results of this study are encouraging. An alternative explanation for the results could be that the patients who improved had reversible dyskinesia and that those who did not improve had persistent dyskinesia. Nevertheless, the treatment approach proposed by Jus *et al.* (1979) warrants careful consideration by other investigators and physicians, especially since it is likely to be clinically feasible.

Summary

Neuroleptics have been shown to produce significant improvement (symptom suppression) in about two-thirds of patients with tardive dyskinesia. Neuroleptics seem to possess a specific antidyskinetic action. Usual neuroleptics in equivalent doses have comparable dyskinesia-suppressing effects. The improvement caused by neuroleptics is symptomatic, and eventual withdrawal of the drugs usually results in at least a temporary recurrence of dyskinesia. Administration of neuroleptics in divided daily doses may be preferable to single-daily-dose administration for masking dyskinetic symptoms. Slow, but progressive, reduction in neuroleptic doses over many months to several years may be a treatment method deserving careful consideration, at least for those patients who need neuroleptics for the control of their psychotic symptoms.

OTHER DOPAMINE ANTAGONISTS

Use of nonneuroleptic dopamine antagonists in the treatment of tardive dyskinesia is of clinical as well as theoretical interest.

Oxypertine

This dopamine-depleting agent was first tried successfully in three patients by Eckman in 1968. In a later double-blind study, Chien, Jung, and Ross-Townsend (1978) found significant improvement in two of their five patients. These investigators reported that oxypertine was superior to sodium valproate and deanol. Freeman and Soni (1980) also observed significant improvement with oxypertine in some dyskinetic patients.

Methyldopa

Methyl-3, 4-dihydroxyphenylalanine, or methyldopa, is a commonly prescribed antihypertensive drug. There are two suggested mechanisms for its antidopamine action: It competitively inhibits dopa decarboxylase and thus prevents conversion of dopa to dopamine, and it may be decarboxylated into methyldopamine and α-methylnorepinephrine, which may then act as false neurotransmitters. Villeneuve and Boszormenyi (1970) and Viukari and Linnoila (1975) obtained encouraging results with methyldopa, whereas Kazamatsuri, Chien, and Cole (1972c) noticed no significant effect of the drug on symptoms of tardive dyskinesia. The latter investigators also reported exacerbation of psychosis in two patients.

α-Methyl-p-tyrosine (AMPT)

This drug inhibits tyrosine hydroxylase, the rate-limiting enzyme in the synthesis of dopamine. Two studies found that AMPT, given alone (Gerlach, Reisby, & Randrup, 1974; Gerlach, 1977) or in combination with reserpine (Fahn, 1978) was useful in reducing dyskinetic symptoms.

Papaverine

This is a smooth-muscle relaxant frequently used in the treatment of conditions associated with vascular or visceral spasm. Prompted by reports of dopamine antagonist actions of papaverine in animal and clinical studies, Gardos and Cole (1975), Gardos, Cole, and Sniffin (1976), and Cole, Gardos, Tarsy, *et al.* (1980) tried papaverine in patients with tardive dyskinesia and obtained modest improvement in some cases.

Apomorphine

Apomorphine is presumed to have a dose-related, dual effect on dopaminergic neurons. In large doses it acts as a direct, but partial, postsynaptic dopamine receptor agonist. In smaller doses it is believed to stimulate presynaptic dopaminergic autoreceptors, which are inhibitory in nature; it may thus have an antidopaminergic action. In a study of guinea pigs, Costall and Naylor (1975) observed that apomorphine reduced the intensity of dyskinesias induced by local, intracranial injections of dopamine, but that the dosage of apomorphine was critical. Intermediate doses of apomorphine had antidyskinetic effects, whereas lower and higher doses were ineffective. In an experiment on another animal model of tardive dyskinesia, Christensen and Nielsen (1979) noted that apomorphine administration (5 mg/kg) reversed neuroleptic-induced dopaminergic supersensitivity in mice. Clinical studies on the treatment of tardive dyskinesia with apomorphine have yielded variable results. Whereas Crayton et al. (1977b), Cole, Gardos, Tarsy, et al. (1980) Ettigi et al. (1976), and Meltzer et al. (1976) reported no marked effect, Carroll et al. (1977) and Tolosa (1978a) noted significant improvement in dyskinesia following subcutaneous injections of apomorphine. The patient of Carroll et al., however, seemed to develop tolerance to apomorphine after 1 week of treatment. In a double-blind study, we found no significant change in tardive dyskinesia in three patients treated with small doses (.2 ± .4 mg) of apomorphine (Jeste, Zalcman, Weinberger, et al., 1981).

Droperidol

Casey (1976) and Casey and Denney (1977) used droperidol, a parenterally administered, short acting, and highly sedative dopamine antagonist, and obtained transient improvement in dyskinesia in two of their six patients.

Bromocriptine

Bromocriptine, an ergot derivative, is generally considered to be a partial dopamine agonist and to have a biphasic effect that depends on the dose. Bromocriptine may thus be similar to apomorphine. Pöldinger (1978) gave bromocriptine to three patients with neuroleptic-induced oropharyngoglossal dyskinesia who had not responded to amantadine. Two of these patients had moderate to good improvement with bromocriptine. Tamminga and Chase (1980), however, found no significant effects of low doses (up to 10 mg daily) of bromocriptine on tardive dyskinesia.

CF 25-397

This ergot derivative is a partial dopamine receptor agonist believed to have more specific effects on D_1 receptor and thus different from bromocriptine, which supposedly has selective effects on D_2 receptor. It is possible, but unproven, that CF 25-397, too, acts as a dopamine antagonist when administered in small doses. Used in doses varying from 10 to 60 mg daily, two studies found no marked improvement in tardive dyskinesia with CF 25-397 (Frattola, Albizzati, Bassi, *et al.*, 1980; Tamminga & Chase, 1980).

Substituted Benzamides

Tiapride, sulpiride, and oxiperomide are substituted benzamides. They are presumed to be specific D_2 receptor blockers without noticeable antipsychotic activity. Lutrand and Duncamin (1978) reported success with tiapride in some patients with tardive dyskinesia and certain other movement disorders. The authors also noted that the drug had anxiolytic and antidepressant properties. Casey, Gerlach, and Simmelsgaard (1979) and Casey and Gerlach (1980) found significant improvement in tardive dyskinesia with sulpiride and oxiperomide.

Metoclopramide

This drug is also thought to be a selective D_2 receptor blocker without clinically apparent antipsychotic action. (A recent study by Stanley, Lautin, Rotrosen, *et al.*, 1980, however, reported that metoclopramide, administered in doses indicated by its *in vivo* effect on dopamine turnover, was an effective antipsychotic.) Bateman *et al.* (1979) found that single intravenous injections of metoclopramide suppressed dyskinesia, but the investigators felt that the drug had to be given in such high doses (40 mg) that adverse reactions might neutralize its value as a treatment for tardive dyskinesia.

Table 10-3 summarizes studies on the treatment of tardive dyskinesia with nonneuroleptic dopamine antagonists. The overall weighted mean improvement rate was 46%. Most of the trials were short-term ones. The possibility that some of these drugs might be acting as nonspecific sedatives (e.g., apomorphine, droperidol) remains to be excluded.

Summary

Nonneuroleptic dopamine antagonists have been found to be useful in about one-half of patients with tardive dyskinesia treated for a few days to a few weeks. There is, however, no evidence that these drugs act specifically on dyskinesia, or that they are beneficial over long periods of time.

CHOLINERGIC DRUGS

Deanol, physostigmine, choline, and lecithin have been tried in the treatment of tardive dyskinesia.

Deanol

Deanol (2-dimethylaminoethanol) was probably the single most extensively tried drug in the treatment of tardive dyskinesia during the 1970s. More than 40 reports on the use of deanol in tardive dyskinesia were published between 1974 and 1980. Yet, the value of deanol in treating this condition continues to be uncertain.

History. In 1946, Du Vigneaud, Chandler, Simmonds, *et al.* reported dimethylaminoethanol (DMAE) to be a precursor of choline in rat tissues. Following a 3-week administration of deuterium-labeled DMAE, they demonstrated the presence of deuteriated choline in rat liver. Pfeiffer, Jenney, Gallagher, *et al.* (1957) were the first to suggest that DMAE was a precursor of acetylcholine. Studies using ^{14}C-labeled deanol indicated that deanol crossed the blood–brain barrier and probably was converted intracellularly to acetylcholine (Groth, Bain, & Pfeiffer, 1958). In open clinical studies, Pfeiffer, Broth, and Bain (1959) found deanol to exert stimulant and antidepressant effects. Subsequent studies suggested some similarities between the clinical actions of amphetamine and those of deanol. Deanol was, however, noted to be devoid of several major side ef-

Table 10-3. Treatment with Other Dopamine Antagonists

Investigators	Study design	Dose (mg/24 h)	Length of treatment	Number of patients		
				Improved	Not improved	Total
		Oxypertine				
Eckman (1968)	Open	120–180	NS[a]	3	0	3
Chien, Jung, and Ross-Townsend (1978)	Double-blind	120–160	3 weeks	2	3	5
Freeman and Soni (1980)	Double-blind	NS	4 weeks	NS	NS	10
Kazamatsuri (1980) and four other studies (cited by Freeman & Soni, 1980)	Open	NS	NS	29	21	50
		α-Methyldopa				
Villeneuve and Boszormenyi (1970)	Open	750	4–8 weeks	2	1	3
Kazamatsuri, Chien, and Cole (1972c)	Open	250–1000	6 weeks	NS	NS	9
Viukari and Linnoila (1975)	Double-blind	750	2 weeks	8	7	15
Huang, Wang, Hasegawa, et al. (1980)	Double-blind	750–1500	2 weeks	NS	NS	10
		AMPT				
Gerlach, Reisby, and Randrup (1974)	Blind ratings	3000	3 days	8	0	8
Gerlach and Thorsen (1976); Gerlach (1977)	Double-blind	1400	3 days	10	14	24
Fahn (1978)	Open	Up to 1500 (with reserpine)	NS	7	Probably 0	7

(continued)

Table 10-3. (continued)

Investigators	Study design	Dose (mg/24 h)	Length of treatment	Number of patients		
				Improved	Not improved	Total
Papaverine						
Gardos and Cole (1975)	Open	300–600	3 weeks	2	1	3
Gardos, Cole, and Sniffin (1976)	Blind ratings	600	3–6 weeks	2	7	9
Cole, Gardos, Tarsy, et al. (1980)	Blind ratings	300–600	6 weeks	6	35	41
Apomorphine (s.c.)						
Ettigi, Nair, Cerbantes, et al. (1976)	Open	.75	1–3 times	0	4	4
Meltzer, Goode, Fang, et al. (1976)	Open	.75–1.5	Twice	0	2	2
Carroll, Curtis, and Kokmen (1977)	Open	2.6 mg every 2–6 h	2–4 weeks	1	0	1
Crayton, Smith, Klass, et al. (1977)	Open	4 mg (i.v.)	Once	0	1	1
Tolosa (1978a)	Double-blind	.1–1.5	NS	5	0	5
Smith, Oswald, Kucharski, et al. (1978)	Double-blind	.75–6	Several days	NS	NS	8
Cole, Gardos, Tarsy, et al. (1980)	Open	Probably 1–1.5 (with L-dopa)	NS	1	6	7
Jeste, Zalcman, Weinberger, et al. (1981)	Double-blind	.2–.4	Once	0	3	3
Droperidol						
Casey and Denney (1977); also, Casey (1976)	Single-blind	2.5 (i.v.)	Given once	2	4	6

	Bromocriptine					
Pöldinger (1978)	Open	15	Several weeks	2	1	3
Ringwald (1978)	Single-blind	32	2 months	NS	NS	16
Tamminga and Chase (1980)	Double-blind	10	3 weeks	0	7	7
	Metoclopramide (i.v.)					
Bateman, Dutta, McClelland, et al. (1979)	Double-blind	10	Once	3	5	8
		40	Once	8	0	8
	Tiapride					
Lutrand and Duncamin (1978)	Open	400–800	15–90 days	6	8	14
	Sulpiride					
Casey, Gerlach, and Simmelsgaard (1979)	Double-blind	400–1200 (mean 847)	6 weeks	10	1	11
	Oxiperomide					
Casey and Gerlach (1980)	Double-blind	10–24	6 weeks	6	4	10
	CF 25-397					
Frattola, Albizzati, Bassi, et al. (1980)	Probably double-blind	10–20	NS	0	4	4
Tamminga and Chase (1980)	Double-blind	60	3 weeks	2	6	8

[a]NS = not stated.

fects associated with amphetamine, such as anorexia, anxiety, and rise in blood pressure. In view of its low toxicity, deanol was tried and found to be useful in the treatment of some cases of hyperkinetic behavior problems and learning disorders in children. Miller (1974a, 1974b) was the first to report successful use of deanol in L-dopa-induced dyskinesia and neuroleptic-induced tardive dyskinesia.

Mechanism of Action. The modes of action of deanol in various clinical conditions are still largely speculative. Deanol is usually classified as a cholinergic drug. Yet, the animal studies have provided conflicting answers to the question of whether deanol is a precursor of acetylcholine. For example, Haubrich, Wang, Clody, *et al.* (1975) found increased levels of striatal choline and acetylcholine following deanol administration in rats, whereas Zahniser, Chou, and Hanin (1977) found no such change in brain acetylcholine with deanol. Summing up the various animal studies, Goldberg (1977) concluded that pathways for synthesis of acetylcholine from deanol did exist, but that the significance and magnitude of these potential routes were unclear. He suggested three possible metabolic pathways for the conversion of deanol to acetylcholine:

(1) Deanol + Methyl group → Choline
     Choline + Acetyl coenzyme A → Acetylcholine
(2) Deanol + Acetyl coenzyme A → Acetyl deanol
     Acetyl deanol + Methyl group → Acetylcholine
(3) Deanol + Phosphate group → Deanol phosphate
     Deanol phosphate + Methyl group → Choline phospate
     Choline phosphate → Choline + Phosphate
     Choline + Acetyl coenzyme A → Acetylcholine

In an interesting experiment employing simultaneous intracarotid administration of ^{14}C-labeled choline and deanol in rats, Millington, McCall, and Wurtman (1978) found opposite effects of deanol on blood and brain concentrations of choline. Although deanol increased blood choline concentrations, it suppressed the brain uptake of choline by competitive inhibition. It is possible that such discrepant actions of deanol on blood and brain concentrations of choline might be partly responsible for the differences in clinical effects of deanol seen in different patients.

It should be added that most of the animal studies on the mode of action of deanol have been acute or short-term studies and may therefore have limited application to the clinical use of deanol. Clinical data on cholinergic actions of deanol have been variable and inconsistent. Stafford and Fann (1977) found no increase in plasma choline levels in nine patients with tardive dyskinesia following a daily administration of 1200 mg deanol for 2 weeks. Whereas Casey and Denney (1977) noted a positive correlation between reponses to deanol and physostigmine, Davis, Berger, and Hollister (1975) and Lindeboom and Lakke (1978) failed to find such a correlation. Nesse and Carroll (1976) reported cholinergic side effects—namely, rhinorrhea, sialorrhea, tachycardia, tachypnea, and diffuse rhonchi—in one patient given deanol. These symptoms disappeared 2 days after stopping the drug. Such cholinergic reactions are, however, uncommon during deanol therapy. De Montigny, Chouinard, and Annable (1979) observed worsening of schizaphrenic symptoms with deanol. Casey (1979) noted mood alterations in 8 of the 38 patients taking high doses of deanol. Five patients became depressed, and three became hypomanic, making any simple interpretation of the biochemical effects of deanol rather difficult. It is possible that deanol affects catecholamine systems, too, directly or indirectly. The nature of these actions remains to be determined.

Effects of Deanol on Animal Models of Tardive Dyskinesia. Christensen and Nielsen (1979) studied the effects of a number of drugs on the supersensitivity (to apomorphine-induced gnawing in mice) caused by pretreatment with teflutixol. Cholinergic treatment did not modify the enhanced receptor response. In the supersensitivity phase deanol had no effect on the supersensitivity. Similarly, Davis, Hollister, Vento, *et al.* (1979) found that deanol did not reduce apomorphine-induced stereotypy in rats pretreated with haloperidol. They suggested that choline might be more effective than deanol in augmenting striatal cholinergic activity. Thus the available data do not indicate any effect of deanol on at least one animal model of tardive dyskinesia.

Deanol in the Treatment of Various Movement Disorders. It may be instructive to review briefly the clinical trials of deanol in movement disorders, such as chorea in Huntington's disease and L-dopa-induced dyskinesias, which are presumed to have some neurochemical similarities with neuroleptic-induced tardive dyskinesia. Until 1972, deanol was used mainly in children with learning disorders and hyperkinetic behavior problems. In 1972, Klawans and Rubovits reported that physostigmine was effective in reducing symptoms of Huntingtons's chorea in some patients, whereas anticholinergic drugs worsened the symptoms. The investigators suggested a central cholinergic–anticholinergic imbalance in this disorder. Later, Walker, Hoehn, Sears, *et al.* (1973) found that deanol was beneficial in five of seven patients with Huntington's chorea. Amsterdam and Dubin (1978) also reported successful use of deanol in one case of Huntington's chorea. Two other studies (Laterre & Fortemps, 1975; Reibling, Reyes, & Jameson, 1975), however, showed that deanol was of no benefit in this disorder.

Miller (1974a) first reported successful results with deanol in the treatment of 9 of 11 patients with L-dopa-induced dyskinesias. Her trial was prompted by Birkmayer and Neumayer's (1972) suggestion that stimulation of the cholinergic system may alleviate dyskinesia induced by L-dopa and by a report by Tarsy, Leopold, and Sax (1973) that physostigmine improved such dyskinesias. Birkmayer (cited by Re, 1975; and Casey, 1977) found that 79% of patients treated with deanol had good improvement in their dyskinesias. Studies by Laterre and Fortemps (1975) and Klawans, Topel, and Bergen (1975), however, failed to find significant efficacy of deanol in L-dopa-induced dyskinesia. In a carefully designed double-blind, crossover study, Lindeboom and Lakke (1978) noted that deanol produced improvement in symptoms in 50% of cases of L-dopa-induced dyskinesias, but that placebo was also effective in 50% of cases. The authors attributed the improvement with deanol to a placebo effect.

Deanol has also been tried in several other movement disorders and has usually been found to be ineffective. Although Miller (1973) reported deanol to be useful in two patients with blepharospasm, Dahadelah, Small, and Thomas (1975) showed, in a double-blind trial, that the drug was of little value in the treatment of blepharospasm and hemifacial spasms. Similar negative results with deanol were reported in congenital athetosis and torticollis (Laterre & Fortemps, 1975) and in Gilles de la Tourette's syndrome (Sweet, Bruun, Shapiro, *et al.*, 1976).

One may conclude from all these studies that the value of deanol in the various movement disorders considered here remains doubtful. Attempts to explain failures with deanol on the basis of improper dosages, inadequate length of treatment, or chronicity of the disease process (Casey, 1977; Re, 1975) have also been largely unsuccessful. It remains to be demonstrated that deanol is significantly more useful than placebo in any of these movement disorders.

Deanol in the Treatment of Tardive Dyskinesia. Table 10-4 summarizes 42 studies on deanol in tardive dyskinesia. Of a total of 246 patients treated with deanol, only 34% were reported to have improved. Further analysis of the studies shows a progressive decline in "positive" reports on deanol (Figure 10-1) as well as the following trends:

1. Design of study. There are 29 open and single-blind studies and 13 double-blind studies. (The study by Stafford & Fann, 1977, used both methods, whereas Casey, 1979, gave combined results employing open and blind designs.) In the 29 open and single-blind studies reported, 42% of the 92 patients treated improved. In the 13 double-blind studies, only 24% of the 123 patients treated improved significantly. Open studies are known to involve bias on the part of the subjects as well as the investigators and are useful only as a preliminary trial. Miller (1974b) and other earlier investigators believed that the chronic, unremitting nature of the symptoms in tardive dyskinesia made a "cure" by chance unlikely and therefore saw no need for conducting placebo-controlled trials in the treatment of tardive dyskinesia. Subsequent work has shown that the course of tardive dyskinesia is variable over time and that the symptoms respond to placebo in a sizable proportion of patients. The low rate of success with deanol in double-blind studies argues against a specific therapeutic action of deanol in mitigating symptoms of tardive dyskinesia.

2. Daily dose of deanol. Of the 29 open and single-blind studies, 10 employed a mean daily dose of less than 900 mg, whereas in 15 studies the drug was given at a mean daily dose of 900 mg or more. (Betts *et al.,* 1979, and Pickar & Davies, 1978, did not specify the dose used. Lambert *et al.,* 1978, gave variable doses.) Of the 25 patients treated with less than 900 mg/day, 72% improved, whereas only 25% of the 60 given higher doses improved. The overall rate of improvement in the double-blind studies was so low that an analysis of results by daily dose was not meaningful. On the basis of the open and single-blind trials, we can state that deanol at 900 mg or higher daily doses is usually of little value in tardive dyskinesia. Side effects with higher doses may be thought to be partly responsible for the clinical ineffectiveness of deanol. A number of studies, however, did not report significant side effects with deanol at doses exceeding 900 mg/day. It is therefore possible that the effectiveness of deanol in smaller doses might have been at least partly related to a placebo action.

3. Length of treatment. Most studies that reported successful results with deanol found that the drug produced significant improvement

Table 10-4. Treatment with Cholinergic Drugs

Investigators	Study design	Dose (mg/24 h)	Length of treatment	Improved	Not improved	Total
		Deanol				
Miller (1974b)	Open	600	1 week	2	0	2
Casey and Denney (1974, 1975)	Open	1600	8 weeks	1	0	1
Escobar and Kemp (1975)	Open	1200	2 weeks	0	2	2
Crane (1975)	Open	1200–1600	18 weeks	1	10	11
Curran, Nagaswami, and Mohan (1975)	Open	500	8 weeks	1	0	1
Fann, Sullivan, Miller, et al. (1975)	Open	500	5 days	10	0	10
DeSilva and Huang (1975)	Open	800–1000	1–2 weeks	4	0	4
Laterre and Fortemps (1975)	Open	225–900	14 weeks	1	0	1
Widrowe and Heisler (1976)	Open	200–300	3–8 weeks	1	1	2
Nesse and Carroll (1976); Carroll, Curtis, and Kokmen (1977)	Open	1500	19 days	0	1	1
Cole, Gardos, and Granacher (1976)	Double-blind	1500	5 weeks	0	12	12
Kumar (1976)	Open	1200	12 weeks	1	0	1
Bockenheimer and Lucius (1976)	Double-blind	1500	5 weeks	7	4	11
Mehta, Mehta, and Mathew (1976)	Open	600–800	3–5 months	0	2	2
Casey (1976); Casey and Denney (1977)	Double-blind	900–1250	2–3 weeks	0	6	6
Davis, Berger, and Hollister (1977b)	Double-blind	1600–2000	3–8 weeks	0	3	3
Tamminga, Smith, Ericksen, et al. (1977)	Single-blind	800–1200	4 weeks	3	3	6
Simpson, Voitaschevsky, Young, et al. (1977)	Double-blind	800–1200	8 weeks	7	3	10

Ray (1977)	Open	200–600	Several weeks	1	0	1
Rosenbaum, Niven, Hanson, et al. (1977)	Open	400–1800	1–2 weeks	1	0	1
Tarsy and Bralower (1977)	Double-blind	1000–2000	8 weeks	1	4	5
Stafford and Fann (1977)	Single-blind	1200	30 days	3	7	10
Crayton, Smith, Klass, et al. (1977)	Double-blind	1200	2 weeks	1	8	9
Crews and Carpenter (1977)	Open	900; 300 (with lithium)	3 weeks	0	1	1
Chien, Jung, and Ross-Townsend (1978)	Double-blind	1200–1600	3 weeks	1	6	7
Penovich, Morgan, Kerzner, et al. (1978)	Double-blind	2000	4 weeks	6	8	14
Pickar and Davies (1978)	Open	NS[a]	NS	0	1	1
McLean and Casey (1978)	Open	300–2700	Several months	1	0	1
Jus, Villeneuve, Gautier, et al. (1978)	Double-blind	Average 900 (500–1000)	8 weeks	3	23	26
Lambert, Wolff, DeManimy, et al. (1978)	Open	Variable	Weeks	4	0	4
Jeste, Potkin, Sinha, et al. (1979)	Open	Average 900 (200–1200)	6 weeks	0	7	7
Casey (1979)	Variable	400–6000	1–14 months	14	17	31
Amsterdam and Mendels (1979)	Open	1250	4 weeks	0	1	1
Paulson (1979)	Open	400–1200	NS	1	3	4
Betts, Johnston, and Pratt (1979)	Open	NS	NS	0	1	1
De Montigny, Chouinard, and Annable (1979)	Double-blind	1500	3 weeks	NS	NS	10
Lonowski, Sterling, and King (1979)	Double-blind	300–1800 (average 1800)	3 weeks or more	1	3	4

(continued)

Table 10-4. (continued)

Investigators	Study design	Dose (mg/24 h)	Length of treatment	Number of patients		
				Improved	Not improved	Total
Deanol (continued)						
Tamminga, Smith, and Davis (1980)	Double-blind	500–1250	3 weeks	0	6	6
Amsterdam and Mendels (1980)	Open	2000	NS	0	1	1
Weiss, Ciraulo and Shader (1980)	Open	2000	NS	0	1	1
Moore and Bowers (1980)	Open	600–1800	Several weeks	3	7	10
Singh, Nasrallah, Lal, et al. (1980)	Open	800–1200	Several weeks	0	3	3
TOTAL				81 (34.3%)	155	236 (+10[b])
Physostigmine (i.v.)						
Tarsy, Leopold, and Sax (1974)	Open	1–1.5		0	7	7
Fann, Lake, Gerber, et al. (1974); Fann, Sullivan, Miller, et al. (1975)	Blind ratings	40μg/kg		6	1	7
Klawans and Rubovits (1974)	Single-blind	1		10	2	12
Gerlach, Reisby, and Randrup (1974)	Blind ratings	1		5	3	8
Davis, Berger, and Hollister (1975, 1976; Davis, Hollister, Vento, et al. (1978)	Blind ratings	3		5	0	5
Carroll, Curtis, and Kokmen (1977)	Open	1		0	1	1
Tamminga, Smith, Ericksen, et al. (1977)	Double-blind	.5–2		5	1	6
Casey and Denney (1977); also, Casey (1976)	Double-blind	1		3	3	6
Tarsy and Bralower (1977)	Double-blind	1		0	5	5

Study	Design	Dose	Duration			
Crayton, Smith, Klass, et al. (1977)	Open	5		1	0	1
Weiss, Ciraulo, and Shader (1980)	Open	1-2		NS	NS	2
Nasrallah (1980)	Open	2		0	1	1
Moore and Bowers (1980)	Probably single-blind	2		1	9	10
TOTAL				36 (52.2%)	33	69 (+ 2[c])

Choline

Study	Design	Dose	Duration			
Davis, Berger, and Hollister (1975)	Open	Up to 1600	8 days	1	0	1
Davis and Berger (1978); Davis, Hollister, Barchas, et al. (1976); Davis, Berger, Hollister, et al. (1977a)	Probably single-blind	4000-20,000	5-11 weeks	4	1	5
Tamminga, Smith, Ericksen, et al. (1977); Tamminga, Smith, and Davis (1980)	Open	3000-18,000	NS	1	3	4
Growdon, Hirsch, Wurtman, et al. (1977)	Double-blind	150-200 mg/kg	2 weeks	9	11	20
Gelenberg, Doller-Wojcik, and Growdon (1979)	Open	150-200 mg/kg	6-8 weeks	1	4	5
Rosenbaum, O'Connor, and Duane (1980)	Open	200 mg/kg	NS	0	1	1
TOTAL				16 (44.4%)	20	36

(continued)

Table 10-4. (continued)

Investigators	Study design	Dose (mg/24 h)	Length of treatment	Improved	Not improved	Total
		Lecithin				
Growdon, Gelenberg, Doller, *et al.* (1978)	Open	40,000–80,000	NS	3	0	3
Barbeau (1978)	Open	3600–49,000	NS	2	0	2
Gelenberg, Doller-Wojcik, and Growdon (1979)	Open	21,000–105,000	2–6 months	1	3	4
Jackson, Nuttali, Ibe, *et al.* (1979)	Double-blind	50,000	2 weeks	Probably 6	0	6
Branchey, Branchey, Bark, *et al.* (1979)	Double-blind	25,000[d]	2 weeks	0	8	8
Singh, Nasrallah, Lal, *et al.* (1980)	Open	20,000	2 weeks	0	1	1
Jeste (unpublished data)	Double-blind	15,000–30,000[e]	3 weeks	0	1	1
TOTAL				12 (48%)	13	25

[a]NS = not stated.

[b]For ten patients, the numbers improved and not improved were not known.

[c]For two patients, the numbers improved and not improved were not known.

[d]25,000 mg of this 60% pure lecithin is equivalent to 100,000 mg of type 11-5 lecithin (from soya) used by several other investigators. Contains 3000 mg of choline base.

[e]94% pure.

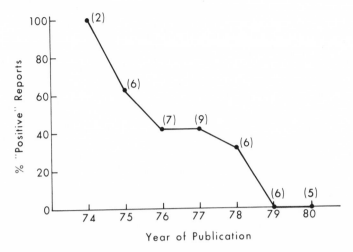

Figure 10-1. Progressive decline in "positive" reports with deanol in tardive dyskinesia. (Numbers in parentheses represent total numbers of studies done.)

within 1 or 2 weeks of starting the treatment. By contrast, the longer-term studies were usually negative.

4. Other factors. No significant relationship was observed between the efficacy of deanol and factors such as the patient's age, the patient's gender, and the severity or duration of dyskinesia.

Summary. The value of deanol in the treatment of tardive dyskinesia (and other movement disorders) is unproven. It is usually no more effective than placebo. It probably has some cholinergic effects; the extent of such effects is, however, variable. Administration of deanol in doses exceeding 900 mg/day is usually not recommended on the basis of the available data. Deanol should be used cautiously in patients with a past history or a family history of affective disorders.

Physostigmine

Physostigmine is a cholinesterase inhibitor that is usually administered parenterally (intramuscularly or intravenously), although an oral form is currently under investigation.

Effects on Animal Model of Tardive Dyskinesia. Christensen and Nielsen (1979) studied the effects of physostigmine on teflutixol-induced supersensitivity to apomorphine actions in mice. They found that physostigmine, injected during the receptor-blocking phase of teflutixol, did not modify the apomorphine-induced gnaw compulsion—that is, physostigmine had no effect on this animal model of tardive dyskinesia.

Clinical Studies. We found 13 studies with physostigmine in the treatment of tardive dyskinesia. Of the total 71 patients given physostigmine, 52% improved. In these studies the drug was usually administered on a single occasion, and its effects were observed for 2 to 24 hours. Using a dose of 40µg/kg of physostigmine along with methscopolamine (to block the peripheral cholinergic effects), Fann *et al.* (1974) noted maximum improvement 24 hours after the injection. In contrast, Davis, Hollister, Barchas, *et al.* (1976) found that significant effects of 3 mg/kg physostigmine along with methscopolamine lasted for less than 90 minutes. Most investigators have reported that the effects of physostigmine tend to be very brief. Recently, Weiss, Ciraulo, and Shader (1980) suggested that acute effects of physostigmine might be helpful in distinguishing tardive dyskinesia from rabbit syndrome, since the former would be expected to improve, and the latter to worsen, with this drug.

In a double-blind study, Tamminga *et al.* (1977) observed improvement in five of the six patients with tardive dyskinesia who were given physostigmine. Interestingly, methohexital, a sedative, also produced improvement, which was comparable to that seen with physostigmine. Neostigmine, a peripheral cholinomimetic agent, was ineffective. The investigators concluded that the sedative action of physostigmine might be responsible for the antidyskinetic effect seen in some patients. Supporting this view is an observation by Tarsy and Bralower (1977). Of their five patients, only one had brief improvement, and this, too, while the patient appeared sedated; when alerted, he had a prompt return of dyskinesia to the predrug levels. Thus it remains to be demonstrated that physostigmine reliably improves dyskinesia (even temporarily) and that this effect is due to its cholinergic action.

Summary. Studies of the acute effects of parenteral physostigmine do not offer convincing evidence of the usefulness of this drug in the treatment of tardive dyskinesia. The possibility that oral physostigmine may have a place in the therapy of some dyskinetic patients has not yet been explored.

Choline

Choline is a naturally occurring precursor of acetylcholine. Choline is normally present in such foods as soybeans, liver, fish, meat, eggs, and products containing lecithin (phosphatidyl choline). The brain cannot synthesize choline. The main source of brain choline is free choline taken up from the bloodstream at the blood–brain barrier. Administration of choline raises blood choline, brain choline, and brain acetylcholine concentrations in rats (Cohen & Wurtman, 1975), and blood and CSF choline levels in humans (Growden et al., 1977). Acetylcholine is synthesized from choline and acetyl coenzyme A in the presence of choline acetyltransferase.

Davis et al. (1978) reported interesting effects of choline chloride on an animal model of tardive dyskinesia. The animal model involved supersensitivity to the effect (stereotypy) of apomorphine following long-term pretreatment with haloperidol in rats. The investigators noted that acute administration of choline at the time of apomorphine challenge had no effect on the stereotypy; however, chronic treatment with choline either during or after induction of supersensitivity significantly reduced apomorphine-induced stereotypy. The suggestion was that prolonged, but not acute, treatment with choline might be helpful in treating tardive dyskinesia.

For clinical trials, choline chloride needs to be administered in relatively large doses (4 to 20 g daily). It is bitter tasting and produces a body odor that is best described as "dead fish." This odor is presumed to be caused by trimethylamine, a metabolite of choline formed in the gut (Davis, Hollister, Barchas, et al., 1976). Cholinergic reactions such as lacrimation, blurred vision, anorexia, and diarrhea may occur. Tamminga, Smith, Ericksen, et al. (1977) reported depression severe enough to warrant discontinuation of medication in two of their four patients receiving choline; depression remitted on stopping choline. Thus the use of choline on a routine clinical basis is inconvenient and unpleasant and has a potentiality for side effects.

We found six published reports on choline in tardive dyskinesia. Of the total 36 patients treated with choline, 44% improved. Growdon et al. (1977) found marked improvement in five patients, 25% to 50% improvement in four, no change in ten, and worsening in one patient. Thus only one-fourth of the total 20 patients had 50% or greater improvement. The investigators noted a significant increase in plasma choline levels in all the patients whether or not they improved. The clinical improvement, therefore, could not be correlated with an increase in plasma choline. In another study in which plasma choline was measured, Davis, Hollister, Barchas, *et al.* (1976) reported an increase in plasma choline levels in their patients. Three of their four patients improved. On discontinuing choline, plasma choline levels returned to almost normal levels within 48 hours, although clinical relapse was delayed for up to 2 weeks. Thus the investigators did not obtain an apparent correlation between rise in plasma choline and clinical improvement.

Summary. Administration of choline in adequate doses reliably increases plasma choline levels. Such an increase in plasma choline is, however, not necessarily related to clinical improvement in tardive dyskinesia. Therapeutic effects of choline are variable. Choline needs to be given in relatively high doses and has a number of side effects. The present value of choline in the treatment of tardive dyskinesia is still experimental.

Lecithin

Lecithin is the naturally occurring source of dietary choline. Lecithin is phosphatidyl choline, which is metabolized to choline in the intestine and liver. In rats, oral administration of lecithin increases brain choline and acetylcholine levels (Hirsch & Wurtman, 1978). In normal humans, oral lecithin raises blood choline concentrations to a greater extent than an equimolar dose of choline (Wurtman, Hirsch, & Growdon, 1977). Lecithin does not produce a bitter taste or a fishy body odor, which is often caused by ingestion of choline. Growdon, Gelenberg, Doller, *et al.* (1978) were the first to report successful use of lecithin in patients with tardive dyskinesia. Of the seven published studies of lecithin, four were open and three double-blind. Six of the 10 patients in open studies and 6 of the 15 patients in double-blind studies improved with lecithin. The overall improvement rate was 48%. Lecithin carries problems of the variable purity of available supplies and weight gain due to the high caloric value of the large amounts of the drug that need to be administered daily.

Summary. The clinical value of lecithin in the treatment of tardive dyskinesia is unclear, although it may be a useful research tool for investigating cholinergic mechanisms in movement disorders.

Other Cholinergic Agents

Davis *et al.* (1978) reported that oxotremorine, a central muscarinic agonist, was effective in inhibiting methylphenidate-induced stereotypy in mice. The authors suggested that this drug deserved a trial in the treatment of movement disorders such as tardive dyskinesia.

Summary

Available data do not support routine use of cholinomimetic agents in long-term treatment of tardive dyskinesia. The overall improvement rate with cholinergic drugs is 39% (Table 10-10). It is possible, however, that potent cholinergic drugs without troublesome side effects may have a place in the management of subgroups of patients with tardive dyskinesia.

PUTATIVE GABA'ERGIC DRUGS

Benzodiazepines (e.g., diazepam) are the most commonly prescribed putative GABA'ergic drugs in medicine. Although the mechanism of action of benzodiazepines is not yet known, available evidence generally favors a specific facilitatory action of these drugs on GABA'ergic synapses in the central nervous system (Haefely, 1978). Benzodiazepines were initially employed in tardive dyskinesia because of their sedative and anxiolytic effects; it was hoped that reducing patients' anxiety would also cause a reduction in dyskinesia. There were a number of isolated case reports (mostly with negative results), but no controlled studies, on the treatment of tardive dyskinesia with benzodiazepines during the 1960s. Experimental demonstrations that GABA was an inhibitory neurotransmitter linked with nigrostriatal dopaminergic functions (Stevens, Wilson, & Foote, 1974) led to a renewed interest in the use of presumptively GABA'ergic drugs, such as benzodiazepines, in treating tardive dyskinesia.

Animal Studies

The effects of GABA'ergic drugs on animal models of tardive dyskinesia have been variable. Christensen and Nielsen (1979) found that administration of diazepam and muscimol during the dopaminergic supersensitivity phase (induced by pretreatment with teflutixol) *increased* the supersensitivity. In another experiment, Christensen, Arnt, and Scheel-Kruger (1980) noted that repeated administration of a GABA agonist, THIP (tetrahydroisoxazolopyridin), potentiated stereotyped gnawing induced by dopaminergic drugs such as methylphenidate. These data do not support the rationale for using GABA agonists in disorders presumably associated with dopaminergic hyperactivity. In contrast, Lloyd, Worms, Zivkovic, *et al.* (1980) found that coadministration of SL76-002, another GABA agonist, with haloperidol greatly reduced the development of supersensitivity to haloperidol. Reasons for such discrepant findings are not obvious.

Clinical Studies

We found 19 studies (Table 10-5) on the treatment of tardive dyskinesia with drugs that are supposedly GABA'ergic. We excluded individual case reports on the use of commonly prescribed benzodiazepines, investigations on the acute effects of intravenous diazepam, and studies with drugs such as baclofen, the GABA'ergic activity of which is controversial.

Of the 204 patients treated, 54% improved significantly. Caution is necessary in interpreting the results of trials with GABA'ergic drugs. Most of the studies done were relatively short-term. Furthermore, Linnoila *et al.* (1976) found that improvement with a putative GABA'ergic drug, sodium valproate, was not related to blood levels of the drug. Little attempt has been made to separate the antidyskinetic effect of benzodiazepines from their other effects, such as sedation and muscle relaxation. (Singh *et al.*, 1980, reported, however, that diazepam, administered in doses that did not cause sedation, was effective in suppressing tardive dyskinesia.) Jus *et al.* (1974) gave intravenous diazepam (10 mg) to 14 patients with tardive dyskinesia and 6 with rabbit syndrome, a disorder related to parkinsonism. The investigators had equally good results in both syndromes. The current biochemical theories of the extrapyramidal disorders make it difficult to explain how a drug could be equally effective in two antagonistic conditions, unless it acted nonspecifically (e.g., as a sedative). Similar considerations probably apply to the observation of Linnoila *et al.* (1976) that sodium valproate relieved symptoms of tardive dyskinesia as well as those of akathisia and dystonia.

Drug Combinations

As mentioned earlier, Nair *et al.* (1978) suggested that the combined use of haloperidol and sodium valproate might be more beneficial than using either drug alone. This is contrasted by an observation by Linnoila and Viukari (1979) that sodium valproate was effective only when used in combination with "low-potency" neuroleptics such as chlorpromazine and was ineffective when given along with "high-potency" neuroleptics. Casey, Gerlach, Magelund, *et al.* (1980) reported that acetylenic GABA was useful in dyskinesia patients who were also receiving neuroleptics. Acetylenic GABA has been found to increase brain GABA by inhibiting GABA-T and to decrease dopamine turnover in rodents. Further clinical as well as basic research on neuroleptic–GABA'ergic drug combinations is warranted.

Side Effects

A number of authors have reported side effects with GABA'ergic drugs. Singh *et al.* (1980) noted behavior problems, such as impulsiveness and belligerence, in two of their patients treated with diazepam. Sedman (1976) encountered a high incidence of side effects with clonazepam; these included drowsiness, which sometimes progressed to confusion and ataxia, especially in elderly patients. Tamminga *et al.* (1979) found a 5-day trial of muscimol useful in patients with tardive dyskinesia, but added that this drug would be of little practical value because of its behavioral side effects, such as worsening of psychosis. Kaplan and Murkofsky (1978) and Rosenbaum and De La Fuente (1979) have even described cases of tardive dyskinesia presumably induced by benzodiazepine treatment.

Summary

There is as yet no convincing evidence to suggest that the putative GABA'ergic drugs exert a specific antidyskinetic effect. The possibility that their nonspecific actions, such as sedation, might be temporarily beneficial in some patients remains to be ruled out. Yet, GABA'ergic drugs are more effective than most nonneuroleptic agents in the suppression of tardive dyskinesia and therefore deserve a trial in cases of persistent dyskinesia.

DOPAMINERGIC DRUGS

Tardive dyskinesia is generally thought to be associated with, if not a result of, dopaminergic hyperactivity. It is therefore intriguing that dopaminergic drugs have been tried in the treatment of this disorder. The absence of a satisfactory treatment for, and the presumed extrapyramidal

Table 10-5. Treatment with GABA'ergic Drugs

Investigators	Study design	Dose (mg/24 h)	Length of treatment	Number of patients		
				Improved	Not improved	Total
		Diazepam				
Godwin-Austen and Clark (1971)	Double-blind	2–4	1 week	5	1	6
Bullock (1972)	Open	NS[a]	NS	0	3	3
Singh (1976)	Open	7–30	3 weeks to 6 months	3	0	3
Singh, Nasrallah, Lal, *et al.* (1980)	Open and single-blind	15–30	3 weeks	9	5	14
		Clorazepate				
Itil, Unverdi, and Mehta (1974)	Open	15–45	6 weeks	7	5	12
		Clonazepam				
O'Flanagan (1975)	Open	1–3	NS	42	0	42
Sedman (1976)	Open	1–4	Probably weeks	2	16	18
Jeste (unpublished data)	Double-blind	.5–8	4 weeks	0	2	2
Cole, Gardos, Tarsy, *et al.* (1980)	Open	1.5–6	NS	NS	NS	6

Sodium valproate

Linnoila, Viukari, and Hietala (1976)	Double-blind	900	2 weeks	14	17	31
Chien, Jung, and Ross-Townsend (1978)	Double-blind	1200–1600	3 weeks	0	5	5
Gibson (1978b)	Blind ratings	600	4 weeks	8	17	25
Nair, Yassa, Ruiz-navarro, et al. (1978)	Double-blind	600–1400	3 weeks	NS	NS	10
Casey and Hammerstad (1979)	Open	900–3000	9 weeks	1	0	1
Nagao, Ohshimo, Mitsunobu, et al. (1979)	Probably open	400–600	3 weeks	3	4	7
Singh, Nasrallah, Lal, et al. (1980)	Open	600	1 month	0	1	1
Pandurangi, Devi, and Channabasavanna (1980)	Open	NS	NS	0	2	2

Muscimol

Tamminga, Crayton, and Chase (1976)	Double-blind	3–9	Up to 5 days	NS	NS	7

γ-Acetylenic GABA

Casey, Gerlach, Magelund, et al. (1980)	Double-blind	75–225	8 weeks	4	6	10

[a] NS = not stated.

pathogenesis of, tardive dyskinesia have led to studies on its treatment with drugs such as amantadine and L-dopa (Table 10-6). These drugs are useful in Parkinson's disease, another extrapyramidal system disorder. Parkinsonism and tardive dyskinesia are, however, considered to be clinical and pharmacologic opposites; predictably, dopaminergic agents have proved to be of little value in treating dyskinesia.

Amantadine

l-Amantadine hydrochloride is an antiparkinsonian, antiviral agent. It has been shown to cause an increase in the release of dopamine (as well as norepinephrine) in the animal brain. Vale and Espejel (1971) first reported successful use of amantadine in two patients with tardive dyskinesia. This study was criticized by Kazamatsuri (1971) and by Ringel and Klawans (1971) for a probable misdiagnosis of parkinsonian patients as having tardive dyskinesia.

There are nine reports on the use of amantadine in dyskinesia. In six of these trials, including a double-blind one, not a single patient treated with amantadine improved. Combining all nine studies, the overall weighted mean improvement rate with amantadine was 22%.

L-Dopa

Levodopa, or L-dopa, is the levorotatory isomer of dihydroxyphenylalanine (DOPA), a metabolic precursor of dopamine. Unlike dopamine, L-dopa does cross the blood–brain barrier and is presumably converted into dopamine in the basal ganglia.

We found 11 studies on the effects of oral administration of L-dopa in tardive dyskinesia. Only 33% of the patients treated had improvement; the others were either unimproved or had a worsening of dyskinesia. In another study Hippius and Longemann (1970) reported that slow intravenous administration of 100 mg of L-dopa produced aggravation of dyskinesia in 12 of their 40 patients; the rest of the subjects were not significantly affected.

A different approach to the treatment of tardive dyskinesia with L-dopa has been suggested by Alpert and Friedhoff (1980). It is based on the hypothesis that temporarily increasing dopamine levels by treatment with L-dopa would reduce dopamine receptor supersensitivity. Experiments by Friedhoff *et al.* (1978) indicated that a combination of L-dopa and carbidopa reversed the manifestations of haloperidol-induced dopamine receptor supersensitivity in rats.[2] In their clinical trial, Alpert and Friedhoff (1980) found improvement in three of their seven patients treated with L-dopa. Earlier, these patients had not responded to neuroleptic withdrawal for at least 3 months. Two other patients had to be taken off L-dopa because of side effects such as a grand mal seizure and allergic rash, while two more patients showed no signs of adaptation to L-dopa during a week of treatment at the maximal dose, before they were removed from the study for administrative reasons. The hypothesis of receptor sensitivity modification by L-dopa administration is attractive; however, the incidence of various side effects (including worsening of psychosis) with L-dopa is rather high. Hence further experimental work is necessary before this potentially promising approach can be recommended for routine clinical use.

Other Catecholaminergic Drugs

Fann *et al.* (1973) tried caffeine, amphetamine, and methylphenidate in a pilot study in dyskinetic patients. There was no response to caffeine and amphetamine, while methylphenidate induced modest improvement. A double-blind trial of methylphenidate showed, however, that the drug was of little value in the treatment of tardive dyskinesia. Carroll *et al.* (1977) and Crayton *et al.* (1977b) reported worsening of dyskinesia with *d*-amphetamine. Roccatagliata *et al.* (1977) studied the effect of trazadone, a new antidepressent of the triazolopyridine type, on tardive dyskinesia. The symptoms of dyskinesia improved on intravenous administration of the drug. The mechanism of action of trazadone is not yet well established, although it is thought to have adrenolytic, dopaminergic, and serotonergic actions.

The most frequently employed animal model of tardive dyskinesia involves demonstation of increased responsiveness to dopaminergic drugs following neuroleptic treatment. Hence the use of the same drugs to treat dyskinesia may be hard to justify. Combining all the studies with catecholaminergic drugs, the overall improvement rate is 25%. It is possible that at least some of the patients who improved had parkinsonism rather than tardive dyskinesia.

---

[2]Recently, Weiner, Carvey, Nausieda, *et al.* (1981) have confirmed this observation using guinea pigs.

Table 10-6. Treatment with Dopaminergic Drugs

Investigators	Study design	Dose (mg/24 h)	Length of treatment	Improved	Not improved	Total
					Number of patients	
Amantadine						
Dynes (1970)	Open	50–200	2 weeks	0	22	22
Vale and Espejel (1971)	Probably single-blind	4 mg/kg	NS[a]	2	0	2
Decker, Davis, Janowsky, et al. (1971)	Open	300	1 week	6	0	6
Crane (1971b)	Open	200–400	2 weeks	0	9	9
Janowsky, El-Yousef, Davis, et al. (1972)	Double-blind	300	10 days	0	12	12
Merren (1972)	Open	200–300	1–2 months	0	3	3
Ehrensing (1974)	Open	NS	NS	0	1	1
Pöldinger (1978)	Open	200	Probably several weeks	6	3	9
Weiss, Ciraulo, and Shader (1980)	Open	200	NS	0	1	1
L-Dopa						
Klawans and McKendall (1971)	Open	NS	2 weeks	0	1	1
Gerlach, Thorsen, and Munkvad (1974)	Blind ratings	600–1200 (+ peripheral decarboxylase inhibitor)	2 weeks	0	5	5
Ehrensing (1974)	Open	NS	NS	0	1	1
Carroll, Curtis, and Kokmen (1977)	Open	Up to 6000	3 weeks	1	0	1
Casey and Denney (1977)	Single-blind	500	1 dose	0	6	6
Tolosa (1978b)	Open	Up to 4000	Up to 13 months	3	1	4

Reference	Design	Dose	Duration			
Ringwald (1978)	Single-blind	Up to 3000	2 months	NS	NS	16
Betts, Johnston and Pratt (1979)	Open	NS (with carbidopa)	NS	0	1	1
Alpert and Friedhoff (1980)	Open	Up to 6000	Several weeks to months	3	0	3
Pandurangi, Devi, and Channabasavanna (1980)	Open	NS	NS	0	1	1
Cole, Gardos, Tarsy, et al. (1980)	Open	200–1000[b]	NS	4	5	9
	Open	200–400 (with fusaric acid)	NS	0	3	3
Methylphenidate						
Fann, Davis, and Wilson (1973)	Double-blind	20–80	6 weeks	3	14	17
d-Amphetamine						
Carroll, Curtis, and Kokmen (1977)	Open	10	Once	0	1	1
Crayton, Smith, Klass, et al. (1977)	Open	15	Once	0	1	1
Smith, Tamminga, and Davis (1980)	Double-blind	20 (p.o.) and 15–20 (i.v.)	Once each	0	8	8
Trazadone						
Roccatagliata, Albano, Cocito, et al. (1977)	Probably open	50 (i.v.)	Once	4	0	4

[a]NS = not stated.

[b] The actual doses of L-dopa (50 to 250 mg daily) given in combination with carbidopa were equivalent to 200 to 1000 mg of L-dopa given alone.

Summary

Amantadine, L-dopa (except, possibly, given in the manner of Alpert & Friedhoff, 1980), and other dopaminergic drugs are of little benefit in treating tardive dyskinesia. The improvement rate with catecholaminergic drugs is only 8.1% (Table 10-10). They may aggravate dyskinetic and psychotic symptoms in some patients and also have a number of other side effects.

ANTICHOLINERGIC DRUGS

Anticholinergic drugs such as trihexyphenidyl are useful in the treatment of neuroleptic-induced parkinsonism. Sometimes these drugs are prescribed routinely in combination with neuroleptics. Hence the number of patients with tardive dyskinesia who have received antiparkinsonian medication at one time or another is quite large. There is a near unanimity among clinicians and investigators that the anticholinergic agents are of little or no benefit in the treatment of tardive dyskinesia. A number of other authors commented in the 1960s on the lack of response of dyskinesia to antiparkinsonian medications (Druckman, Seelinger, & Thulin 1962; Evans, 1965; Hunter et al., 1964; Schmidt & Jarcho, 1966). It was only during the 1970s, however, that systematic studies on the effects of these drugs on tardive dyskinesia were reported.

Animal Studies

The effects of anticholinergic drugs on animal models of tardive dyskinesia have been contradictory. Christensen and Nielsen (1979) and Tarsy and Baldessarini (1974) concluded that anticholinergic treatment did not modify neuroleptic-induced dopamine receptor supersensitivity. Smith and Davis (1975) reported that chronic administration of benztropine mesylate concomitant with haloperidol reduced behavioral supersensitivity in rats to apomorphine and amphetamine. In contrast, Borison et al. (1979) found that rats pretreated with a haloperidol–benztropine combination showed more intense stereotypy in response to apomorphine as compared to the animals treated with haloperidol alone. (Long-term pretreatment with benztropine alone did not result in dopamine receptor supersensitivity.)

Clinical Studies

There are 14 studies on the treatment of tardive dyskinesia with anticholinergic drugs (Table 10-7). They include only those investigations in which the effects of these agents were studied in a rather systematic manner in several or many patients. Table 10-10 shows that 7.3% of the patients were described as having improved with anticholinergic drugs. Four studies in which results were not given in terms of numbers of patients improved and unimproved also reported negative effects of treatment with anticholinergic agents. It is interesting to note that in only two studies even a small proportion of patients improved. In both these reports, the medication was injected intravenously on a single occasion, and only the acute effects were studied.

Klawans (1976) and others have suggested that anticholinergic agents may not only aggravate preexisting dyskinesia, but may also predispose to the development of tardive dyskinesia in individuals receiving neuroleptics. Although worsening of tardive dyskinesia with anticholinergic medication is well documented, there is as yet no convincing evidence to indicate that these drugs predispose to tardive dyskinesia. Chouinard, De Montigny, Annable, *et al.* (1979) and Gerlach and Simmelsgaard (1978) found that short-term treatment with biperiden and procyclidine, respectively, increased severity of dyskinesia, but had no significant influence on the syndrome after discontinuation of that treatment. Although there are isolated case reports of tardive dyskinesia induced by anticholinergic drugs (see Chapter 4), most of the epidemiologic studies of neuroleptic-induced tardive dyskinesia have not found any significant association between past use of antiparkinsonian agents and prevalence of tardive dyskinesia.

Side Effects

A number of untoward reactions have been reported with anticholinergic drugs. These vary from minor discomforts such as dryness of the mouth to serious reactions such as anticholinergic delirium. Interference with gastrointestinal absorption of neuroleptics is believed to result in a lowering of serum neuroleptic concentrations; consequently, the clinician may be required to increase the dose of neuroleptics in order to obtain therapeutic effects. (A recent study by Simpson, Cooper, Bark, *et al.*, 1980, however, found no significant effect of antiparkinsonian medication on plasma

Table 10-7. Treatment with Anticholinergic Drugs

Investigators	Study design	Dose (mg/24 h)	Length of treatment	Number of patients		
				Improved	Not improved	Total
Benzotropine (p.o.)						
Dynes (1970)	Open	1–5	2 months	0	22	22
Benzotropine (i.v.)						
Jus, Jus, Gautier, et al. (1974)	NS[a]	2	Once	5	9	14
Casey and Denney (1977); also, Casey (1976)	Single-blind	2	Once	3	3	6
Tarsy and Bralower (1977)	Probably open	2	Once	0	5	5
Moore and Bowers (1980)	Probably single-blind	2	Once	0	10	10
Trihexyphenidyl						
Dynes (1970)	Open	2–10	2 months	0	22	22
Turek, Kurland, Hanlon, et al. (1972)	Double-blind	Individualized	12 weeks (plus 20 weeks with neuroleptics)	NS	NS	16

Study	Design	Dose	Duration			
Ringwald (1978)	Single-blind	27	2 months	NS	NS	16
Burnett, Prange, Wilson, *et al.*(1980)	Blind ratings	4-15 (average 6)	1 month Twice	0	7	7
Biperiden						
Gerlach, Reisby, and Randrup (1974)	Blind ratings	18	2 weeks	0	7	7
Gerlach and Simmelsgaard (1978); Gerlach (1977)	Blind ratings	6 (plus halo-peridol)	4 weeks	NS	NS	16
Procyclidine						
Chouinard, De Montigny, and Annable (1979)	Probably open	30	1 week	NS	NS	20
Scopolamine (i.v.)						
Klawans and Rubovits (1974)	Single-blind	1	Once	NS	NS	10
Various anticholinergic drugs						
Burnett, Prange, Wilson, *et al.* (1980)	Blind ratings	Individualized	8 weeks	NS	NS	10

[a]NS = not stated.

levels of chlorpromazine.) Occasionally, anticholinergic drugs may produce symptoms of an organic mental syndrome.

Summary

Anticholinergic drugs are of little, if any, benefit in the treatment of tardive dyskinesia. Indeed, nonresponse to anticholinergic agents may be one of the criteria for a diagnosis of tardive dyskinesia (Chapter 3).

MISCELLANEOUS DRUGS

A number of miscellaneous drugs have been tried in the treatment of tardive dyskinesia for various reasons (Table 10-8).

Pyridoxine

Yahr and Duvoisin (1969) observed that pyridoxine (vitamin B_6) antagonized the therapeutic effects of L-dopa in patients with parkinsonism. Since there is some evidence for a reciprocal relationship between tardive dyskinesia and parkinsonism, Crane, Turek, and Kurland (1970) used pyridoxine in dyskinetic patients, but obtained disappointing results. Dynes (1970) also saw no benefit with pyridoxine treatment, whereas Prange et al. (1973) found a combined administration of pyridoxine and L-tryptophan useful. DeVeaugh-Geiss and Manion (1978) employed high doses (1000 to 1400 mg daily) of pyridoxine; yet, only one of their five patients had more than 50% improvement in dyskinetic symptoms.

Lithium

Dalen (1973) and Prange et al. (1973) first reported successful use of lithium in three patients with dyskinesia. Subsequent trials have yielded conflicting data. In a double-blind study, Gerlach, Thorsen, and Munkvad (1975) found that the overall improvement with lithium was statistically significant, although only 3 of the 15 patients had more than 50% improvement in severity of dyskinesia. The overall improvement rate with lithium is only 27%.

In separate animal experiments Klawans, Weiner, and Nausieda (1977) and Pert, Rosenblatt, Sivit, et al. (1978) found that concurrent treatment with lithium and haloperidol prevented development of dopamine receptor supersensitivity, which would have developed following long-term treatment with haloperidol alone. This suggested a possible use of lithium to prevent tardive dyskinesia, although there has been little clinical evidence supporting this suggestion. Indeed there are at least three case reports of tardive dyskinesia induced or aggravated by lithium (Crews & Carpenter, 1977; Beitman, 1978; Stancer, 1979). Klawans, Weiner, and Nausieda (1977) also reported that treatment with lithium, after chronic pretreatment with haloperidol had already produced dopamine receptor supersensitivity, was of no value in reducing the supersensitivity. These investigators therfore predicted that lithium would have no role in the treatment of tardive dyskinesia.

Estrogens

Reports of a high prevalence of tardive dyskinesia in postmenopausal women provided a rationale for trying estrogens in the treatment of tardive dyskinesia. Bedard *et al.* (1977) first reported clinically apparent antidopaminergic effects of estrogens in patients with tardive dyskinesia. Later, Villeneuve *et al.* (1980) conducted an open trial of the effects of conjuated estrogens in 20 male patients and observed significant reduction in tardive dyskinesia in some cases. On the other hand, Koller *et al.* (1979) have reported induction of choreiform movement disorders in patients who received estrogens for prolonged periods. Animal studies suggest that long-term treatment with estradiol, either alone or in combination with haloperidol, increases dopamine receptor supersensitivity (Gordon *et al.*, 1980; Nausieda *et al.*, 1979), whereas administration of estradiol following haloperidol pretreatment tends to reduce such supersensitivity (Gordon *et al.*, 1980). It thus appears that estrogens may have some dyskinesia-suppressing action, although long-term use of estrogens may aggravate underlying pathology in neuroleptic-treated patients.

Tryptophan

Prange, Wilson, Morris, *et al.* (1973) first tried L-tryptophan in tardive dyskinesia. They had observed that combined use of L-tryptophan and pyridoxine caused rapid deterioration in patients with Parkinson's disease and therefore reasoned that L-tryptophan might be helpful in tardive dyskinesia (thought to be a biochemical opposite of parkinsonism). The investi-

Table 10-8. Treatment with Miscellaneous Drugs

Investigators	Study design	Dose (mg/24 h)	Length of treatment	Number of patients		
				Improved	Not improved	Total
Pyridoxine						
Crane, Turek, and Kurland (1970)	Open	300	10–14 days	1	10	11
Dynes (1970)	Open	50–200	2 weeks	0	22	22
Prange, Wilson, Morris, et al. (1973)	Single-blind	50 (with L-tryptophan)	1–2 months	4	0	4
DeVeaugh-Geiss and Manion (1978)	Blind ratings	1000–4000	Probably weeks	1	4	5
Lithium						
Prange, Wilson, Morris, et al. (1973)	Double-blind	NS[a]	NS	2	0	2
Dalen (1973)	Open	NS	NS	1	0	1
Ehrensing (1974)	Open	900–1200 (with doxepin)	1 year	1	0	1
Reda, Escobar, and Scanlan (1975)	Open	600–1200	4 weeks	NS	NS	6
Gerlach, Thorsen, and Munkvad (1975)	Double-blind	12–24 mEq	3 weeks	3	12	15
Simpson, Branchey, Lee, et al. (1976)	Single-blind	300–1800	3 months	0	10	10
	Double-blind	300–1200	6 weeks	0	10	10
Pickar and Davies (1978)	Open	NS	NS	Probably 1	0	1
Jus, Villeneuve, Gautier, et al. (1978)	Double-blind	200–500	8 weeks	5	18	23
Ereshefsky, Rubin, and Friedman (1979)	Open	600–900	3 weeks	1	0	1
Rosenbaum, Maruta, Duane, et al. (1980); Rosenbaum, O'Connor, and Duane (1980)	Open	225–1200 (with amitriptyline)	1 month (or longer)	9	11	20

Tryptophan						
Prange, Wilson, Morris, et al. (1973)	Single-blind	Up to 6000 (with pyridoxine)	4–8 weeks	4	0	4
Jus, Jus, Gautier, et al. (1974)	Double-blind	6000	4 weeks	0	3	3
	Open	120 mg/kg	NS	0	8	8
MIF-1						
Ehrensing (1974)	Open	150	6 days	1	0	1
Ehrensing, Kastin, Larsons, et al. (1977)	Open	50–250	7 weeks	NS	NS	13
Diphenylhydantoin						
Jus, Jus, Gautier, et al. (1974)	Probably open	100 mg (i.v.)	Once	8	6	14
Manganese						
Kunin (1976a, 1976b)	Open	15–80	Days to weeks	4	1	5
Norris and Sams (1977)	Open	NS	NS	6	0	6
Niacin						
Kunin (1976b)	Open	100–500	Days to weeks	1	1	2
Cyproheptadine						
Goldman (1976)	Open	4–8	6–12 months	3	0	3
Gardos and Cole (1978)	Open	8	3–6 weeks	0	5	5
Nagao, Ohshimo, Mitsunobu, et al. (1979)	Open	8–24	3 weeks	1	4	5

(continued)

Table 10-8. (continued)

Investigators	Study design	Dose (mg/24 h)	Length of treatment	Number of patients		
				Improved	Not improved	Total
Baclofen						
Korsgaard (1976)	Double-blind	15–60	2 weeks	15	5	20
Gerlach, Rye, and Kristjansen (1978)	Double-blind	20–120	3 weeks	9	9	18
Simpson, Lee, Shrivastava, et al. (1978)	Single-blind	20–120	7 weeks	NS	NS	4
Nair, Yassa, Ruiz-navarro, et al. (1978)	Double-blind	30–90	3 weeks	NS	NS	10
Amsterdam and Mendels (1979)	Open	Up to 60	2 months	1	0	1
Amsterdam and Mendels (1979)	Open	NS	NS	0	1	1
Feder and Moore (1980)	Open	60–120	Several months	1	0	1
Fusaric acid						
Viukari and Linnoila (1977)	Open	150–450	3 weeks	NS	NS	14
Propranolol						
Carroll, Curtis, and Kokmen (1977)	Open	160	8 days	0	1	1
Moreira and Karnio (1979)	Open	800	NS	1	0	1
Bacher and Lewis (1980)	Open	20–40	Weeks to months	7	3	10
Kulik and Wilbur (1980)	Open	30–40	3 months	3	0	3

Reference	Design	Dose (mg)	Duration			
Tricyclic antidepressant—amitriptyline						
Rosenbaum, Maruta, Duane et al. (1980); Rosenbaum, O'Connor, and Duane (1980)	Open	20-125 (with lithium)	1 month or longer	9	11	20
Conjugated estrogens						
Villeneuve, Cazejust, and Cote (1980)	Open	1.25 / 2.5	6 weeks / 6 weeks	6 / 4	4 / 6	10 / 10
Enkephalin—FK33-824						
Bjørndal, Casey, and Gerlach (1980)	Single-blind	1-3	Single i.m. injections	2	6	8
Morphine						
Bjørndal, Casey, and Gerlach (1980)	Single-blind	10	Single s.c. injections	NS	NS	8
Naloxone						
Bjørndal, Casey, and Gerlach (1980)	Single-blind	8	Single i.m. injections	1	7	8
Clonidine						
Freedman, Bell, and Kirch (1980)	Open / Open	.3 / .4-.7	2 weeks / Several weeks	0 / 1	1 / 0	1 / 1

[a]NS = not stated.

gators noted that, although a combination of L-tryptophan and pyridoxine was beneficial, L-tryptophan alone was of no value in patients with dyskinesia. Later, Jus *et al.* (1974) reported negative results with D,L-tryptophan.

MIF-1

Prompted by an observation that MIF-1 (chemically, prolyl-leucyl-glycin-amide) reduced L-dopa-induced dyskinesias in parkinsonian patients, Ehrensing (1974) used MIF-1 in a depressive patient with tardive dyskinesia and saw significant improvement in dyskinesia. A subsequent trial on 13 patients, however, showed no significant improvement in dyskinesia after 7 weeks of treatment with MIF-1 (Ehrensing *et al.*, 1977). In a recent study of an animal model of tardive dyskinesia, Davis, Kastin, Beilstein, *et al.* (1980) found that MIF-1 increased apomorphine-induced stereotypy in rats pretreated with haloperidol, suggesting that MIF-1 might not be useful in patients with tardive dyskinesia.

Diphenylhydantoin

Jus *et al.* (1974) studied acute effects of intravenous diphenylhydantoin in 14 patients with tardive dyskinesia. The investigators had been encouraged by reports that this well-known anticonvulsant was also useful in some cases of chorea minor (probably Sydenham's chorea) and was of controversial value in the treatment of parkinsonism. Eight of the 14 patients with tardive dyskinesia had transient improvement (on polygraphic and clinical assessment) following an injection of phenytoin. The improvement was, however, less dramatic than that following diazepam.

Manganese

Kunin (1976a, 1976b) was probably the first investigator to report treatment of tardive dyskinesia with manganese chelate. His rationale was as follows: Phenothiazines are potent chelators of manganese, and manganese is found in high concentrations in the extrapyramidal system. It is possible that phenothiazines might chelate manganese and thus make it unavailable for some presumed function, such as an enzyme activation. Providing additional dietary manganese might therefore correct the manganese deficiency and improve dyskinesia. Of the 15 patients treated by Kunin, 14 were reportedly "cured" or much improved. Only five of Kunin's patients, however, appear to be probable cases of tardive dyskinesia; the others had symptoms that are not typical of tardive dyskinesia, such as rigidity, akathisia, and tremors. Norris and Sams (1977) also found manganese to be useful in dyskinetic patients. Controlled trials with manganese in tardive dyskinesia are, however, lacking. Moreover, the rationale for using manganese in this disorder is open to some question. Weiner, Nausieda, and Klawans (1980) have reported that long-term treatment of guinea pigs with chlorpromazine results in significant increases in managanese concentrations in the caudate nucleus. In view of the reports of potentially irreversible neurological disorders, including movement disorders, caused by chronic manganese intoxication (Cook, Fahn, & Brait, 1974), it is difficult to suggest treatment of tardive dyskinesia with manganese.

Niacin

Theorizing that niacin or nicotinamide (vitamin B_3) has antihistaminic and prostaglandin-stimulating activity and that the latter may augment cholinergic function, Kunin (1976b) gave niacin to patients with dyskinesia and obtained "cure" or marked improvement in most of them. However, only 2 of his 10 patients treated with niacin seemed to have tardive dyskinesia.

Cyproheptadine

Cyproheptadine (4-amino-3-p-chlorphenylbutyric acid) is an antihistaminic, antiserotonergic compound with sedative properties, used mainly in allergic conditions. Goldman (1976) reported improvement with cyproheptadine in all three of his dyskinetic patients, whereas Gardos and Cole (1978) and Nagao et al. (1979) had negative results in their subjects.

Baclofen

Korsgaard (1976) first used baclofen as a GABA'ergic drug in the treatment of tardive dyskinesia. Subsequent work has shown, however, that, although baclofen is a GABA analogue, it may not be a GABA agonist. Rather, it may act as an antagonist of substance P, a putative modulator of neuronal transmission. Recently, Moore and Demarest (1980) reported a dose-related increase in brain dopamine concentrations with systemic administration of baclofen. Nair *et al.* (1978) and Simpson, Lee, Shrivastava, *et al.* (1978) found that baclofen did not produce significant improvement in dyskinesia. Interestingly, combined use of baclofen and haloperidol (Nair *et al.*, 1978) or baclofen and deanol (Amsterdam & Mendels, 1979) was observed to be more beneficial in some patients with tardive dyskinesia.

Fusaric Acid

This is an inhibitor of DBH and reduces noradrenaline synthesis. Its effects on brain dopamine and serotonin concentrations are variable. Viukari and Linnoila (1977) found significant improvement in tardive dyskinesia with fusaric acid treatment. This report assumes added significance in view of our finding of high plasma DBH activity in patients with tardive dyskinesia (see Chapter 5). Another DBH inhibitor, disulfiram, was successfully tried in patients with L-dopa-induced dykinesia and deserves careful experimental study in tardive dyskinesia.

Propranolol

This is a specific β-adrenergic receptor blocker. Bacher and Lewis (1980) reported that low doses of propranolol were useful in significantly reducing dyskinesia in seven of their ten patients, whereas Moreira and Karnio (1979) observed improvement with high doses of propranolol in one case. These findings are consistent with the possibility of noradrenergic hyperactivity in tardive dyskinesia (see Chapter 5). At the same time, some alternative explanations should also be considered. The possibility of nonspecific sedative effects of propranolol on abnormal movements cannot be ruled out. Indeed, Kulik and Wilbur (1980) found that this drug was useful in reducing simultaneously both tardive dyskinesia and parkinsonian tremors in three patients. Peet, Middlemiss, and Yates (1981) recently found that plasma concentrations of chlorpromazine and its metabolites were significantly increased by concomitant administration of propranolol. Increased blood levels of neuroleptics would be expected to suppress dyskinetic symptoms. More work is therefore warranted to understand the mechanism of action of propranolol in tardive dyskinesia.

Clonidine

This imidazoline derivative is believed ot act, when given in small doses, by inhibiting central noradrenergic function, probably by stimulating the inhibitory α_1-noradrenergic autoreceptors. Freedman *et al.* (1980) found that clonidine, .3 to .4 mg/day, reduced both psychotic and dyskinetic symptoms in two patients. Further work with the drug would be particularly interesting in view of the likelihood of noradrenergic pathology in at least a subtype of tardive dyskinesia (see Chapter 5).

Barbiturates

Barbiturates have been given as sedatives to a large number of psychiatric patients, including some with tardive dyskinesia. Although Lipsius (1977) reported improvement in dyskinesia in one patient treated with phenobarbital, most clinicians have found barbiturates to be of little benefit in this disorder (Betts *et al.*, 1979; Druckman *et al.*, 1962; Evans, 1965; Sovner & Loadman, 1978). In animal experiments Costall and Naylor (1975) observed that sodium pentobarbital had no effect on dopamine-induced dyskinesias in guinea pigs, whereas Christensen and Nielsen (1979) noticed an increase in neuroleptic-induced dopaminergic supersensitivity following phenobarbital administration.

Other Drugs

Recently, Rosenbaum, Maruta, Duane, *et al.* (1980) reported successful treatment of some depressed and dyskinetic patients with an amitriptyline–lithium combination. In another study Bjørndal *et al.* (1980) tried three drugs: FK33-824 (a synthetic met-enkephalin analogue), morphine, and naloxone. Of these, only FK33-824 had some beneficial effect on tardive dyskinesia in patients who were receiving high-dose neuroleptic therapy.

Summary

It is apparent that most of these miscellaneous drugs have not been found to be of significant value in the treatment of tardive dyskinesia. The combined overall rate of improvement with these drugs is 36% (Table 10-10).

Further studies on certain types of drugs, for example, noradrenergic inhibitors such as clonidine or DBH inhibitors such as disulfiram, may be of interest.

NEUROLEPTIC WITHDRAWAL

It is logical to expect that withdrawal of neuroleptics may be considered the first line of treatment for tardive dyskinesia. We found 23 treatment studies in which neuroleptics were withdrawn for periods varying from 1 or 2 weeks to 3 years (Table 3-4). Of the patients withdrawn from neuroleptics, 37% had a remission of dyskinetic symptoms – that is, they had reversible dyskinesia (see Chapter 3). Most of the patients whose dyskinesia improved following neuroleptic withdrawal had symptom relief within 3 months of the discontinuation of neuroleptics. Of the patients who were taken off neuroleptics, 33.5% improved significantly within 3 months. Only 3% of the patients had remission more than 3 months after discontinuation of neuroleptics. This suggests that, for research purposes, presence of tardive dyskinesia 3 months after neuroleptic withdrawal may be taken as a reasonably valid criterion for persistence of dyskinesia. For clinical purposes, however, it should be stressed that the longer the period of neuroleptic withdrawal, the greater the likelihood of remission of dyskinesia.

Neuroleptic withdrawal usually results in an initial aggravation of dyskinesia, which reaches its peak intensity within 1 or 2 weeks (Crane *et al.*, 1969; Jeste, Potkin, Sinha, *et al.*, 1979). The severity of dyskinesia then decreases. The dyskinesia either continues to lessen progressively and disappears (in 37% patients) or persists at a plateaued level of severity (in the remaining 63% patients).

Of the various factors studied in relation to persistence of dyskinesia, aging and brain damage are the most commonly implicated. Degkwitz (1969), Uhrbrand and Faurbye (1960), and Yagi *et al.* (1976) found that the persistent dyskinesia group was significantly older than the reversible dyskinesia group. The highest rate of reversibility (over 90%) was seen in a study on a sample with a mean age of 36.9 years with most patients under 50 (Quitkin *et al.*, 1977). Combining various studies, Smith and Baldessarini (1980) noted an inverse correlation between age and spontaneous remission of tardive dyskinesia.

An association between brain damage and persistent dyskinesia was reported by Uhrbrand and Faurbye (1960) and Yagi *et al.* (1976). A number of studies in which there was a preponderance of brain-damaged patients also found a high rate of persistence of dyskinesia (Edwards, 1970; Hunter *et al.*, 1964; Paulson, 1968; Pryce & Edwards, 1966). The criteria for a diagnosis of brain damage were, however, not specified in most of these surveys.

Quitkin *et al.* (1977) suggested that the duration of tardive dyskinesia might be an important determinant of reversibility. Discontinuation of neuroleptics soon after tardive dyskinesia was detected resulted in remission of symptoms in over 90% of their patients. As stated earlier, most of the patients in this investigation were under 50. In our study (Jeste, Potkin, Sinha, *et al.*, 1979), duration of dyskinesia was shorter in reversible dyskinesia patients; yet, it was not a statistically significant variable on multivariate analysis. A number of other investigators have pointed out the difficulty in assessing the exact duration of tardive dyskinesia since its symptoms usually have an insidious onset.

Degkwitz (1969) and Jeste, Potkin, Sinha, *et al.* (1979) reported that patients with a history of interrupted neuroleptic treatment were more likely to have persistent dyskinesia compared to patients with almost continuous drug therapy. Recently, McCreadie *et al.* (1981) observed a higher incidence of tardive dyskinesia in patients receiving intermittent pimozide as compared with those being treated regularly with fluphenazine. In experiments with animal models of tardive dyskinesia, Weiss and Santelli (1978) found that some monkeys who did not develop dyskinesia with continuous administration of haloperidol did so when switched to intermittent treatment. Two studies with the supersensitivity model in rodents (Bannet *et al.*, 1980; Jeste, Stoff, Potkin, *et al.*, 1979) concluded that intermittent administration of a neuroleptic did not prevent or reduce development of dopaminergic supersensitivity.

Thus there is little clinical or experimental evidence to support the notion that drug interruptions lower the incidence of persistent tardive dyskinesia. Intermittent treatment either may have no specific effect on the occurrence of tardive dyskinesia or sometimes may even increase the likelihood of developing persistent dyskinesia through a possible kindling effect (Jeste, Potkin, Sinha, *et al.*, 1979; Post, 1980). Simpson believes that the reported high prevalence of tardive dyskinesia among certain patients with affective disorders might be attributable to the intermittent neuroleptic treatment of these patients. Crane *et al.* (1969) noted that patients who were receiving higher doses of neuroleptics prior to withdrawal benefited most. Longer duration of neuroleptic therapy was found to be significantly associated with persistent dyskinesia in two studies (Jeste, Potkin, Sinha, *et al.*, 1979; Yagi *et al.*, 1976). In the various studies on neuroleptic withdrawal, no relationship was noted between persistence of dyskinesia and factors such as patients' gender, primary psychiatric diagnosis, and type of neuroleptic given.

Summary

Withdrawal of neuroleptics results in remission of dyskinesia in a little over one-third of all patients. In a large number of patients with reversible dyskinesia, the symptoms remit within 3 months of discontinuing the drugs, although, for individual patients, the chances of symptom relief increase with longer periods of neuroleptic withdrawal. Aging, brain damage, and, sometimes, intermittent neuroleptic treatment have been found to be associated with persistent dyskinesia.

NONDRUG TREATMENTS

A number of psychological, surgical, electrical, dental, and other treatments have been tried in individual cases (Table 10-9).

Prosthodontia

Dental or denture problems may be caused by abnormal involuntary movements of the tongue, jaw, and lips or may make such movements worse. Using well-fitting dentures may help such patients (Evans, 1965; Lauciello & Appelbaum, 1977).

Surgery

Druckman *et al.* (1962) reported temporary relief of tardive dyskinesia in one patient who underwent bilateral thalamotomy. Nashold (1969) used bilateral stereotaxic procedures and obtained improvement in dyskinesia in one patient. The follow-up, however, suggested a likelihood of recurrence of limb dyskinesia. Heath (1977) observed remission of tardive dyskinesia in a young patient following cerebellar stimulation through an implanted pacemaker.

Table 10-9. Nondrug Treatments

Investigators	Treatment	Number of patients		
		Improved	Not improved	Total
Evans (1965)	Prosthodontia	1	0	1
Lauciello and Appel-baum (1977)	Prosthodontia	1	0	1
Kline (1968b)	Deconditioning	1	0	1
Druckman, Seelinger, and Thulin (1962)	Bilateral thalamotomy	1	0	1
Nashold (1969)	Bilateral stereotaxic lesions in tegmentum of midbrain	1	0	1
Heath (1977)	Cerebellar stimulation	1	0	1
Albanese and Gaarder (1977)	Biofeedback	2	0	2
Sherman (1979)	Biofeedback	1	0	1
Price and Levin (1978)	ECT	1	0	1
Asnis and Leopold (1978)	ECT	0	4	4
Rosenbaum, O'Connor, and Duane (1980)	ECT	1	0	1
Betts, Johnston, and Pratt (1979)	Transcutaneous nerve stimulation	1	0	1

Deconditioning

Kline (1968b) reasoned that oral dyskinesia might result from stereotyped mouth movements in response to drug-induced dryness of the mouth and successfully used a deconditioning technique in one patient.

Biofeedback

The abnormal movements in tardive dyskinesia can be controlled voluntarily by many patients, although only for brief periods. This fact, and reports of the use of biofeedback in certain other movement disorders, prompted Albanese and Gaarder (1977) to attempt biofeedback in two patients with oral dyskinesia. Ten sessions of electromyographic feedback to the masseter muscles resulted in symptom relief in the two patients, both of whom were well motivated for the treatment. Sherman (1979) also found that electromyographic feedback from the masseters was effective in controlling tardive dyskinesia in one patient; such feedback from the frontalis muscles and verbal muscle relaxation training were, however, ineffective.

Electroconvulsive Therapy

Price and Levin (1978) gave seven sessions of ECT to a depressed patient with tardive dyskinesia and noted improvement in depression as well as in dyskinesia. A similar result was reported by Rosenbaum, O'Connor, and Duane (1980), whereas Asnis and Leopold (1978) found no significant change in dyskinesia with ECT. Possible effects of ECT on tardive dyskinesia deserve to be studied carefully for clinical as well as theoretical reasons.

Transcutaneous Nerve Stimulation

Betts *et al.* (1979) used transcutaneous nerve stimulation for pain relief in a patient with severe dyskinesia. The investigator noted that the treatment also alleviated the abnormal movements.

Summary

Of the various nondrug treatments, prosthodontia should receive consideration in patients with ill-fitting dentures. Although it is not related to the central pathophysiology of tardive dyskinesia, any symptomatic improvement obtained by local procedures such as prosthodontia may be of value to the patient. Stereotaxic surgery has to be ruled out as a treatment procedure in tardive dyskinesia until the knowledge of neuropathology and the techniques in neurosurgery have advanced considerably. Behavioral methods, such as deconditioning and biofeedback, may be of some use in isolated instances. The effects of ECT on tardive dyskinesia need to be studied carefully. The various nonpharmacologic treatments have only a limited application in the specific treatment of tardive dyskinesia.

GENERAL DISCUSSION: METHODS

DIAGNOSIS OF TARDIVE DYSKINESIA

As discussed in Chapter 3, the diagnosis of tardive dyskinesia is based on clinical history and examination. Two ways of increasing the reliability of diagnosis are to specify the diagnostic criteria used and to have two or more investigators agree on the diagnosis in each patient in the study. Unfortunately, these procedures have not been commonly employed. Several studies have been questioned because of a doubt about the diagnosis of tardive dyskinesia. For example, Vale and Espejel's (1971) report of successful treatment of dyskinesia with amantadine has been criticized by Kazamatsuri (1971) and by Ringel and Klawans (1971) for questionable diagnosis. The critics wondered whether Vale and Espejel's patients had pseudoparkinsonism rather than tardive dyskinesia.

CHARACTERISTICS OF PATIENTS

Most reported studies mention patients' age, gender, and psychiatric diagnosis. In view of the suggestion that dyskinesia tends to be reversible in younger and non-brain-damaged subjects, such information may be necessary for comparing different treatment trials. It would also be useful to have some description of the evidence for or against brain damage in a given patient population.

CHARACTERISTICS
OF TARDIVE DYSKINESIA

Several investigators have found that oral dyskinesia responds to treatment better than limb or trunk dyskinesia (Bucci, 1971; Gardos & Cole, 1975; Jeste et al., 1977). Gibson (1979), however, came to the opposite conclusion with pimozide and fluspirilene treatments. Similarly, it has been mentioned that the longer the duration of dyskinesia, the more it is likely to be persistent. This remains to be demonstrated satisfactorily. Furthermore, many estimates of duration of tardive dyskinesia are rather imprecise because of the typically insidious onset of symptoms.

STUDY DESIGN

Many earlier studies on the treatment of dyskinesia were nonblind. It was thought that this disorder was an irreversible condition and that therefore any type of intervention that reduced or relieved dyskinesia must be of use in its treatment (Kunin, 1976b; Miller, 1974b; Vale & Espejel, 1971). It is now apparent, however, that there is a significant proportion of patients with dyskinesia who are placebo responders. Two well-conducted double-blind crossover studies (Penovich *et al.*, 1978; Simpson *et al.*, 1977) illustrate the need for considering nonpharmacologic factors in drug trials. In the first study all ten patients (seven on deanol and three on placebo) improved during the first of the two treatment phases, but none showed further improvement during the second phase. Penovich *et al.* (1978) noted that, of the six patients who improved with deanol, all but one also responded to placebo. Therefore the need for double-blind, placebo-controlled crossover studies is as strong for tardive dyskinesia as it is for most psychiatric disorders. That a large number of apparently unrelated treatments produce improvement in over one-third of the patients (Table 10-10) also indicates a significant percentage of placebo responders among cases of this syndrome.

The highest rate of improvement in double-blind studies is seen with neuroleptic treatment (67%). Similarly, 72% of the treatment trials with neuroleptics could be said to have "positive" results — that is, 50% or more of the patients treated (with at least four subjects in each study) improved (Table 10-11). Most treatments had less satisfactory results in double-blind studies as compared to open and single-blind trials. One exception[3] to this rule was treatment with nonneuroleptic dopamine antagonists. The latter group of drugs produced better results in double-blind studies than in open and single-blind ones. This finding is difficult to explain and may be an artifact.

SELECTION OF PATIENTS

Some investigators may select only those patients who have not responded to conventional treatments (e.g., Dynes, 1970), whereas other researchers may exclude, for practical reasons, patients with any major medical or active psychiatric problems and thus may include "more easily treatable" patients. The response rate might vary according to the method of patient selection.

---

[3]With miscellaneous drugs, there were 17 open and only 5 double-blind studies that met the criteria for inclusion in Table 10-11. Hence a comparison of the two types of studies for miscellaneous drug treatments was not particularly meaningful.

Table 10-10. Improvement Rates with Various Treatments

Treatment	Number of studies	Number of patients	Percentage of patients improved in various studies[a]		
			Open	Double-blind	Total
Neuroleptics	50	501	69	63	66.9
Other dopamine antagonists	32	323	43.8	50	46.3
Cholinergic drugs	68	379	47	30	39
GABA'ergic drugs	19	204	58.6	42.6	53.8
Dopaminergic drugs	25	146	31	8.1	24.8
Anticholinergic drugs	14	177	7.3	—	7.3
Neuroleptic withdrawal	23	1019	37	—	37
Miscellaneous drugs	57	350	42.7	34.3	40.5
TOTAL[b]	285	3099	44.5	41.7	43.8

[a] The figures represent the mean percentage of patients (weighted by the total number of patients in individual studies) who had at least moderate (50%) improvement in their symptoms.

[b] These numbers include some repeats with different treatments.

Table 10-11. Percentage of "Positive" Studies

Treatment	Open studies		Double-blind studies		Combined	
	Total	Percentage positive	Total	Percentage positive	Total	Percentage positive
Neuroleptics	17	76	12	67	29	72
Other dopamine antagonists	9	33	10	40	19	37
Cholinergic drugs	17	47	18	28	36[a]	36
GABA'ergic drugs	6	50	4	25	10	40
Dopaminergic drugs	9	44	3	0	12	25
Anticholinergic drugs	8	13	—	—	8	13
Neuroleptic withdrawal	19	37	—	—	19	37
Miscellaneous drugs	17	35	5	40	23[a]	39
TOTAL[b]	102	45	52	38	156	42

Note. Only those studies that included four or more patients and that gave results in terms of the number of patients improved were considered. "Positive" studies were the ones in which at least 50% of the patients had moderate to marked improvement.

[a] Includes one study with design not stated or mixed.

[b] Includes some repeats with different treatments.

ASSESSMENT OF SEVERITY OF SYMPTOMS

Many studies, particularly recent ones, specify the methods used for assessing severity of dyskinetic symptoms. These usually include use of various clinical rating scales. Jus *et al.* (1974) combined such a clinical assessment with a polygraphic one to make it more objective. Because of the influence of various subjective and environmental factors on the severity of dyskinesia, keeping the time and place of ratings constant throughout the experimental period and making unobtrusive observations are to be preferred. Having at least two "blind" raters and/or using devices such as videotapes or films for recording patients' symptoms also help to increase the reliability of the ratings. Klawans and Rubovits (1974) used an interesting technique of recording movement of a torch held by the patient to judge the severity of dyskinesia involving upper limbs. In view of the possible confusion of dyskinetic symptoms with those of other extrapyramidal disorders, such as drug-induced pseudoparkinsonism, a rating scale for the latter, too, has been included in some drug trials. Furthermore, some investigators also have studied changes in the severity of psychopathology during the treatment period, so as to evaluate their relationship to the severity of dyskinesia.

SEPARATING DYSKINESIA FROM OTHER INVOLUNTARY MOVEMENTS

Drugs with sedative and muscle relaxant properties may reduce the overall severity of abnormal movements without affecting dyskinesia per se. We thus noticed that one patient whose symptoms of tardive dyskinesia were coupled with those of dystonias and schizophrenic mannerisms was helped by clonazepam. An analysis of the symptomatic improvement revealed, however, that clonazepam had reduced dystonias and mannerisms only and had had little effect on the typical signs of tardive dyskinesia.

LENGTH OF STUDY

It is interesting that a number of the "positive" studies report that the patients improve within a few days of starting treatment. This again raises the possibility of a placebo effect. Some longer term studies (Ehrensing *et al.*, 1977; Kazamatsuri, Chien, & Cole 1973) reported that the improvement in tardive dyskinesia usually reached its peak by the second week of treatment, after which the severity of dyskinesia increased again and remained at that level unless the dose of the drug was increased. It appears that sudden changes in treatment often produce a short-lasting improvement in symptoms, but that the severity of dyskinesia soon increases. It may be that the initial beneficial effect was a psychogenic one and/or there was subsequent development of tolerance to the effects of the new treatment. Gardos and Cole (1978) and Simpson *et al.* (1976) have commented on fluctuations in severity of tardive dyskinesia over time. This calls for long-term studies of any treatment for tardive dyskinesia before proclaiming its efficacy. Claims of "cure" of tardive dyskinesia within 1 day of starting a treatment such as manganese chelate (Kunin, 1976b) are rather difficult to accept.

A long-term study may help reveal the influence of various unexpected endogenous and exogenous factors on treatment outcome. For example, Bedard *et al.* (1977) observed that their dyskinetic patient, being treated with reserpine and deanol, improved during a 4-month period of amenorrhea and became worse when her gynecologist put her on estrogens. If not for this observation, they might have attributed their patient's response to reserpine and deanol.

DRUG DOSAGE

Most studies on relatively larger samples of patients have employed fixed dosage schedules. Although this is more practicable, it does not take into account quantitative differences in individual patients' needs for a drug, based on differences in their weight, severity of symptoms, etc.

CONCURRENT MEDICATIONS, ESPECIALLY NEUROLEPTICS

This is an important issue in considering any treatment study for tardive dyskinesia. In about two-thirds of patients, dyskinetic symptoms are masked or reduced by neuroleptics, whereas in about one-third of patients, withdrawal of neuroleptics relieves dyskinesia. Furthermore, there is a possibility of an interaction between the experimental drug and neuroleptic, so that in a patient who is receiving both drugs simultaneously, the resultant effect on the symptoms may be due to such an interaction. Thus evaluation of the presumably specific antidyskinetic effects of a drug poses many problems. One of the better ways to avoid these would be to stop the neuroleptics at least 3 months before the study. This would serve to exclude cases of tardive dyskinesia that respond to neuroleptic withdrawal and also to avoid the question of the effects of neuroleptics on dyskinesia. In those patients in whom such a neuroleptic withdrawal is not feasible because of the risk of psychotic relapse, the neuroleptics should be continued at a stable dose for at least 1 month before and throughout the study period.

STATISTICAL ANALYSIS OF DATA

Studies on small numbers of patients have usually reported the results in terms of the numbers of patients improved or not improved. The degree of improvement is sometimes specified as minimal, mild, moderate, and marked. Placebo-controlled experiments involving large numbers of patients have analyzed the results in one of two ways—comparing the average degree of improvement obtained with the drug and with the placebo or comparing the numbers of patients improved with the two treatments. Although the former method may seem more accurate in considering the "amount" of improvement, it has a serious drawback. With a sufficient number of patients, an average drop in severity of symptoms from 80% to 50%, for example, may show that the treatment effect is statistically significant. Yet, the fact remains that the patients still have 50% of their symptoms. Given that the severity of tardive dyskinesia varies over time without any change in treatment, a statistically significant effect may be clinically nonsignificant. Simpson *et al.* (1976) have referred to this distinction between statistically and clinically significant improvement. This point is well illustrated in a study by Gardos, Cole, and Sniffin (1976) on the value of papaverine in tardive dyskinesia. The investigators observed a statistically significant reduction in the overall rating scale scores of nine patients treated with papaverine. Yet, a clinically significant improvement (50% or greater improvement) was seen in only two patients, the others showing less than a 33% drop in the severity of dyskinesia.

PRESUMED SPECIFICITY OF TREATMENT EFFECTS

Even when a particular treatment is shown to be effective for relief of tardive dyskinesia, the underlying mechanism of action remains uncertain. Most drugs have multiple actions, and the possibility remains that a drug may not owe its efficacy to the specific action in which the investigator is interested. Thus a number of investigators found physostigmine to have a transitory ameliorating effect on dyskinesia and attributed this to its cholinergic action. Yet, Tamminga, Smith, Ericksen, et al. (1977), who also noted a significant response to physostigmine, found a comparable improvement with methohexital, a sedative; they therefore entertained the possibility that physostigmine might owe its antidyskinetic effect to its sedative property rather than to its cholinergic action. It is well known that dyskinesia disappears during sleep and is aggravated by anxiety. Thus it is advisable, in conducting double-blind trials on drugs that also have sedative properties, to use an active placebo with similar sedative action. Neuroleptics are probably the only known major class of drugs that may have specific antidyskinetic effect.

SIDE EFFECTS OF THE EXPERIMENTAL TREATMENT

Deanol has been reported to produce peripheral cholinergic side effects in some patients (Rosenbaum et al., 1977). Emergence of such symptoms during a double-blind trial is likely to make the study nonblind unless the placebo also produces similar side effects.

ANALYSIS OF DROPOUTS

Several studies on relatively large numbers of patients report a significant proportion of dropouts from the experiment (Fann et al., 1973; Gerlach, Thorsen, & Munkvad, 1975; Reda et al., 1975; Simpson et al., 1976). The reasons for dropping out are protean—for example, side effects, lack of responsiveness, worsening of symptoms, or practical problems such as a family crisis. Unless the reasons for dropping out, when known, are specified, it may sometimes be difficult to interpret the overall effects of the experimental treatment.

REPORTING STUDIES

It is probably a universal phenomenon that positive results of a treatment are reported more often than negative ones. This may serve to skew literature reviews in favor of the "positive" studies.

POSSIBLE SUBTYPES OF TARDIVE DYSKINESIA

Casey (1976) suggested that there may be at least two subtypes of tardive dyskinesia, one of which responds to cholinergic drugs and the other to antidopaminergic agents. Some studies using various drugs on the same patients (Casey & Denney, 1977; Nesse & Carroll, 1976) are quoted as favoring this hypothesis. Mackay and Sheppard (1979) proposed the strategy of acute drug challenge for defining pharmacologic subtypes and thus for choosing the optimal treatment for individual patients.

We have classified tardive dyskinesia into persistent and reversible types. Response to withdrawal of neuroleptics for at least 3 months may be used as a criterion for judging reversibility of tardive dyskinesia. It is probable that patients with reversible dyskinesia respond to many nonspecific treatments, whereas persistent dyskinesia is resistant to most of the available treatments. It is interesting to note that about 35% to 45% of patients respond to many different types of drugs with dissimilar mechanisms of action (Table 10-10). This suggests that, in at least some of these cases, the positive results with the treatments given might not have been due to the specific actions of the drugs, but could have been due to such nonspecific factors as placebo response, spontaneous remission, raters' bias, and concomitant treatments, including milieu therapy, psychotherapy, or environmental manipulations. These cases probably belong to the subgroup of reversible dyskinesia. It is also possible that neuroleptic-withdrawal-induced dyskinesia may be more easily reversible than the dyskinesia that develops during the course of neuroleptic treatment, although this remains to be studied.

WELL-DESIGNED TREATMENT STUDIES

Following are suggestions for well-designed treatment studies:

1. Diagnosis of tardive dyskinesia should be based on strict criteria (see Chapter 3). It should be confirmed by at least two investigators independently and should be made by repeated, unobtrusive observations.

2. If possible, neuroleptics and other psychotropic medications should be withdrawn for at least 3 months before the study. Most cases of reversible dyskinesia can thus be excluded. If this is not feasible, neuroleptics and other drugs should be maintained at a stable dose level for at least 1 month before the study and throughout the trial period.

3. Patients with persistent tardive dyskinesia should then be assigned to two or more treatment groups. All the groups should be comparable, particularly in terms of age, psychiatric diagnosis (especially with respect to organic mental syndrome), length of neuroleptic treatment, and localization and duration of dyskinesia.

4. Double-blind crossover designs should preferably use active placebo.

5. Dosage should be flexible, according to a patient's individual needs as determined (by a nonrating clinician) on the basis of the patient's age, weight, medical and psychiatric status, and past history of drug response. Blood concentrations of the drug should be analyzed, if available.

6. Severity of symptoms of dyskinesia, other extrapyramidal symptoms, and psychopathology should be assessed by at least two independent raters. Standardized rating scales for these purposes—for example, the AIMS (see Appendix)—should be used. Videotaping or filming, and employing objective methods for assessment of tardive dyskinesia are also recommended. The evaluations of patients should be done at the same time (of the day and the week) and at the same place throughout the experiment. These should be carried out at least once a week.

7. Long-term trials are preferred to short-term ones.

8. Data should be analyzed in terms of both the average change in scores (absolute, as well as percentage, change) and the number of patients showing 50% or greater improvement.

9. Reasons for dropouts should be analyzed.

10. Among the large number of potentially useful lines of research, the following seem to be more pragmatic at present:

a. Effects of continued neuroleptic administration in dyskinetic patients who require neuroleptics for the control of their psychotic symptoms. Such patients should be carefully monitored for various behavioral, biochemical, and neuropathological changes.

b. Specificity of drug actions. If patients responding to a certain drug also respond similarly to other drugs of the same family (e.g., cholinergic), but not to different types of drugs (e.g., dopamine-blocking), the specificity of drug actions would be supported. It will also favor the possibility of subtypes of tardive dyskinesia on a biochemical basis (Casey & Denney, 1977; Mackay & Sheppard, 1979).

c. The desensitization technique of Jus *et al.* (1979), treatment with DBH inhibitors such as fusaric acid (Viukari & Linnoila, 1977) or disulfiram, treatment with noradrenergic blockers such as propanolol or clonidine, receptor sensitivity modification with chronic L-dopa treatment (Alpert & Friedhoff, 1980), or use of drugs (such as carbamazepine) that retard kindling (Post, 1980) have considerable potential theoretical and clinical value. The latter suggestion is based on the possibility that persistent dyskinesia in some patients may be associated with repeated, lengthy drug interruptions during chronic neuroleptic treatment and that these drug interruptions may have a kindling effect (Jeste, Potkin, Sinha, *et al.*, 1979) similar to the postulated kindling effect of alcohol withdrawal (Ballenger & Post, 1978).

GENERAL DISCUSSION: RESULTS

Tables 10-10 and 10-11 summarize the results of various studies. It is apparent that there is no single treatment modality that can be called "the most effective treatment" for tardive dyskinesia.

Probably the greatest number of dyskinetic patients reported in these studies have been "treated" by withdrawal of neuroleptics. Most of the investigators conclude that tardive dyskinesia is more likely to disappear on withdrawing neuroleptics in younger and non-brain-damaged patients (Degkwitz, 1969; Dynes, 1970; Edwards, 1970; Hunter *et al.*, 1964; Paulson, 1968b; Pryce & Edwards, 1966; Turunen & Achte, 1967; Uhrbrand & Faurbye, 1960; Yagi *et al.*, 1976). The criteria for brain damage have, however, been different in different studies. Two studies found a high proportion of cases of persistent dyskinesia in patients given interrupted treatment (Degkwitz, 1969; Jeste, Potkin, Sinha, *et al.*, 1979).

Taken as a group, neuroleptics have been the most effective drugs for suppressing dyskinesia. This creates an ethical dilemma in that the drugs used for treating tardive dyskinesia are the same that probably caused it in the first place. There is a concern that continued administration of neuroleptics may make dyskinesia irreversible (Hollister, 1975) and/or more severe. Several long-term trials of neuroleptics have found no evidence of ill effects of the neuroleptic treatment on dyskinesia. In one long-term study comparing the effects of neuroleptic administration versus neuroleptic withdrawal, Turek *et al.* (1972) noted significant improvement in tardive dyskinesia during the periods of neuroleptic administration and worsening with neuroleptic withdrawal. The use of neuroleptics for treating dyskinesia may be compared to the use of opiates in the treatment of opiate dependence, although the two situations have some obvious differences. Another possibility, which has not been explored carefully, is that of development of tolerance to nigrostriatal catecholaminergic hyperactivity with continued neuroleptic treatment. Tolerance is known to develop for most other extrapyramidal, autonomic, and sedative side effects of neuroleptics (Davis, 1980). It is conceivable that similar tolerance to tardive dyskinesia may develop in at least some patients.

Although more studies have been done on deanol than on any other single drug for treating tardive dyskinesia, the value of deanol still remains questionable. Significant improvement in dyskinesia was reported in a majority of studies using physostigmine. However, these trials employed intravenous administration of the drug on a single occasion and studied its short-lasting effects. There is uncertainty about the duration of the effects of physostigmine on dyskinesia. With comparable doses of the drug, Davis, Hollister, Barchas, *et al.* (1976) found that the effects lasted for 2 hours, whereas Fann *et al.* (1974) noted maximum improvement 24 hours after the injection. Furthermore, Tamminga, Smith, Ericksen, *et al.* (1977) have attributed the salutary effects of physostigmine to its sedative action. The hope of a successful cholinergic drug for tardive dyskinesia has not yet materialized. Choline and lecithin are still to be considered experimental treatments for tardive dyskinesia.

Putative GABA'ergic drugs, such as benzodiazepines, have been reported to reduce symptoms of dyskinesia in some studies. Most of these investigations, however, were carried out in a nonblind design. There is a possibility that these drugs may exert their effects on tardive dyskinesia as sedatives and not necessarily through their central GABA'ergic action. Well-designed studies on large patient populations are needed for assessing the exact value of GABA agonist agents in the treatment of tardive dyskinesia. The same holds true for nonneuroleptic dopamine antagonists.

There is a general consensus that antiparkinsonian agents—both anticholinergic (e.g., trihexyphenidyl) and dopaminergic (e.g., amantadine or L-dopa in the usual doses for the treatment of Parkinson's disease—do not help, and indeed may aggravate, the symptoms of tardive dyskinesia.

SUMMARY

There is still no satisfactory treatment for the majority of patients with neuroleptic-induced tardive dyskinesia. Paradoxically, neuroleptics are the most effective and the most specific dyskinesia-suppressing agents. Studies have shown that administration of neuroleptics for weeks or months to patients with dyskinesia does not result in a worsening of the dyskinesia; however, longer term studies are lacking, and therefore caution should be used in prescribing neuroleptics to dyskinetic patients for long periods. Withdrawal of neuroleptics leads to reversal of dyskinesia in a little over one-third of all patients. GABA'ergic agents are more effective than most other nonneuroleptic drugs in suppressing dyskinesia. Anticholinergic and dopaminergic drugs should be avoided in patients with dyskinesia. Other drugs, including cholinergic agents, may be useful in certain patients, but the overall efficacy of these drugs in treating tardive dyskinesia is uncertain.

CHAPTER XI

Suggestions for Clinical Use of Neuroleptics

MAIN ISSUES

The need for weighing benefits and risks associated with potent drugs is not restricted to the use of neuroleptics. As Koch-Weser (1974) asserted, "Few drugs that help anybody will not hurt somebody, and all potent drugs, no matter how skillfully used, can cause serious untoward effects in some patients." That neuroleptics can produce serious side effects such as tardive dyskinesia is hardly surprising. The reasons for the concern caused by persistent tardive dyskinesia include the magnitude of the problem (see Chapter 2) and the lack of effective alternatives to neuroleptics in the treatment of the majority of chronic schizophrenic patients.

There are no known ways of preventing tardive dyskinesia in patients who receive long-term treatment with neuroleptics, nor are there satisfactory methods of managing the syndrome once it develops. A clinician is therefore caught on the horns of a dilemma. A fear of tardive dyskinesia may lead to withholding neuroleptics from a number of patients who would not respond to any other available treatment; this may constitute a serious clinical error because of the resultant aggravation or recurrence of psychosis, with damaging consequences for the patients, their families, and society. On the other hand, with long-term use of neuroleptics, there is a clinical and medicolegal risk of producing persistent tardive dyskinesia in some patients. This situation may improve in the near future as more knowledge is gained about the pathophysiology and treatment of tardive dyskinesia, schizophrenia, and other psychiatric disorders. At present, however, there is no simple solution to the problem of preventing and managing tardive dyskinesia. Two ways of coping with this problem are flexibility in the overall treatment approach and sharing the dilemma with the patients and his or her family so that they, too, have an input into decisions about the management.

One of the many unfortunate aspects of tardive dyskinesia is that there is no available method of predicting the risk of persistent tardive dyskinesia in a particular patient. Although some variables (e.g., aging) have been found to be associated with an increased prevalence of the disorder, it is not yet possible to judge the risk in an individual case. When this type of information about risk prediction becomes available, it not only may help in preventing dyskinesia in (at least some of) the high-risk subjects, but also may enable physicians to treat the low-risk patients with relatively less fear of inducing the iatrogenic syndrome.

Most of the age-old and often-repeated suggestions about treatment of patients are as applicable to tardive dyskinesia as they are to any other disorder. The primary principle of therapy is to treat the whole patient and not merely his or her present symptoms. Tardive dyskinesia is one, albeit important, aspect of treatment with neuroleptics. Ignoring tardive dyskinesia would be as inexcusable as being obsessed by a fear of dyskinesia and banishing neuroleptics from psychiatric treatment. It is the physician's responsibility to try to find the most practical approach to the management of an individual patient. The treatment strategy that is worked out may not always be the ideal one; however, with the patient and his or her family contributing to the decision-making process, the clinician's burden will be lightened.

The issue of obtaining "informed consent" from patients who are to be treated with neuroleptics is controversial. The various medicolegal issues involved have been discussed by Ayd (1977), Brooks (1981), Jaffe (1981), Stone (1979, 1981), and others. According to DeVeaugh-Geiss (1979) and Sovner, DiMascio, Berkovitz, et al. (1978), a written informed consent for neuroleptic treatment is necessary. However, a questionnaire survey completed by senior psychiatrists from 42 institutions in the United States and Canada (Baldessarini et al., 1980) showed that only 11% of the respondents favored a written consent for prolonged neuroleptic treatment. It is likely that future court decisions may dictate procedures such as obtaining consent from patients.

Some suggestions for prevention and management of tardive dyskinesia are discussed in the remainder of this chapter. Epidemiologically, prevention is of three types. Primary prevention (which is the type commonly referred to simply as "prevention") of tardive dyskinesia would aim at reducing the *incidence* of the disorder (i.e., occurrence of new cases of dyskinesia). Secondary prevention is the early detection and treatment of tardive dyskinesia, aimed at lowering the *prevalence* of the disorder (i.e., the total number of cases at a given time). Tertiary prevention is the treatment of complications of tardive dyskinesia so as to reduce the misery and dysfunction of patients in whom the disorder itself is irreversible. Secondary and tertiary prevention are often included under the term "management."

There are three types of clinical situations that need to be discussed with reference to prevention and management of tardive dyskinesia:

1. Patients presenting for the first time as possible candidates for neuroleptic therapy.
2. Patients who are already receiving neuroleptics and who do not have dyskinesia.
3. Patients who have developed tardive dyskinesia.

The first two situations call for a consideration of primary prevention of tardive dyskinesia, whereas the last one warrants secondary or tertiary prevention.

PATIENTS AT COMMENCEMENT OF NEUROLEPTIC TREATMENT

When patients present themselves or are brought for psychiatric treatment, the first step for the physician to perform is a thorough psychiatric and physical evaluation. This is based primarily on history taking and clinical examination, aided, when necessary, by psychological and laboratory tests. The clinician should make at least a tentative diagnosis before deciding about possible treatments.

According to the American Psychiatric Association Task Force on Tardive Dyskinesia (Baldessarini *et al.,* 1980), long-term use of neuroleptics is primarily indicated in schizophrenia, paranoia, childhood psychoses, and certain neuropsychiatric disorders such as Gilles de la Tourette's syndrome and Huntington's disease. Short-term administration (for less than 6 months) of neuroleptics is also justifiable in many cases of acute psychotic episodes, manic excitement, agitated depression, certain organic mental disorders, and medical conditions including intractable hiccoughs, nausea, and vomiting.

Development of persistent tardive dyskinesia within 3 months of beginning neuroleptic therapy is rare. Therefore it should not be necessary at this stage of treatment to have a detailed discussion with the patient and his or her family about the risk of tardive dyskinesia. The goal of the initial treatment in acutely psychotic patients is to provide symptom relief. There is little justification for withholding the use of neuroleptics in such cases until an "informed consent" is obtained.

PATIENTS ALREADY RECEIVING NEUROLEPTICS

A clinician frequently encounters patients without dyskinesia who have been receiving neuroleptics for more than 3 months. Assuming that the physician has already completed a thorough physical and psychiatric evaluation and has arrived at a diagnosis, two additional steps are warranted at this phase of treatment: (1) assessment and documentation of the need to continue neuroleptics and (2) discussion with the patient and his or her family about the risk of tardive dyskinesia.

ASSESSMENT AND DOCUMENTATION OF THE NEED FOR CONTINUING NEUROLEPTICS

Primary indications for long-term use of neuroleptics have already been enumerated.[1] In other patients an attempt should be made, after 3 months of neuroleptic therapy, to reduce the dosage and, preferably, to discontinue neuroleptics. If this maneuver leads to an unacceptable level of severity of symptoms, and if both the physician and the patient explicitly agree to resume neuroleptics despite a possible risk of tardive dyskinesia, the drugs may be resumed. Documentation of the reasons for continuing neuroleptics in such patients should be made.

The role of neuroleptics in the maintenance therapy of schizophrenia is well established. On reviewing the literature on this subject, Davis (1980) concludes that there is a 50% relapse rate among moderately ill

---

[1]The efficacy of neuroleptics in the long-term management of two of these primary indications, paranoia and childhood psychoses, remains to be established satisfactorily with the help of controlled studies (Baldessarini *et al.,* 1980). Furthermore, not all schizophrenic patients benefit from or need maintenance treatment with neuroleptics. Also, neuroleptics are more effective in relieving "positive" symptoms of schizophrenia (e.g., hallucinations, delusions) than "negative" symptoms such as emotional blunting.

schizophrenics within 6 months of discontinuation of their medication. Hogarty and Goldberg (1973) studied the value of maintenance therapy with neuroleptics in schizophrenic patients discharged from hospitals. The investigators found that about two-thirds of the patients maintained on placebo relapsed within a year, while only 16% of those who took neuroleptics regularly relapsed during that period. In view of the serious impact of a relapse on the patient and his or her family, Davis recommends that most schizophrenics be maintained on neuroleptics for 3 months to a year after the control of acute symptoms and that treatment thereafter be individualized. Severity of illness and past history of a recurrence on discontinuing medication or reducing dosage suggest a relatively high risk of relapse. In any case, once the patient has recovered from an acute psychotic episode and has remained in a stable psychiatric condition, the psychiatrist should begin to reduce the neuroleptic dosage. He or she may do so gradually over a period of several months; this may enable the psychiatrist to detect early signs of relapse. If the patient shows signs of a recurrence, the physician may reinstitute the medication or increase the dose.

An essential part of the maintenance therapy with neuroleptics is evaluation and documentation of the need for continuing the medication. Routinely and blindly prescribing neuroleptics on a long-term basis without ever assessing and documenting a need for the same is indefensible. This does not mean that the clinician has to stop the medication for prolonged periods in every patient. If the clinician finds that a mere reduction of dose results in a marked aggravation of psychotic symptoms in a patient, he or she may be justified in raising the dose immediately. However, this fact should be recorded in the patient's chart.

Neuroleptics should be administered in the lowest effective doses. A review of the studies of neuroleptics in the long-term treatment of schizophrenia (Baldessarini & Davis, 1980) suggested that the maintenance doses required by many patients might be low. The authors found no significant difference in relapse rates at doses higher than versus lower than 310 mg equivalents of chlorpromazine. Also, there was no significant correlation between reduction of relapse rates and neuroleptic doses ranging from 100 to more than 2000 mg equivalents of chlorpromazine. Thus it appears that many chronic schizophrenic patients do not need more than 300 mg equivalents of chlorpromazine daily to prevent exacerbations; the necessary dose may sometimes be as low as 100 mg per 24 hours.

In Chapter 4 a reference was made to the issue of frequent and lengthy drug-free periods. Some psychopharmacologists recommend prolonged drug interruptions in order to reduce the incidence of persistent tardive dyskinesia. There is, however, little evidence to indicate that intermittent neuroleptic therapy prevents persistent tardive dyskinesia; in a subgroup of patients, it might even increase the likelihood of development of persistent dyskinesia (Degkwitz, 1969; Jeste, Potkin, Sinha, *et al.*, 1979). Furthermore, routine use of lengthy drug interruptions may result in psychotic relapses in a number of patients. This is not to suggest continuous long-term administration of neuroleptics to all patients, but to advocate that the treatment be individualized to suit each patient's requirements, including that of avoiding a relapse or exacerbation of psychotic symptoms, and that the physician record the rationale for his or her decisions in every case.

DISCUSSION WITH THE PATIENT AND HIS OR HER FAMILY ABOUT THE RISK OF TARDIVE DYSKINESIA

It is advisable, both for ethical and medicolegal reasons, that the clinician discuss with patients who have been receiving neuroleptics for 3 months and their families the possible risk of development of tardive dyskinesia. Three main aspects should be brought to their attention: possible benefits from the use of neuroleptics, the possibility of developing tardive dyskinesia, and treatment alternatives (to neuroleptics), with their own advantages and disadvantages. The discussion will, of course, vary, depending on the individual patient and on the kind of patient–therapist relationship. Following is a brief outline of the salient points that the patient may be made aware of.

Benefits of Neuroleptic Treatment

Neuroleptics have been shown to be the most effective treatment for schizophrenia. They are useful not only for relieving acute psychotic symptoms, but also for preventing relapses in schizophrenic patients. Whereas four of six schizophrenics would relapse within a year of discontinuing neuroleptics, only one of six patients taking neuroleptics regularly would have a recurrence of illness within a year. A psychotic relapse may have a serious impact on the patient and his or her family.

Risk of Developing Tardive Dyskinesia

Treatment with neuroleptics for months and years has been known to produce tardive dyskinesia in a variable proportion of patients. Old persons are more likely to develop this complication than young patients. The dyskinesia consists of abnormal movements, usually of the tongue, lips, and jaws, and sometimes of the upper limbs, lower limbs, and trunk. The risk of developing tardive dyskinesia cannot be estimated for an individual patient. There are no known ways of preventing the disorder in patients who are treated with neuroleptics for prolonged periods. Early detection of dyskinesia is advisable; it is, however, made difficult by the slow evolution and the painless nature of the symptoms. After it is detected, stopping the neuroleptics will result in an eventual disappearance of dyskinesia in over one-third of patients. A number of treatments have been tried for the remaining patients, but none is uniformly satisfactory. In the majority of patients who develop tardive dyskinesia, the symptoms are mild to moderate in intensity; a small proportion of patients have symptoms severe enough to interfere with physical functions, such as swallowing or speaking.

Alternative Treatments

Several forms of alternative treatments for schizophrenia are available—for example, psychotherapy, ECT, or milieu therapy. However, none of them is as effective as neuroleptics for the treatment of the majority of chronic schizophrenic patients. Each of these alternative treatments has its own advantages and disadvantages.

A discussion of all these points may enable the patient and his or her family to arrive at a decision regarding continuation of neuroleptics. The physician should stress that all potent treatments have a risk:benefit ratio and that one may need to choose the lesser of the two evils (e.g., tardive dyskinesia vs. psychotic relapse). It may also be clarified that, whatever decision the patient makes, it is not an irrevocable one and that later experience may result in either reinstitution or discontinuation of the medication.

At present, most clinicians do not require a written consent from patients who do not have dyskinesia and who are to be maintained on neuroleptics. It should, however, be documented that the risk of tardive dyskinesia was discussed with the patient and his or her family and that a verbal assent for neuroleptic administration was obtained. (For legally incompetent patients without close relatives, such discussion should be held with the patients and their legally authorized guardians or representatives.)

Other Considerations

Today most (but not all) psychopharmacologists agree that antiparkinsonian medications should be restricted to the treatment of parkinsonian symptoms and should not be prescribed prophylactically as a routine accompaniment to neuroleptics.

The clinician should be alert to the possibility that any patient on long-term neuroleptic therapy may develop tardive dyskinesia. Routine evaluations for abnormal involuntary movements of the mouth, limbs, and trunk are necessary. Keeping in mind the early manifestations and the diagnostic criteria for tardive dyskinesia (see Chapter 3) and being familiar with the AIMS are helpful. (It should be added that the AIMS is meant for judging the severity of the abnormal movements and is not a test for diagnosing tardive dyskinesia.)

PATIENTS WITH TARDIVE DYSKINESIA

When a physician diagnoses or even suspects tardive dyskinesia in a patient, the following sequential procedure for management may be recommended. This is, of course, a general outline, and variations in the treatment plan may be warranted according to specific needs of the individual patient.

DIAGNOSIS OF TARDIVE DYSKINESIA

A diagnosis of tardive dyskinesia may be made on the basis of certain diagnostic criteria and after excluding conditions in the differential diagnosis (see Chapter 3). Repeated clinical examinations for the abnormal movements and neurological and dental evaluations may be required for making a diagnosis of tardive dyskinesia. A second opinion from a colleague may be advisable in doubtful cases.

INFORMING THE PATIENT AND HIS OR HER FAMILY

Once the clinician has arrived at a definite diagnosis of tardive dyskinesia, this should be conveyed to the patient and his or her family or legally authorized guardian. The relevant aspects of this syndrome, described earlier, should be explained, including the fact that the symptoms are usually not incapacitating and that they are reversible on discontinuing neuroleptics in over one-third of patients with dyskinesia. The diagnosis of tardive dyskinesia and the duration (if known) and severity of symptoms should be recorded in the patient's chart.

TRIAL OF NEUROLEPTIC WITHDRAWAL

After tardive dyskinesia is diagnosed, the clinician should attempt to discontinue the neuroleptics gradually. He or she need not do so immediately if the patient has active psychotic symptoms, but should try to begin lowering the neuroleptic dose as soon as the patient's psychiatric condition improves sufficiently. Possible exceptions to this trial of neuroleptic withdrawal or dose reduction in dyskinesia are (1) patients who continue to be actively psychotic and in whom any dose reduction is likely to result in further worsening of mental symptoms and (2) patients who refuse to have any lowering of the dose in spite of the presence of tardive dyskinesia. In both these situations, the physician should record the reasons for not reducing the medication and should have consent from the patient and his or her family or guardian for continuing neuroleptics.

A trial of neuroleptic withdrawal in patients with tardive dyskinesia is important for assessing the need for continuing the drugs as well as for reversing the dyskinesia in over one-third of the patients. The physician may often wish to add sedatives such as benzodiazepines during this period of neuroleptic withdrawal so as to reduce the intensity of psychiatric and dyskinetic symptoms in at least some patients. If there still results an aggravation of the symptoms that is of an unacceptable severity, the clinician may return to the previous dosage of the neuroleptics. He or she should, however, document this experience in the patient's chart.

Treatment without neuroleptics may be difficult in a number of patients, especially schizophrenics. Various other forms of therapy (psychotherapy, ECT, sedatives, milieu therapy, etc.) may be considered.

DISCONTINUING ANTIPARKINSONIAN DRUGS

Drugs such as trihexyphenidyl, biperiden, benztropine, and orphenadrine, which are all anticholinergic agents used to treat parkinsonian symptoms, may aggravate tardive dyskinesia. There is little justification for maintaining dyskinetic patients on these drugs, unless their withdrawal is found to produce marked and persistent aggravation of dyskinesia in a particular patient.

ADMINISTERING NEUROLEPTICS TO PATIENTS WHO NEED THEM

Patients with tardive dyskinesia may need to be treated with neuroleptics under the following specific circumstances:

1. If neuroleptic reduction produces a significant aggravation of psychiatric symptoms that does not respond to other forms of treatment.
2. If past history suggests a high risk of psychotic relapse on discontinuing neuroleptics.
3. If neuroleptic withdrawal results in a marked and persistent worsening of dyskinesia, which does not improve with sedatives and other treatments.
4. If the patient and his or her family (or guardian) refuse to allow lowering of the medication.

In these cases, administering neuroleptics will be justified. The clinician may, however, be advised to follow certain suggestions:

1. The reasons for prescribing neuroleptics to dyskinetic patients should be documented.
2. A consent should be obtained from the patient and his or her family or guardian.
3. A type of neuroleptic that was not given to a particular patient in the past may be preferred. Although all of the currently available neuroleptics carry some risk of inducing tardive dyskinesia, specific neuroleptics could be better or worse for individual patients.

4. The lowest dose of the drug that is effective for the particular patient should be used.
5. The drug may be given in a divided daily dose schedule rather than in a single large daily dose. Jeste *et al.* (1977) noted that in some patients the dyskinetic symptoms were controlled better by administering a neuroleptic in small divided doses.
6. A periodic and careful review of the patient's mental status and the severity of his or her dyskinesia should be done and the findings recorded.

As stressed in Chapter 10, neuroleptics are the most effective temporary suppressors of dyskinesia. However, since these drugs have been responsible for tardive dyskinesia, their use in patients with dyskinesia must be cautious. The desensitization technique of Jus *et al.* (1979), employing slow and progressive reduction of neuroleptic dosage over several years, may be of value in some patients.

OTHER TREATMENTS FOR DYSKINESIA

A number of pharmacologic and other treatments have been tried in dyskinetic patients. Of these, anticholinergic and dopaminergic drugs have no place in the clinical treatment of tardive dyskinesia. Sedatives such as benzodiazepines may have a beneficial effect in some patients. Dental prosthetic therapy may be helpful when indicated. Other treatments may still be considered experimental.

SUMMARY

There are no known ways of preventing tardive dyskinesia in patients who receive long-term treatment with neuroleptics, nor is there a generally satisfactory treatment for the disorder. The clinician can best deal with the dilemma associated with the chronic administration of neuroleptics by using a flexible approach, assessing and documenting the need for continuing neuroleptics, making the patient and his or her family partners in decisions about the treatment, avoiding all unnecessary medications, and being alert to the risk of tardive dyskinesia. Long-term use of neuroleptics is primarily indicated in those patients with schizophrenia, paranoia, childhood psychoses, and neuropsychiatric disorders (such as Tourette's syndrome) in whom a discontinuation of the medication is likely to result in a relapse or a significant exacerbation of symptoms. Neuroleptics should be administered in the lowest effective doses. In patients with tardive dyskinesia, withdrawal of neuroleptics should be attempted.

Appendix

ABNORMAL INVOLUNTARY MOVEMENT SCALE (AIMS)

EXAMINATION PROCEDURE

Either before or after completing the examination procedure, observe the patient unobtrusively at rest (e.g., in waiting room).

The chair to be used in this examination should be a hard, firm one without arms.

1. Ask patient whether there is anything in mouth (gum, candy, etc.), and if there is, to remove it.
2. Ask patient about the *current* condition of his or her teeth. Ask if patient wears dentures. Do teeth or dentures bother patient *now*?
3. Ask whether patient notices any movements in mouth, face, hands, or feet. If yes, ask to describe and to what extent they *currently* bother patient or interfere with activities.
4. Have patient sit in chair with hands on knees, legs slightly apart, and feet flat on floor. (Look at entire body for movements while in this position.)
5. Ask patient to sit with hands hanging unsupported—if male, between legs, and if female and wearing a dress, hanging over knees. (Observe hands and other body areas.)
6. Ask patient to open mouth. (Observe tongue at rest within mouth.) Do this twice.
7. Ask patient to protrude tongue. (Observe abnormalities of tongue movement.) Do this twice.
8. Ask patient to tap thumb, with each finger, as rapidly as possible for 10 to 15 seconds —first with right hand, then with left hand. (Observe facial and leg movements.)
9. Flex and extend patient's left and right arms (one at a time). (Note any rigidity separately.)
10. Ask patient to stand up. (Observe in profile. Observe all body areas again, hips included.)
11. Ask patient to extend both arms outstretched in front with palms down. (Observe trunk, legs, and mouth.)
12. Have patient walk a few paces, turn, and walk back to chair. (Observe hands and gait.) Do this twice.

DEPARTMENT OF HEALTH, EDUCATION, AND WELFARE
PUBLIC HEALTH SERVICE
ALCOHOL, DRUG ABUSE, AND MENTAL HEALTH ADMINISTRATION
NATIONAL INSTITUTE OF MENTAL HEALTH

ABNORMAL INVOLUNTARY
MOVEMENT SCALE
(AIMS)

	STUDY	PATIENT	FORM	PERIOD	RATER	HOSPITAL
			117			
	(1-6)	(7-9)	(10-12)	(13-15)	(16-17)	(79-80)

PATIENT'S NAME

RATER

DATE

INSTRUCTIONS: Complete Examination Procedure before making ratings.   Code:

MOVEMENT RATINGS: Rate highest severity observed.
Rate movements that occur upon activation one _less_ than
those observed spontaneously.

0 = None
1 = Minimal, may be extreme normal
2 = Mild
3 = Moderate
4 = Severe

CARD 01
(18-19)

(Circle One)

FACIAL AND ORAL MOVEMENTS:	1. **Muscles of Facial Expression** e.g., movements of forehead, eyebrows, periorbital area, cheeks; include frowning, blinking, smiling, grimacing	0	1	2	3	4	(20)
	2. **Lips and Perioral Area** e.g., puckering, pouting, smacking	0	1	2	3	4	(21)
	3. **Jaw** e.g., biting, clenching, chewing, mouth opening, lateral movement	0	1	2	3	4	(22)
	4. **Tongue** Rate only increase in movement both in and out of mouth, NOT inability to sustain movement	0	1	2	3	4	(23)
EXTREMITY MOVEMENTS:	5. **Upper** _(arms, wrists, hands, fingers)_ Include choreic movements, (**i.e.**, rapid, objectively purposeless, irregular, spontaneous), athetoid movements (i.e., slow, irregular, complex, serpentine). Do NOT include tremor (i.e., repetitive, regular, rhythmic)	0	1	2	3	4	(24)
	6. **Lower** _(legs, knees, ankles, toes)_ e.g., lateral knee movement, foot tapping, heel dropping, foot squirming, inversion and eversion of foot	0	1	2	3	4	(25)

		0	1	2	3	4	
TRUNK MOVEMENTS:	7. Neck, shoulders, hips e.g., rocking, twisting, squirming, pelvic gyrations						(26)
	8. Severity of abnormal movements	None, normal — 0 Minimal — 1 Mild — 2 Moderate — 3 Severe — 4					(27)
GLOBAL JUDGMENTS:	9. Incapacitation due to abnormal movements	None, normal — 0 Minimal — 1 Mild — 2 Moderate — 3 Severe — 4					(28)
	10. Patient's awareness of abnormal movements Rate only patient's report	No awareness — 0 Aware, no distress — 1 Aware, mild distress — 2 Aware, moderate distress — 3 Aware, severe distress — 4					(29)
DENTAL STATUS:	11. Current problems with teeth and/or dentures	No — 0 Yes — 1					(30)
	12. Does patient usually wear dentures?	No — 0 Yes — 1					(31)

MH-9—117
11-74

Abnormal Involuntary Movement Scale developed by the Psychopharmacology Research Branch; National Institute of Mental Health; Alcohol, Drug Abuse, and Mental Health Administration; Public Health Service; U.S. Department of Health, Education, and Welfare. (From *Early Clinical Drug Evaluation Unit Intercom*, 1975, *4*, 3–6.)

ROCKLAND RESEARCH INSTITUTE (SIMPSON)
ABBREVIATED DYSKINESIA RATING SCALE

Patient _____ # _____ Date _____ Time _____ A.M./P.M.
Setting _____ Study # _____ Rater # _____ Period _____

	Rating*
Facial and oral movements	
1. Periocular area (blinking of eyes, tremor of eyelids)	1 2 3 4 5 6
2. Movements of the lips (pouting, puckering, smacking)	1 2 3 4 5 6
3. Chewing movements	1 2 3 4 5 6
4. Bonbon sign	1 2 3 4 5 6
5. Tongue protrusion	1 2 3 4 5 6
6. Tremor and/or choreoathetoid movements of the tongue	1 2 3 4 5 6
7. Other (describe) _____	1 2 3 4 5 6
Neck and trunk	
8. Axial hyperkinesis (patient standing)	1 2 3 4 5 6
9. Rocking movements	1 2 3 4 5 6
10. Torsion movements	1 2 3 4 5 6
11. Other (describe) _____	1 2 3 4 5 6
Extremities	
12. Movements of fingers and wrists	1 2 3 4 5 6
13. Movements of ankles and toes	1 2 3 4 5 6
14. Stamping movements	1 2 3 4 5 6
15. Other (describe) _____	1 2 3 4 5 6
Entire body	
16. Akathisia	1 2 3 4 5 6
17. Other (describe) _____	1 2 3 4 5 6

*Rating   1 – absent   4 – moderate   Total score:
        2 – questionable   5 – moderately severe
        3 – mild   6 – severe

From "A Rating Scale for Tardive Dyskinesia" by G. M. Simpson, J. H. Lee, B. Zoubok, *et al.*, *Psychopharmacology*, 1979, *64*, 171–179. Reprinted with the permission of the publishers.

References

Adams, R. D., & Victor, M. *Principles of neurology.* New York: McGraw-Hill, 1977.

Adamson, L., Curry, S. H., Bridges, P. K., *et al.* Fluphenazine decanoate trial in chronic inpatient schizophrenics failing to absorb oral chlorpromazine. *Diseases of the Nervous System,* 1973, *34,* 181–191.

Ahmad, S., Laidlaw, J., Houghton, G. W., *et al.* Involuntary movements caused by phenytoin intoxication in epileptic patients. *Journal of Neurology, Neurosurgery and Psychiatry,* 1975, *38,* 225–231.

Akindele, M. O., & Odejide, A. O. Amodiaquine-induced involuntary movements. *British Medical Journal,* 1976, *2,* 214–215.

Albanese, H., & Gaarder, K. Biofeedback treatment of tardive dyskinesia: Two case reports. *American Journal of Psychiatry,* 1977, *134,* 1149–1150.

Alexopoulos, G. S. Lack of complaints in schizophrenics with tardive dyskinesia. *Journal of Nervous and Mental Disease,* 1979, *167,* 125–127.

Allen, R. E., & Stimmel, G. L. Neuroleptic dosage, duration, and tardive dyskinesia. *Journal of Clinical Psychiatry,* 1977, *38,* 385–387.

Alpert, M., & Friedhoff, A. J. Clinical application of receptor modification. In W. E. Fann, R. C. Smith, J. M. Davis, *et al.* (Eds.), *Tardive dyskinesia: Research and treatment.* New York: SP Medical & Scientific Books, 1980.

Altrocchi, P. H. Spontaneous oral-facial dyskinesia. *Archives of Neurology,* 1972, *26,* 506–512.

American College of Neuropsychopharmacology–FDA Task Force. Neurological syndromes associated with antipsychotic drug use. *Archives of General Psychiatry,* 1973, *28,* 463–467.

Amsterdam, J. D., & Dubin, W. Huntington's chorea and dimethylaminoethanol (deanol). *Journal of Clinical Psychiatry,* 1978, *39,* 626–628.

Amsterdam, J., & Mendels, J. Treatment-resistant tardive dyskinesia: A new therapeutic approach. *American Journal of Psychiatry,* 1979, *136,* 1197–1198.

Amsterdam, J., & Mendels, J. Baclofen and tardive dyskinesia. *American Journal of Psychiatry,* 1980, *137,* 634.

Ananth, J. V., Ban, T. A., & Lehmann, H. E. An uncontrolled study with thiopropazate in the treatment of persistent dyskinesia. *Psychopharmacology Bulletin,* 1977, *13*(3), 9.

Anden, N. E., & Grabowska-Anden, M. Contributions of adrenoreceptor blockage to extrapyramidal effects of neuroleptic drugs. *Journal of Neural Transmission,* 1980, Suppl. 16, 83–93.

Appleton, W. S. Skin and eye complications of psychoactive drug therapy. In A. DiMascio & R. I. Shader (Eds.), *Clinical handbook of psychopharmacology.* New York: Science House, 1970.

Arnfred, T., & Randrup, A. Cholinergic mechanisms in brain inhibiting amphetamine induced stereotyped behavior. *Acta Pharmacologica et Toxicologica,* 1968, *26,* 384–394.

Ashcroft, G. W., Eccleston, D., & Waddell, J. L. Recognition of amphetamine addicts. *British Medical Journal,* 1965, *1,* 57.

Asnis, G. M., & Leopold, M. A. A single-blind study of ECT in patients with tardive dyskinesia. *American Journal of Psychiatry,* 1978, *135,* 1235–1237.

Asnis, G. M., Leopold, M. A., Duvoisin, R. C., *et al.* A survey of tardive dyskinesia in psychiatric outpatients. *American Journal of Psychiatry,* 1977, *134,* 1367–1370.

Asnis, G. M., Sachar, E. J., Langer, G., *et al.* Normal prolactin responses in tardive dyskinesia. *Psychopharmacology,* 1979, *66,* 247–250.

Ayd, F. J., Jr. A survey of drug-induced extrapyramidal reactions. *Journal of the American Medical Association,* 1961, *175,* 1054–1060.

Ayd, F. J., Jr. Prevention of recurrence (maintenance therapy). In A. DiMascio & R. I. Shader (Eds.), *Clinical handbook of psychopharmacology.* New York: Science House, 1970.

Ayd, F. J., Jr. Ethical and legal dilemmas posed by tardive dyskinesia. *International Drug Therapy Newsletter,* 1977, *12,* 29–36.

Ayd, F. J., Jr. Respiratory dyskinesias in patients with neuroleptic-induced extrapyramidal reactions. *International Drug Therapy Newsletter,* 1979, *14,* 1–3.

Bacher, N. M., & Lewis, H. A. Low-dose propranolol in tardive dyskinesia. *American Journal of Psychiatry,* 1980, *137,* 495–497.

Baker, A. B. Discussion. In G. E. Crane & R. Gardner, Jr. (Eds.), *Psychotropic drugs and dysfunctions of the basal ganglia* (U.S. Public Health Service Publication No. 1938). Washington, D.C.: U.S. Government Printing Office, 1969.

Baldessarini, R. J. The pathophysiological basis of tardive dyskinesia. *Trends in Neurosciences,* 1979, *2,* 133–135.

Baldessarini, R. J. Personal communication, 1981.

Baldessarini, R. J., Cole, J. O., Davis, J. M., *et al. Tardive dyskinesia: A task force report of the American Psychiatric Association.* Washington, D.C.: American Psychiatric Association, 1980.

Baldessarini, R. J., & Davis, J. M. What *is* the best maintenance dose of neuroleptics in schizophrenia? *Psychiatry Research,* 1980, *3,* 115–122.

Baldessarini, R. J., & Fischer, J. E. Biological models in the study of false neurochemical synaptic transmitters. In D. J. Ingle & H. M. Shein (Eds.), *Model systems in biological psychiatry.* Cambridge, Mass.: MIT Press, 1975.

Baldessarini, R. J., & Tarsy, D. Tardive dyskinesia. In M. A. Lipton, A. DiMascio, & K. F. Killam (Eds.), *Psychopharmacology: A generation of progress.* New York: Raven Press, 1978.

Baldessarini, R. J., & Tarsy, D. Relationship of the actions of neuroleptic drugs to the pathophysiology of tardive dyskinesia. *International Review of Neurobiology,* 1979, *21,* 1–45.

Ballenger, J. C., & Post, R. M. Kindling as a model for the alcohol withdrawal syndromes. *British Journal of Psychiatry,* 1978, *133,* 1–14.

Ban, T. A. Adverse effects in maintenance therapy. *International Pharmacopsychiatry,* 1978, *13,* 217–229.

Bannet, J., Belmaker, R. H., & Ebstein, R. P. The effect of drug holidays in an animal model of tardive dyskinesia. *Psychopharmacology,* 1980, *69,* 223-224.

Barany, S., & Gunne, L. M. Pharmacologic modification of experimental tardive dyskinesia. *Acta Pharmacologica et Toxicologica,* 1979, *45,* 107-111.

Barany, S., Ingvast, A., & Gunne, L. M. Development of acute dystonia and tardive dyskinesia in cebus monkeys. *Research Communications in Chemical Pathology and Pharmacology,* 1979, *25,* 269-279.

Barbeau, A. Lecithin in neurologic disorders. *The New England Journal of Medicine,* 1978, *299,* 200-201.

Barbeau, A., Mars, H., Gillo-Joffrey, L., *et al.* A proposed classification of dopa-induced dyskinesias. In A. Barbeau & F. H. McDowell (Eds.), *L-Dopa and parkinsonism.* Philadelphia: F. A. Davis, 1970.

Barnes, T. R. E., & Kidger, T. The concept of tardive dyskinesia. *Trends in Neurosciences,* 1979, *2,* 135-136.

Bartholini, G., & Pletscher, A. Atropine-induced changes of cerebral dopamine turnover. *Experientia,* 1971, *27,* 1302.

Bartholini, G., & Stadler, H. Cholinergic and GABAergic influence on the dopamine release in extrapyramidal centers. In O. Almgren, A. Carlsson, & J. Engel (Eds.), *Chemical tools in catecholamine research* (Vol. 2). Amsterdam: North-Holland, 1975.

Bateman, D. N., Dutta, D. K., McClelland, H. A., *et al.* Metoclopramide and haloperidol in tardive dyskinesia. *British Journal of Psychiatry,* 1979, *135,* 505-508.

Bedard, P., Langelier, P., & Villeneuve, A. Oestrogen and extrapyramidal system. *Lancet,* 1977, *2,* 1367-1368.

Beitman, B. D. Tardive dyskinesia reinduced by lithium carbonate. *American Journal of Psychiatry,* 1978, *135,* 1229-1230.

Bell, R. C. H., & Smith, R. C. Tardive dyskinesia: Characterization and prevalence in a statewide system. *Journal of Clinical Psychiatry,* 1978, *39,* 39-47.

Berger, P. A. Biochemistry and the schizophrenias: Old concepts and new hypotheses. *Journal of Nervous and Mental Disease,* 1981, *169,* 90-99.

Betts, W. C., Johnston, F. S., & Pratt, M. J. An effective palliative treatment for phenothiazine-induced tardive dyskinesia. *North Carolina Medical Journal,* 1979, *40,* 286.

Bird, E. D. The clinical significance of disturbances in the central GABA system. In H. M. van Praag & J. Bruinvels (Eds.), *Neurotransmission and disturbed behavior.* New York: SP Medical & Scientific Books, 1978.

Birket-Smith, E. Abnormal involuntary movements induced by anticholinergic therapy. *Acta Neurologica Scandinavica,* 1974, *50,* 801-811.

Birket-Smith, E., & Andersen, J. V. Treatment of side effects of levodopa. *Lancet,* 1973, *1,* 431.

Birkmayer, W., & Neumayer, E. Die Moderne Medikamentoese Behandlung des parkinsonismus. *Zeitschrift für Neurologie,* 1972, *202,* 257-280.

Bjørndal, N., Casey, D. E., & Gerlach, J. Enkephalin, morphine, and naloxone in tardive dyskinesia. *Psychopharmacology,* 1980, *69,* 133-136.

Blackwell, B. Drug therapy: Patient compliance. *The New England Journal of Medicine,* 1973, *289,* 249-252.

Blombery, P. A., Kopin, I. J., Gordon, E. K., *et al.* Conversion of MHPG to vanillylmandelic acid. *Archives of General Psychiatry,* 1980, *37,* 1095-1098.

Bloom, F. E., Costa, E., & Salmoiraghi, S. C. Anesthesia and the responsiveness of individual neurons of the caudate nucleus of the cat to acetylcholine, norepinephrine and dopamine administered by microelectrophoresis. *Journal of Pharmacology and Experimental Therapeutics,* 1965, *150,* 244-252.

Bockenheimer, S., & Lucius, G. Zur Therapie mit Dimethylaminoethanol (Deanol) bei neuroleptikainduzierten extrapyramidalen Hyperkinesen. *Archiv für Psychiatrie und Nervenkrankheiten (Berlin)*, 1976, *222*, 69–75.

Borison, R. L., & Diamond, B. I. A new animal model for schizophrenia: Interactions with adrenergic mechanisms. *Biological Psychiatry*, 1978, *13*, 217–225.

Borison, R. L., Havdala, H. S., & Diamond, B. I. *Anticholinergic promotion of tardive dyskinesia*. Paper presented at the annual meeting of the American Psychiatric Association, May 1979.

Bourgeois, M., Bouilh, P., Tignol, J., et al. Spontaneous dyskinesias vs. neuroleptic-induced dyskinesias in 270 elderly subjects. *Journal of Nervous and Mental Disorders*, 1980, *168*, 177–178.

Bowers, M. B., Jr., Moore, D., & Tarsy, D. Tardive dyskinesia: A clinical test of the supersensitivity hypothesis. *Psychopharmacology*, 1979, *61*, 137–141.

Branchey, M. H., Branchey, L. B., Bark, N. M., et al. Lecithin in the treatment of tardive dyskinesia. *Communications in Psychopharmacology*, 1979, *3*, 303–307.

Brandon, S. Unusual effect of fenfluramine. *British Medical Journal*, 1969, *4*, 557–558.

Brandon, S., McClelland, H. A., & Protheroe, C. A study of facial dyskinesia in a mental hospital population. *British Journal of Psychiatry*, 1971, *118*, 171–184.

Brandrup, E. Tetrabenazine treatment in persisting dyskinesia caused by psychopharmacy. *American Journal of Psychiatry*, 1961, *118*, 551–552.

Brody, J. Personal communication, 1981.

Brooks, A. D. *The constitutional right to refuse antipsychotic medications*. Lecture delivered at the Staff College of the National Institute of Mental Health, Rockville, Md., February 1981.

Browning, D. H., & Ferry, P. C. Tardive dyskinesia in a ten-year-old boy. *Clinical Pediatrics*, 1976, *15*, 955–957.

Bucci, L. The dyskinesias: A new therapeutic approach. *Diseases of the Nervous System*, 1971, *32*, 324–327.

Bullock, R. J. Efficacy of thiopropazate dihydrochloride (Dartalan) in treating persisting phenothiazine-induced choreoathetosis and akathisia. *The Medical Journal of Australia*, 1972, *2*, 314–316.

Bunney, B. S., & Aghajanian, G. K. Dopaminergic influence in the basal ganglia: Evidence for striatonigral feedback regulation. In M. D. Yahr (Ed.), *The basal ganglia*. New York: Raven Press, 1976.(a)

Bunney, B. S., & Aghajanian, G. K. The effect of antipsychotic drugs on the firing of dopaminergic neurons: A reappraisal. In G. Sedvall, B. Urnas, & Y. Zotterman (Eds.), *Antipsychotic drugs: Pharmacodynamics and pharmacokinetics*. New York: Pergamon Press, 1976.(b)

Burki, H. R. Biochemical methods for predicting the occurrence of tardive dyskinesia. *Communications in Psychopharmacology*, 1979, *3*, 7–15.

Burnett, G. B., Prange, A. J., Wilson, I. C., et al. Adverse effects of anticholinergic antiparkinsonian drugs in tardive dyskinesia. *Neuropsychobiology*, 1980, *6*, 109–120.

Burt, D. R., Creese, I., & Snyder, S. H. Antischizophrenic drugs: Chronic treatment elevates dopamine receptor binding in brain. *Science*, 1977, *196*, 326–328.

Buxton, M. Diagnostic problems in Huntington's chorea and tardive dyskinesia. *Comprehensive Psychiatry*, 1976, *17*, 325–333.

Caine, E. D., Margolin, D. I., Brown, G. L., et al. Gilles de la Tourette's syndrome, tardive dyskinesia, and psychosis in an adolescent. *American Journal of Psychiatry*, 1978, *135*, 241–243.

Caine, E. D., Polinsky, R. J., Kartzinel, R., et al. Trial use of clozapine for abnormal involuntary movement disorders. *American Journal of Psychiatry*, 1979, *136*, 317–320.

Calil, H. M., Avery, D. H., Hollister, L. E., et al. Serum levels of neuroleptics measured by

dopamine radioreceptor assay and some clinical observations. *Psychiatry Research,*
1979, *1,* 39–44.

Calne, D. B., Claveria, L. E., Teychenne, P. F., *et al.* Pimozide in tardive dyskinesia. *Transactions of the American Neurological Association,* 1974, *99,* 166–170.

Carlson, K. R. "Tardive dyskinesia" resulting from chronic narcotic treatment. In W. E.
Fann, R. C. Smith, J. M. Davis, *et al.* (Eds.), *Tardive dyskinesia: Research and treatment.* New York: SP Medical & Scientific Books, 1980.

Carlsson, A. Biochemical aspects of abnormal movements induced by L-dopa. In A. Barbeau
& F. H. McDowell (Eds.), *L-Dopa and parkinsonism.* Philadelphia: F. A. Davis, 1970.

Carlsson, A. The impact of catecholamine research on medical science and practice. In E.
Usdin, I. J. Kopin, & J. D. Barchas (Eds.), *Catecholamines: Basic and clinical frontiers.* New York: Pergamon Press, 1979.

Carlsson, A., & Lindqvist, M. Effect of chlorpromazine on formation of 3-methoxytyra-
mine and normetanephrine in mouse brain. *Acta Pharmacologica et Toxicologica,*
1963, *20,* 140–144.

Carpenter, M. B. Anatomical organization of the corpus striatum and related nuclei. In M.
D. Yahr (Ed.), *The basal ganglia.* New York: Raven Press, 1976.

Carroll, B. J., Curtis, G. C., Davies, B. M., *et al.* Urinary free cortisol excretion in depression. *Psychological Medicine,* 1976, *6,* 43–50.

Carroll, B. J., Curtis, G. C., & Kokmen, E. Paradoxical response to dopamine agonists in
tardive dyskinesia. *American Journal of Psychiatry,* 1977, *134,* 785–789.

Carruthers, S. G. Persistent tardive dyskinesia. *British Medical Journal,* 1971, *3,* 572.

Casey, D. E. Tardive dyskinesia: Are there subtypes? *The New England Journal of Medicine,*
1976, *295,* 1078.

Casey, D. E. Deanol in the management of involuntary movement disorders: A review.
Diseases of the Nervous System, 1977, *38*(Suppl.), 7–15.

Casey, D. E. Mood alterations during deanol therapy. *Psychopharmacology,* 1979, *62,* 187–
191.

Casey, D. E., & Denney, D. Dimethylaminoethanol in tardive dyskinesia. *The New England
Journal of Medicine,* 1974, *29,* 797.

Casey, D. E., & Denney, D. Deanol in the treatment of tardive dyskinesia. *American Journal
of Psychiatry,* 1975, *132,* 864–867.

Casey, D. E., & Denney, D. Pharmacological characterization of tardive dyskinesia. *Psychopharmacology,* 1977, *54,* 1–8.

Casey, D. E., & Gerlach, J. Oxiperomide in tardive dyskinesia. *Journal of Neurology, Neurosurgery and Psychiatry,* 1980, *43,* 264–267.

Casey, D. E., Gerlach, J., Magelund, G., *et al.* γ-Acetylenic GABA in tardive dyskinesia.
Archives of General Psychiatry, 1980, *37,* 1376–1379.

Casey, D. E., Gerlach, J., & Simmelsgaard, H. Sulpiride in tardive dyskinesia. *Psychopharmacology,* 1979, *66,* 73–77.

Casey, D. E., & Hammerstad, J. P. Sodium valproate in tardive dyskinesia. *Journal of Clinical Psychiatry,* 1979, *40,* 483–485.

Casey, D. E., & Rabins, P. Tardive dyskinesia as a life-threatening illness. *American Journal
of Psychiatry,* 1978, *135,* 486–488.

Chadwick, D., Reynolds, E. H., Marsden, C. D. Anticonvulsant-induced dyskinesia: A
comparison with dyskinesias induced by neuroleptics. *Journal of Neurology, Neurosurgery and Psychiatry,* 1976, *39,* 1210–1218.

Chase, T. N. Catecholamine metabolism and neurological diseases. In E. Usdin & S. H.
Snyder (Eds.), *Frontiers in catecholamine research.* New York: Pergamon Press,
1973.

Chase, T. N. Rational approaches to the pharmacotherapy of chorea. In M. Yahr (Ed.), *The *basal ganglia.* New York: Raven Press, 1976.

Chase, T. N., Schnur, J. A., & Gordon, E. K. Cerebrospinal fluid monoamine catabolites in drug-induced extrapyramidal disorders. *Neuropharmacology*, 1970, *9*, 265–268.

Chase, T. N., & Tamminga, C. A. GABA system participation in human motor, cognitive, and endocrine function. In P. Korsgaard-Larsen, J. Scheel-Kruger, & H. Kofod (Eds.), *GABA-Neurotransmitters*. New York: Academic Press, 1979.

Chien, C., Jung, K., & Ross-Townsend, A. Efficacies of agents related to GABA, dopamine and acetylcholine in the treatment of tardive dyskinesia. *Psychopharmacology Bulletin*, 1978, *14*, 20–22.

Chien, C., DiMascio, A., & Cole, J. O. Antiparkinsonian agents and a depot phenothiazine. *American Journal of Psychiatry*, 1974, *131*, 86–90.

Chouinard, G., Annable, L., Ross-Chouinard, A., *et al.* Factors related to tardive dyskinesia. *American Journal of Psychiatry*, 1979, *136*, 79–83.

Chouinard, G., De Montigny, C., & Annable, L. Tardive dyskinesia and antiparkinsonian medication. *American Journal of Psychiatry*, 1979, *136*, 228–229.

Chouinard, G., & Jones, B. D. Early onset of tardive dyskinesia: Case report. *American Journal of Psychiatry*, 1979, *136*, 1323–1324.

Chouinard, G., & Jones, B. D. Neuroleptic-induced supersensitivity psychosis: Clinical and pharmacologic characteristics. *American Journal of Psychiatry*, 1980, *137*, 16–21.

Christensen, A. V., Arnt, J., & Scheel-Kruger, J. GABA–dopamine–neuroleptic interaction after systemic administration. *Brain Research Bulletin*, 1980, *5*(Suppl. 2), 885–890.

Christensen, A. V., & Nielsen, I. M. Dopaminergic supersensitivity: Influence of dopamine agonists, cholinergics, anticholinergics, and drugs used for the treatment of tardive dyskinesia. *Psychopharmacology*, 1979, *62*, 111–116.

Christensen, A. V., Fjalland, B., & Nielsen, I. M. On the supersensitivity of dopamine receptors, induced by neuroleptics. *Psychopharmacology*, 1976, *48*, 1–6.

Christensen, E., Moller, J. E., & Faurbye, A. Neurological investigation of 28 brains from patients with dyskinesia. *Acta Psychiatrica Scandinavica*, 1970, *46*, 14–23.

Claveria, L. E., Teychenne, P. F., Calne, D. B., *et al.* Tardive dyskinesia treated with pimozide. *Journal of the Neurological Sciences*, 1975, *24*, 393–401.

Clow, A., Jenner, P., Theodorou, A., *et al.* Striatal dopamine receptors become supersensitive while rats are given trifluoperazine for six months. *Nature*, 1979, *278*, 59–61.

Clow, A., Theodorou, A., Jenner, P., *et al.* Changes in rat striatal dopamine turnover and receptor activity during one year's neuroleptic administration. *European Journal of Pharmacology*, 1980, *63*, 135–144.(a)

Clow, A., Theodorou, A., Jenner, P., *et al.* Cerebral dopamine function in rats following withdrawal from one year of continuous neuroleptic administration. *European Journal of Pharmacology*, 1980, *63*, 145–157.(b)

Cohen, B. M., Herschel, M., & Aoba, A. Neuroleptic, antimuscarinic, and antiadrenergic activity of chlorpromazine, thioridazine, and their metabolites. *Psychiatry Research*, 1979, *1*, 199–208.

Cohen, B. M., Herschel, M., Miller, E., *et al.* Radioreceptor assay of haloperidol tissue levels in the rat. *Neuropharmacology*, 1980, *19*, 663–668.

Cohen, D. J., Detlor, J., Young, G., *et al.* Clonidine ameliorates Gilles de la Tourette syndrome. *Archives of General Psychiatry*, 1980, *37*, 1350–1357.

Cohen, E. L., & Wurtman, R. J. Brain acetylcholine: Increase after systemic choline administration. *Life Sciences*, 1975, *16*, 1095–1102.

Cohen, K. L., Cooper, R. A., & Altshul, S. Prolactin levels in tardive dyskinesia. *The New England Journal of Medicine*, 1979, *300*, 46.

Cole, J. O., Gardos, G., & Granacher, R. *Drug evaluations in tardive dyskinesia.* Paper presented at the annual meeting of the American Psychiatric Association, Miami Beach, Fla., May 1976.

Cole, J. O., Gardos, G., Tarsy, D., *et al.* Drug trials in persistent dyskinesia. In W. E. Fann, R. C. Smith, J. M. Davis, *et al.* (Eds.), *Tardive dyskinesia: Research and treatment.* New York: SP Medical & Scientific Books, 1980.

Commissiong, J. W., Gentleman, S., & Neff, N. H. Spinal cord dopaminergic neurons: Evidence for an uncrossed nigrospinal pathway. *Neuropharmacology,* 1979, *18,* 565–568.

Cook, D. G., Fahn, S., & Brait, K. A. Chronic manganese intoxication. *Archives of Neurology,* 1974, *30,* 59–65.

Cools, A. R., Hendricks, G., & Korten, J. The acetylcholine–dopamine balance in the basal ganglia of rhesus monkeys and its role in dynamic, dystonic, dyskinetic and epileptoid motor activities. *Journal of Neural Transmission,* 1975, *36,* 91–105.

Cooper, J. R., Bloom, F. E., & Roth, R. H. *The biochemical basis of neuropharmacology,* (3rd ed.). New York: Oxford University Press, 1978.

Costall, B., & Naylor, R. J. Neuroleptic antagonism of dyskinetic phenomena. *European Journal of Pharmacology,* 1975, *33,* 301–312.

Costall, B., & Naylor, R. J. Minireview: The hypothesis of different dopamine receptor mechanisms. *Life Sciences,* 1981, *28,* 215–229.

Costall, B., Naylor, R. J., & Olley, J. F. Catalepsy and circling behavior after intracranial injections of neuroleptic, cholinergic and anticholinergic agents into the caudate-putamen, globus pallidus and substantia nigra of rat brain. *Neuropharmacology,* 1972, *11,* 645–663.

Cotzias, G. C., Papavasiliou, P. S., Fehling, C., *et al.* Similarities between neurologic effects of L-dopa and of apomorphine. *The New England Journal of Medicine,* 1970, *282,* 31–33.

Cotzias, G. C., Papavasiliou, P. S., & Gellene, R. Modification of parkinsonism: Chronic treatment with L-dopa. *The New England Journal of Medicine,* 1969, *280,* 337–345.

Cotzias, G. C., Van Woert, W. H., & Schettes, L. M. Aromatic amino acids and modification of parkinsonism. *The New England Journal of Medicine,* 1967, *276,* 374–379.

Coyle, J. T., & Schwarcz, R. Lesion of striatal neurons with kainic acid provides a model for Huntington's chorea. *Nature,* 1976, *263,* 244–246.

Crane, G. E. Dyskinesia and neuroleptics. *Archives of General Psychiatry,* 1968, *19,* 700–703.(a)

Crane, G. E. Tardive dyskinesia in patients treated with major neuroleptics: A review of the literature. *American Journal of Psychiatry,* 1968, *124*(Suppl.), 40–48.(b)

Crane, G. E. Tardive dyskinesia in schizophrenic patients treated with psychotropic drugs. *Agressologie,* 1968, *9,* 209–218.(c)

Crane, G. E. High doses of trifluoperazine and tardive dyskinesia. *Archives of Neurology,* 1970, *22,* 176–180.

Crane, G. E. More on amantadine in tardive dyskinesia. *The New England Journal of Medicine,* 1971, *285,* 1150–1151.(a)

Crane, G. E. Persistence of neurological symptoms due to neuroleptic drugs. *American Journal of Psychiatry,* 1971, *127,* 143–146.(b)

Crane, G. E. Prevention and management of tardive dyskinesia. *American Journal of Psychiatry,* 1972, *129,* 126–127.(a)

Crane, G. E. Pseudoparkinsonism and tardive dyskinesia. *Archives of Neurology,* 1972, *27,* 426–430.(b)

Crane, G. E. Clinical psychopharmacology in its 20th year. *Science,* 1973, *181,* 124–128.(a)

Crane, G. E. Persistent dyskinesia. *British Journal of Psychiatry,* 1973, *122,* 395–405.(b)

Crane, G. E. Rapid reversal of tardive dyskinesia. *American Journal of Psychiatry,* 1973,

130, 1159.(c)

Crane, G. E. Mediocre effects of reserpine on tardive dyskinesia. *The New England Journal of Medicine*, 1973, *288*, 104–105.(d)

Crane, G. E. Factors predisposing to drug-induced neurologic effects. In I. S. Forrest, C. J. Carr, & E. Usdin (Eds.), *The phenothiazines and structurally related drugs*. New York: Raven Press, 1974.

Crane, G. E. Deanol for tardive dyskinesia (cont.). *The New England Journal of Medicine*, 1975, *292*, 926.

Crane, G. E. The prevention of tardive dyskinesia. *American Journal of Psychiatry*, 1977, *134*, 757–759.

Crane, G. E., & Naranjo, E. R. Motor disorders induced by neuroleptics: A proposed new classification. *Archives of General Psychiatry*, 1971, *24*, 179–184.

Crane, G. E., & Paulson, G. W. Involuntary movements in a sample of chronic mental patients and their relation to the treatment with neuroleptics. *International Journal of Neuropsychiatry*, 1967, *3*, 286–291.

Crane, G. E., Ruiz, P., Kernohan, W. J., et al. Effects of drug withdrawal on tardive dyskinesia. *Journal of Neurology, Neurosurgery and Psychiatry*, 1969, *33*, 511–512.

Crane, G. E., & Smeets, R. A. Tardive dyskinesia and drug therapy in geriatric patients. *Archives of General Psychiatry*, 1974, *30*, 341–343.

Crane, G. E., Turek, I. S., & Kurland, A. A. Failure of pyridoxine to reduce drug-induced dyskinesia. *Journal of Neurology, Neurosurgery and Psychiatry*, 1970, *33*, 511–512.

Crayton, J. W., Meltzer, H. Y., & Goode, D. J. Motoneuron excitability in psychiatric patients. *Biological Psychiatry*, 1977, *12*, 545–561.

Crayton, J. W., Smith, R. C., Klass, D., et al. Electrophysiological (H-reflex) studies of patients with tardive dyskinesia. *American Journal of Psychiatry*, 1977, *134*, 775–781.

Creese, I., & Snyder, S. H. A simple and sensitive radioreceptor assay for antischizophrenic drugs in blood. *Nature*, 1977, *270*, 180–182.

Crews, E. L., & Carpenter, A. E. Lithium-induced aggravation of tardive dyskinesia. *American Journal of Psychiatry*, 1977, *134*, 933.

Curran, D. J., Nagaswami, S., & Mohan, K. J. Treatment of phenothiazine-induced bulbar persistent dyskinesia with deanol acetamidobenzoate. *Diseases of the Nervous System*, 1975, *36*, 71–73.

Curran, J. P. Management of tardive dyskinesia with thiopropazate. *American Journal of Psychiatry*, 1973, *130*, 925–927.

Curzon, G. Involuntary movements other than parkinsonism: Biochemical aspects. *Proceedings of the Royal Society of Medicine*, 1973, *66*, 873.

Cutler, N. R., Post, R. M., Rey, A. C., et al. Depression-dependent dyskinesias in two cases of manic–depressive illness. *The New England Journal of Medicine*, 1981, *304*, 1088–1089.

Dahadelah, M. P., Small, M., & Thomas, D. J. Dimethylaminoethanol in blepharospasm and hemifacial spasm. *The New England Journal of Medicine*, 1975, *293*, 98.

Dahlström, A., & Fuxe, K. Evidence for the existence of monoamine-containing neurons in the central nervous system: I. Demonstration of monoamines in the cell bodies of brain stem neurons. *Acta Physiologica Scandinavica*, 1964, *62*(Suppl. 232), 1–55.

Dahlström, A., & Fuxe, K. Evidence for the existence of the monoamine-containing neurons in the central nervous system: II. Experimentally induced changes in the intraneuronal amine levels of bulbospinal neuron systems. *Acta Physiologica Scandinavica*, 1965, *64*(Suppl. 247), 1–36.

Dalen, P. Lithium therapy in Huntington's chorea and tardive dyskinesia. *Lancet*, 1973, *1*, 107–108.

Davis, J. M. Antipsychotic drugs. In H. I. Kaplan, A. M. Freedman, & B. J. Sadock (Eds.), *Comprehensive textbook of psychiatry* (Vol. 3, 3rd ed.). Baltimore: Williams & Wilkins, 1980.

Davis, K. L., & Berger, P. A. Pharmacological investigations of the cholinergic imbalance hypothesis of movement disorders and psychosis. *Biological Psychiatry,* 1978, *13,* 23–49.

Davis, K. L., Berger, P. A., & Hollister, L. E. Choline for tardive dyskinesia. *The New England Journal of Medicine,* 1975, *293,* 152.

Davis, K. L., Berger, P. A., & Hollister, L. E. Tardive dyskinesia and depressive illness. *Psychopharmacology Communications,* 1976, *2,* 125–130.

Davis, K. L., Berger, P. A., Hollister, L. E., *et al.* Choline chloride in the treatment of Huntington's disease and tardive dyskinesia: A preliminary report. *Psychopharmacology Bulletin,* 1977, *13,* 37–38.(a)

Davis, K. L., Berger, P. A., & Hollister, L. E. Deanol in tardive dyskinesia. *American Journal of Psychiatry,* 1977, *134,* 807.(b)

Davis, K. L., Hollister, L. E., Barchas, J. D., *et al.* Choline in tardive dyskinesia and Huntington's disease. *Life Sciences,* 1976, *19,* 1507–1516.

Davis, K. L., Hollister, L. E., Vento, A. L., *et al.* Choline chloride in animal models of tardive dyskinesia. *Life Sciences,* 1978, *22,* 1699–1708.

Davis, K. L., Hollister, L. E., Vento, A. L., *et al.* Dimethylaminoethanol (Deanol): Effect on apomorphine-induced stereotypy and an animal model of tardive dyskinesia. *Psychopharmacology,* 1979, *63,* 143–146.

Davis, K. L., Hollister, L. E., Vento, A. L., *et al.* Cholinergic aspects of tardive dyskinesia: Human and animal studies. In W. E. Fann, R. C. Smith, J. M. Davis, *et al.* (Eds.), *Tardive dyskinesia: Research and treatment.* New York: SP Medical & Scientific Books, 1980.

Davis, K. L., Kastin, A. J., Beilstein, B. A., *et al.* MSH and MIF-I in animal models of tardive dyskinesia. *Pharmacology, Biochemistry and Behavior,* 1980, *13,* 37–40.

Davis, W. A. Dyskinesia associated with chronic antihistamine use. *The New England Journal of Medicine,* 1976, *294,* 113.

Decker, B. L., Davis, J. M., Janowsky, D. S., *et al.* Amantadine hydrochloride treatment of tardive dyskinesia. *The New England Journal of Medicine,* 1971, *285,* 860.

Deckret, J. J., Maany, I., Ramsey, A., *et al.* A case of oral dyskinesia associated with imipramine treatment. *American Journal of Psychiatry,* 1977, *134,* 1297–1298.

Degkwitz, R. Extrapyramidal motor disorders following long-term treatment with neuroleptic drugs. In G. E. Crane & J. R. Gardner, Jr. (Eds.), *Psychotropic drugs and dysfunctions of the basal ganglia* (U.S. Public Health Service Publication No. 1938). Washington, D.C.: U.S. Government Printing Office, 1969.

Degkwitz, R., & Wenzel, W. Persistent extrapyramidal side effects after long-term application of neuroleptis. In H. Brill (Ed.), *Neuro-Psycho-Pharmacology* (International Congress Series No. 129). New York: Excerpta Medica Foundation, 1967.

Delay, J., & Deniker, P. 38 cas de psychoses traités par la cure prolongée et continué de 4568 R. P. *Annales Médico-Psychologique,* 1952, *110,* 364.

Delwaide, P. J., & Desseilles, M. Spontaneous buccolinguofacial dyskinesia in the elderly. *Acta Neurologica Scandinavica,* 1977, *56,* 256–262.

Demars, J. C. A. Neuromuscular effects of long-term phenothiazine medication, electroconvulsive therapy and leucotomy. *Journal of Nervous and Mental Disorders,* 1966, *143,* 73–79.

De Montigny, C., Chouinard, G., & Annable, L. Ineffectiveness of deanol in tardive dyskinesia: A placebo controlled study. *Psychopharmacology,* 1979, *65,* 219–222.

Denckla, M. B., Bemporad, J. R., & Mackay, M. C. Tics following methylphenidate administration. *Journal of the American Medical Association,* 1976, *235,* 1349–1351.

Deneau, G. A., & Crane, G. E. Dyskinesia in rhesus monkeys treated with high doses of chlorpromazine. In G. E. Crane & J. R. Gardner, Jr. (Eds.), *Psychotropic drugs and dysfunctions of the basal ganglia* (U.S. Public Health Service Publication No. 1938). Washington, D.C.: U.S. Government Printing Office, 1969.

Denny-Brown, D., & Yanagisawa, N. The role of the basal ganglia in the initiation of movement. In M. D. Yahr (Ed.), *The basal ganglia.* New York: Raven Press, 1976.

DeSilva, L., & Huang, C. Y. Deanol in tardive dyskinesia. *British Medical Journal,* 1975, *3,* 466.

DeVeaugh-Geiss, J. Aggravation of tardive dyskinesia by phenytoin. *The New England Journal of Medicine,* 1978, *298,* 457–458.

DeVeaugh-Geiss, J. Informed consent for neuroleptic therapy. *American Journal of Psychiatry,* 1979, *136,* 959–962.

DeVeaugh-Geiss, J., & Manion, L. High-dose pyridoxine in tardive dyskinesia. *Journal of Clinical Psychiatry,* 1978, *39,* 573–575.

Diamond, B. I., & Borison, R. L. Enkephalins and nigrostriatal function. *Neurology,* 1978, *28,* 1085–1088.

Diamond, B. I., & Borison, R. L. The role of enkephalins in tardive dyskinesia. *Neurology,* 1979, *29,* 605–606.

Dincmen, K. Chronic psychotic choreo-athetosis. *Diseases of the Nervous System,* 1966, *27,* 399–402.

Doepp, S., & Buddeberg, C. Extrapyramidal symptome unter clozapin. *Nervenarzt,* 1975, *46,* 589–590.

Doongaji, D. R. The treatment of tardive dyskinesia with penfluperidol: A case report. *Neurology India,* 1977, *25,* 244–246.

Dravet, C., Bernardina, B. D., Mesdjian, E., *et al.* Dyskinésies paroxystiques au cours des traitements par la diphénylhydantoine. *Revue Neurologique,* 1980, *136,* 1–14.

Druckman, R., Seelinger, D., & Thulin, B. Chronic involuntary movements induced by phenothiazines. *Journal of Nervous and Mental Diseases,* 1962, *135,* 69–76.

Du Vigneaud, V., Chandler, J. P., Simmonds, S., *et al.* The role of dimethyl and monomethyl amino ethanol in transmethylation reactions *in vivo. Journal of Biological Chemistry,* 1946, *164,* 603–613.

Duvoisin, R. C. Reserpine for tardive dyskinesia (cont.). *The New England Journal of Medicine,* 1972, *286,* 611.

Dynes, J. B. Oral dyskinesias—Occurrence and treatment. *Diseases of the Nervous System,* 1970, *31,* 854–859.

Ebstein, R. P., Biederman, J., Rimon, R., *et al.* Cyclic GMP in the CSF of patients with schizophrenia before and after neuroleptic treatment. *Psychopharmacology,* 1976, *51,* 71–74.

Eckman, F. Problematik von Dauerschaden nach neuroleptischer Langzeitbehandelung. *Therapie der Gegenwart (Berlin),* 1968, *197,* 316–323.

Editorial. Tardive dyskinesia. *Lancet,* 1979, *2,* 447–448.

Edwards, H. Significance of brain damage in persistent oral dyskinesia. *British Journal of Psychiatry,* 1970, *116,* 271–275.

Ehrensing, R. H. Lithium and M.R.I.H. in tardive dyskinesia. *Lancet,* 1974, *2,* 1459–1460.

Ehrensing, R. H., Kastin, A. J., Larsons, P. F., *et al.* Melanocyte-stimulating hormone release-inhibiting factor-1 and tardive dyskinesia. *Diseases of the Nervous System,* 1977, *38,* 303–306.

Eibergen, R. D., & Carlson, K. R. Dyskinesias in monkeys: Interaction of methamphetamine with prior methadone treatment. *Pharmacology, Biochemistry and Behavior,* 1976, *5,* 175–187.

Eldridge, R. The torsion dystonias: Literature review and genetic and clinical studies. *Neurology*, 1970, *20*, 57–78.

Ellison, G., Eison, M. S., Huberman, H. S., *et al.* Long-term changes in dopaminergic innervation of caudate nucleus after continuous amphetamine administration. *Science*, 1978, *201*, 276–278.

Engel, J., Liljequist, S., & Johannessen, K. Behavioral effects of long-term treatment with antipsychotic drugs. In G. Sedvall, B. Uvnas, & Y. Zotterman (Eds.), *Antipsychotic drugs: Pharmacodynamics and pharmacokinetics*. Oxford: Pergamon Press, 1976.

Engelhardt, D. M., Polizos, P., & Waizer, J. CNS consequences of psychotropic drug withdrawal in autistic children: A follow-up report. *Psychopharmacology Bulletin*, 1975, *11*, 6–7.

Ereshefsky, L., Rubin, T. N., & Friedman, S. Treatment of tardive dyskinesia and mania with RBC lithium determinations. *American Journal of Psychiatry*, 1979, *136*, 570–573.

Escobar, J. I., & Kemp, K. F. Dimethylaminoethanol for tardive dyskinesia. *The New England Journal of Medicine*, 1975, *292*, 317–318.

Ettigi, P., Nair, N. P. V., Cerbantes, P. *et al.* Effect of apomorphine on growth hormone and prolactin secretion in schizophrenic patients, with and without oral dyskinesia, withdrawn from chronic neuroleptic therapy. *Journal of Neurology, Neurosurgery and Psychiatry*, 1976, *39*, 870–876.

Ettinger, M., & Curran, J. Liver disease and phenothiazines. *Minnesota Medicine*, 1970, *53*, 731–736.

Evans, J. H. Persistent oral dyskinesia in treatment with phenothiazine derivatives. *Lancet*, 1965, *1*, 458–460.

Eveloff, H. H. A case of amphetamine-induced dyskinesia. *Journal of the American Medical Association*, 1968, *204*, 933.

Fahn, S. Treatment of tardive dyskinesia with combined reserpine and alpha-methyl-tyrosine. *Transactions of the American Neurological Association*, 1978, *103*, 100–103.

Famuyiwa, O. O., Eccleston, D., Donaldson, A. A., *et al.* Tardive dyskinesia and dementia. *British Journal of Psychiatry*, 1979, *135*, 590–594.

Fann, W. E., Davis, J. M., & Janowsky, D. S. The prevalence of tardive dyskinesia in mental hospital patients. *Diseases of the Nervous System*, 1972, 33, 182–186.

Fann, W. E., Davis, J. M., & Wilson, I. C. Methylphenidate in tardive dyskinesia. *American Journal of Psychiatry*, 1973, *130*, 922–924.

Fann, W. E., Lake, C. R., Gerber, C. J., *et al.* Cholinergic suppression of tardive dyskinesia. *Psychopharmacologia (Berlin)*, 1974, *37*, 101–107.

Fann, W. E., Stafford, J. R., Malone, R. L., *et al.* Clinical research techniques in tardive dyskinesia. *American Journal of Psychiatry*, 1977, *134*, 759–762.

Fann, W. E., Sullivan, J. L. III, Miller, R. D., *et al.* Deanol in tardive dyskinesia: A preliminary report. *Psychopharmacologia (Berlin)*, 1975, *42*, 135–137.

Fann, W. E., Sullivan, J. L., & Richman, B. W. Tardive dyskinesia associated with tricyclic antidepressants. *British Journal of Psychiatry*, 1976, *128*, 490–493.

Farley, I. J., Price, K. S., McCullough, E., *et al.* Norepinephrine in chronic paranoid schizophrenia: Above-normal levels in limbic forebrain. *Science*, 1978, *200*, 456–458.

Faurbye, A. The structural and biochemical basis of movement disorders in treatment with neuroleptic drugs and in extrapyramidal diseases. *Comprehensive Psychiatry*, 1970, *11*, 205–225.

Faurbye, A., Rasch, P. J., Petersen, P. B., *et al.* Neurological symptoms in pharmacotherapy of psychoses. *Acta Psychiatrica Scandinavica*, 1964, *40*, 10–27.

Feder, R., & Moore, D. C. Baclofen and tardive dyskinesia. *American Journal of Psychiatry*, 1980, *137*, 633–634.

Forrest, F. M. Evolutionary origin of extrapyramidal disorders in drug-treated mental patients, its significance, and the role of neuromelanin. In I. S. Forrest, C. J. Carr, & E. Usdin (Eds.), *The phenothiazines and structurally related drugs.* New York: Raven Press, 1974.

Forrest, F. M., Forrest, I. S., & Roizin, L. Clinical, biochemical and post-mortem studies on a patient treated with chlorpromazine. *Agressologie,* 1963, *4,* 259-265.

Frangos, E., & Christodoulides, H. Clinical observations on the treatment of tardive dyskinesia with haloperidol. *Acta Psychiatrica Belgica,* 1975, *75,* 19-32.

Frank, S. M., & Djavadi, N. *Tardive dyskinesia in autistic children.* Paper presented at the annual meeting of the American Academy of Child Psychiatry, Chicago, October 1980.

Frattola, L., Albizzati, M. G., Bassi, S., et al. Treatment of dyskinetic and dystonic disorders with CF 25-397: Clinical and pharmacological aspects. In M. Goldstein, D. B. Calne, A. Lieberman, et al. (Eds.), *Ergot compounds and brain function.* New York: Raven Press, 1980.

Freedman, L. S., Roffman, M., & Goldstein, M. Changes in human serum dopamine-β-hydroxylase activity in various physiological and pathological states. In E. Usdin & S. H. Snyder (Eds.), *Frontiers in catecholamine research.* New York: Pergamon Press, 1973.

Freedman, R. Interactions of antipsychotic drugs with norepinephrine and cerebellar neuronal circuitry: Implications for the psychobiology of psychosis. *Biological Psychiatry,* 1977, *12,* 181-197.

Freedman, R., Bell, J., & Kirch, D. Clonidine therapy for coexisting psychosis and tardive dyskinesia. *American Journal of Psychiatry,* 1980, *137,* 629-630.

Freeman, H., & Soni, S. D. Oxypertine for tardive dyskinesia. *British Journal of Psychiatry,* 1980, *137,* 522-523.

Friedhoff, A. J., & Alpert, M. Receptor sensitivity modification as a potential treatment. In M. A. Lipton, A. DiMascio, & K. F. Killam, (Eds.), *Psychopharmacology: A generation of progress.* New York: Raven Press, 1978.

Fuxe, K., Hokfelt, T., & Ungerstedt, U. Morphological and functional aspects of central monoamine neurons. *International Review of Neurobiology,* 1970, *13,* 93-126.

Garber, R. S. Tardive dyskinesia. *Psychiatric News,* 1979, *14*(9), 2.

Gardos, G. Are antipsychotic drugs interchangeable? *Journal of Nervous and Mental Disease,* 1974, *159,* 343-348.

Gardos, G., & Cole, J. O. Papaverine for tardive dyskinesia? *The New England Journal of Medicine,* 1975, *292,* 1355.

Gardos, G., & Cole, J. O. Pilot study of cyproheptadine (Periactin) in tardive dyskinesia. *Psychopharmacology Bulletin,* 1978, *14*(2), 18-20.

Gardos, G., Cole, J. O., & La Brie, R. The assessment of tardive dyskinesia. *Archives of General Psychiatry,* 1977, *34,* 1206-1212.(a)

Gardos, G., Cole, J. O., & La Brie, R. A. Drug variables in the etiology of tardive dyskinesia —Application of discriminant function analysis. *Progress in Neuro-psychopharmacology,* 1977, *1,* 147-154.(b)

Gardos, G., Cole, J. O., & Sniffin, C. An evaluation of papaverine in tardive dyskinesia. *Journal of Clinical Pharmacology,* 1976, *16,* 304-310.

Gardos, G., Cole, J. O., & Sokol, M. *Pitfalls in the assessment of tardive dyskinesia.* Paper presented at the Sixth World Congress of Psychiatry, Honolulu, August 28-September 3, 1977.

Gardos, G., Samu, I., Kallos, M., et al. Absence of severe tardive dyskinesia in Hungarian schizophrenic out-patients. *Psychopharmacology,* 1980, *71,* 29-34.

Gardos, G., Sokol, M., Cole, J. O., et al. Eye color and tardive dyskinesia. Psychopharmacology Bulletin, 1976, 22(2), 7-9.

Gelenberg, A. J. Computerized tomography in patients with tardive dyskinesia. American Journal of Psychiatry, 1976, 133, 578-579.

Gelenberg, A. J., Doller-Wojcik, J. C., & Growdon, J. H. Choline and lecithin in the treatment of tardive dyskinesia: Preliminary results from a pilot study. American Journal of Psychiatry, 1979, 136, 772-776.

Gerbino, L., Shopsin, B., & Collora, M. Clozapine in the treatment of tardive dyskinesia: An interim report. In W. E. Fann, R. C. Smith, J. M. Davis, et al. (Eds.), Tardive dyskinesia: Research and treatment. New York: SP Medical & Scientific Books, 1980.

Gerlach, J. Relationship between tardive dyskinesia and L-dopa-induced hyperkinesia and parkinsonism. Psychopharmacology, 1977, 51, 259-263.

Gerlach, J., Reisby, N., & Randrup, A. Dopaminergic hypersensitivity and cholinergic hypofunction in the pathophysiology of tardive dyskinesia. Psychopharmacologia (Berlin), 1974, 34, 21-35.

Gerlach, J., Rye, T., & Kristjansen, P. Effect of baclofen on tardive dyskinesia. Psychopharmacology, 1978, 56, 145-151.

Gerlach, J., & Simmelsgaard, H. Tardive dyskinesia during and following treatment with haloperidol, haloperidol + biperiden, thioridazine, and clozapine. Psychopharmacology, 1978, 59, 105-112.

Gerlach, J., & Thorsen, K. The movement pattern of oral tardive dyskinesia in relation to anticholinergic and antidopaminergic treatment. International Pharmacopsychiatry, 1976, 11(1), 1-7.

Gerlach, J., Thorsen, K., & Fog, R. Extrapyramidal reactions and amine metabolites in cerebrospinal fluid during haloperidol and clozapine treatment of schizophrenic patients. Psychopharmacologia (Berlin), 1975, 40, 341-350.

Gerlach, J., Thorsen, K., & Munkvad, I. Effect of lithium on neuroleptic-induced tardive dyskinesia compared with placebo in a double-blind cross-over trial. Pharmakopsychiatrie, 1975, 8, 51-56.

Gianutsos, G., & Lal, H. Alteration in the action of cholinergic and anticholinergic drugs after chronic haloperidol: Indirect evidence for cholinergic hyposensitivity. Life Sciences, 1976, 18, 515-520.

Gianutsos, G., & Moore, K. E. Dopaminergic supersensitivity in striatum and olfactory tubercle following chronic administration of haloperidol or clozapine. Life Sciences, 1977, 20, 1585-1592.

Gibbs, E. L., Gibbs, F. A., Tasher, D., et al. An electroencephalographic abnormality correlating with psychosis. Electroencephalography and Clinical Neurophysiology, 1960, 12, 265.

Gibson, A. C. Depot injections and tardive dyskinesia. British Journal of Psychiatry, 1978, 132, 361-365.(a)

Gibson, A. C. Sodium valproate and tardive dyskinesia. British Journal of Psychiatry, 1978, 133, 82.(b)

Gibson, A. C. Questionnaire on severe tardive dyskinesia. British Journal of Psychiatry, 1979, 134, 549-550.

Gilbert, M. M. Haloperidol in severe facial dyskinesia (case report). Diseases of the Nervous System, 1969, 30, 481-482.

Glassman, R. B. A neural systems theory of schizophrenia and tardive dyskinesia. Behavioral Sciences, 1976, 21, 274-288.

Glassman, R. B., & Glassman, H. N. Oral dyskinesia in brain-damaged rats withdrawn from a neuroleptic: Implications for models of tardive dyskinesia. Psychopharmacology,

1980, *69,* 19–25.

Glassman, R. B., Glassman, H. N., & Frew, C. Possible feline analog of tardive dyskinesia. *Neuroscience Abstracts,* 1977, *3,* 1405.

Glazer, W. M., & Moore, D. C. The diagnosis of rapid abnormal involuntary movements with fluphenazine decanoate. *Journal of Nervous and Mental Disease,* 1980, *168,* 439–441.

Gnegy, M., Uzunov, P., Costa, E. Participation of an endogenous Ca^{++}-binding protein activator in the development of drug-induced supersensitivity of striatal dopamine receptors. *Journal of Pharmacology and Experimental Therapeutics,* 1977, *202,* 558–564.

Goddard, G. V. Long-term alterations following amygdala stimulation. In S. Eleftheriou (Ed.), *The neurobiology of the amygdala.* New York: Plenum Press, 1972.

Godwin-Austen, R. B., & Clark, T. Persistent phenothiazine dyskinesia treated with tetrabenazine. *British Medical Journal,* 1971, *4,* 25–26.

Goldberg, A. M. Is deanol a precursor of acetylcholine? *Diseases of the Nervous System,* 1977, *38*(Suppl.), 16–20.

Golden, G. S. Gilles de la Tourette's syndrome following methylphenidate administration. *Developmental and Medical Child Neurology,* 1974, *16,* 76–78.

Goldman, D. Treatment of phenothiazine-induced dyskinesia. *Psychopharmacology,* 1976, *47,* 271–272.

Gordon, J. H., Borison, R. L., & Diamond, B. I. Estrogen in experimental tardive dyskinesia. *Neurology,* 1980, *30,* 551–554.

Gottfries, C. G., Gottfries, I., Johansson, B., *et al.* Acid monoamine metabolites in human cerebrospinal fluid and their relations to age and sex. *Neuropharmacology,* 1971, *10,* 665–672.

Gratton, L. Neuroleptiques, parkinsonisme et schizophrénie. *Union Médicale du Canada,* 1960, *89,* 679–694.

Greenblatt, D. L., Stotsky, B. A., & DiMascio, A. Phenothiazine-induced dyskinesia in nursing home patients. *Journal of the American Geriatric Society,* 1968, *16,* 27–34.

Greiner, A. C., & Berry, K. Skin pigmentation and corneal and lens opacities with prolonged chlorpromazine therapy. *Canadian Medical Association Journal,* 1964, *90,* 663–665.

Gross, H., & Kaltenbach, E. Neuropathological findings in persistent hyperkinesia after neuroleptic long-term therapy. In A. Cerletti & F. J. Bove (Eds.), *The present status of psychotropic drugs.* Amsterdam: Excerpta Medica Foundation, 1969.

Groth, D. P., Bain, J. A., & Pfeiffer, C. C. The comparative distribution of C^{14} labeled 2-dimethylaminoethanol and choline in the mouse. *Journal of Pharmacology and Experimental Therapeutics,* 1958, *124,* 290–295.

Growdon, J. H., Gelenberg, A. J., Doller, J., *et al.* Lecithin can suppress tardive dyskinesia. *The New England Journal of Medicine,* 1978, *298,* 1029–1030.

Growdon, J. H., Hirsch, M. J., Wurtman, R. J., *et al.* Oral choline administration to patients with tardive dyskinesia. *The New England Journal of Medicine,* 1977, *297,* 524–527.

Grunthal, V. E., & Walther-Buhl, H. Uber Schadigung der Oliva inferior durch chlorperphenazin (Trilafon). *Psychiatrie et Neurologie (Basel),* 1960, *140,* 249–257.

Gualtieri, C. T., Barnhill, J., McGimsey, J., *et al.* Tardive dyskinesia and other movement disorders in children treated with psychotropic drugs. *Journal of the American Academy of Child Psychiatry,* 1980, *19,* 491–510.

Gunne, L. M., & Barany, S. A monitoring test for the liability of neuroleptic drugs to induce tardive dyskinesia. *Psychopharmacology,* 1979, *63,* 195–198.

Haddenbrock, S. Prolonged hyperkinetic syndromes following long-term treatment with high doses of neuroleptic agents. In H. Kranz & K. Heinrich (Eds.), *Begleitwirkungen und Misserfolge der psychiatrischen Pharmakotherapie.* Stuttgart: Georg Thieme, 1964.

Haefely, W. E. Central actions of benzodiazepines: General introduction. *British Journal of Psychiatry,* 1978, *133,* 231–238.

Hale, M. S. Reversible dyskinesia caused by haloperidol. *American Journal of Psychiatry,* 1974, *131,* 1413.

Hargreaves, W. A., & Gaynor, J. Risk of tardive dyskinesia: Preliminary hypotheses. *Psychopharmacology Bulletin,* 1980, *16*(2), 48–50.

Haubrich, D. R., Wang, P. F. L., Clody, D. E., *et al.* Increase in rat brain acetylcholine induced by choline or deanol. *Life Sciences,* 1975, *17,* 975–980.

Heath, R. G. Modulation of emotion with a brain pacemaker. *Journal of Nervous and Mental Disease,* 1977, *165,* 300–317.

Heinrich, K., Wagener, I., & Bender, H.-J. Spate extrapyramidal hyperkinesen bei neuroleptischer langzeittherapie. *Pharmakopsychiatrie, Neuro-Psychopharmakologie,* 1968, *1,* 169–195.

Hershon, H. I., Kennedy, P. F., & McGuire, R. J. Persistence of extrapyramidal disorders and psychiatric relapse after withdrawal of long-term phenothiazine therapy. *British Journal of Psychiatry,* 1972, *120,* 41–50.

Hinsie, L. E., & Campbell, R. J. *Psychiatric dictionary* (4th ed.). New York: Oxford University Press, 1974.

Hippius, H., & Lange, J. Zur problematik der spaten extrapyramidalen hyperkinesen nach Langfristiger neuroleptischer Therapie. *Arzneimittel-Forschung,* 1970, *20,* 888–890.

Hippius, H., & Longemann, G. Zur wirkungvon dioxyphenylalanin (L-dopa) auf extrapyramidal motorische hyperkinesen nach langfristiger neuroleptischer therapie. *Arzneimittel-Forschung,* 1970, *20,* 894–896.

Hirsch, M. J., & Wurtman, R. J. Lecithin consumption increases acetylcholine concentrations in rat brain and adrenal gland. *Science,* 1978, *202,* 223.

Hoff, V. H., & Hofmann, G. Das persistierende extrapyramidale syndrom bei neuroleptikatherapie. *Wiener Medizinische Wochenschrift,* 1967, *117,* 14–17.

Hogarty, G. E., & Goldberg, S. E. Drugs and sociotherapy in the aftercare of schizophrenic patients. *Archives of General Psychiatry,* 1973, *28,* 54–59.

Hollister, L. E. New developments in psychotherapeutic drugs. *Psychiatry Digest,* 1975, *3,* 11–22.

Hollister, L. E. Psychotherapeutic drugs. In A. J. Levenson (Ed.), *Neuropsychiatric side effects of drugs.* New York: Raven Press, 1979.

Hong, J. S., Yang, H.-Y.T., Fratti, W., *et al.* Determination of methionine-enkephalin in discrete regions of rat brain. *Brain Research,* 1977, *134,* 383–386.

Hornykiewicz, O. Neurochemical pathology of Parkinson's disease. In F. H. McDowell & C. H. Markham (Eds.), *Recent advances in Parkinson's disease.* Philadelphia: F. A. Davis, 1971.

Hornykiewicz, O. Neurohumoral interactions and basal ganglia function and dysfunction. In M. D. Yahr (Ed.), *The basal ganglia.* New York: Raven Press, 1976.

Huang, C. C., Wang, R. I. H., Hasegawa, A., *et al.* Evaluation of reserpine and alphamethyldopa in the treatment of tardive dyskinesia. *Psychopharmacology Bulletin,* 1980, *16*(3), 41–43.

Hughes, J., Smith, T. W., Kosterlitz, H. W., *et al.* Identification of two related pentapeptides from the brain with potent opiate agonist activity. *Nature,* 1975, *258,* 577–579.

Hunter, R., Blackwood, W., Smith, M. C., *et al.* Neuropathological findings in three cases of persistent dyskinesia following phenothiazines. *Journal of Neurological Sciences,*

1968, *7,* 263–273.

Hunter, R., Earl, C. J., & Thornicroff, S. An apparently irreversible syndrome of abnormal movements following phenothiazine medication. *Proceedings of the Royal Society of Medicine,* 1964, *57,* 758–762.

Itil, T., Unverdi, C., & Mehta, D. Clorazepate dipotassium in tardive dyskinesia. *American Journal of Psychiatry,* 1974, *131,* 1291.

Itoh, H., Miura, S., Yagi, G., *et al.* Irreversible dyskinesia associated with long-term usage of psychotropic drugs. *Annual Reports of the Pharmacopsychiatry Research Foundation,* 1971, *3,* 190–195.

Itoh, H., & Yagi, G. Reversibility of tardive dyskinesia. *Folia Psychiatrica et Neurologica Japonica,* 1979, *33,* 43–54.

Itoh, H., Yagi, G., Ohtsuka, N., *et al.* Serum level of haloperidol and its clinical significance. *Progress in Neuro-psychopharmacology,* 1980, *4,* 171–183.

Ivnik, R. J. Pseudodementia in tardive dyskinesia. *Psychiatric Annals,* 1979, *9,* 211–216.

Jackson, I. V., Nuttali, E. A., Ibe, O. I., *et al.* Treatment of tardive dyskinesia with lecithin. *American Journal of Psychiatry,* 1979, *136,* 1458–1460.

Jackson, I. V., Volavka, J., James, B., *et al.* The respiratory components of tardive dyskinesia. *Biological Psychiatry,* 1980, *15,* 485–487.

Jaffe, R. Informed consent: Recall about tardive dyskinesia. *Comprehensive Psychiatry,* 1981, *22,* 434–437.

Jamielity, F., Kosc, B., & Lukaszewicz, A. Zmiany neuropatologiczne w dyskinezji twarzowojezykowej prawdopodobnie polekowej. *Neurologica i Neurochirurgia Polska,* 1976, *26,* 399–402.

Janowsky, D. S., El-Yousef, M. K., Davis, J. M., *et al.* Effects of amantadine on tardive dyskinesia and pseudoparkinsonism. *The New England Journal of Medicine,* 1972, *286,* 785.

Jellinger, K. Neuropathologic findings after neuroleptic long-term therapy. In L. Roizin, H. Shiraki, & N. Grcevic (Eds.), *Neurotoxicology.* New York: Raven Press, 1977.

Jeste, D. V., De Lisi, L. E., Zalcman, S., *et al.* A biochemical study of tardive dyskinesia in young male patients. *Psychiatry Research,* 1981, *4,* 327–331.

Jeste, D. V., Kleinman, J. E., Potkin, S. G., *et al.* Ex uno multi: Subtyping the schizophrenic syndrome. *Biological Psychiatry,* 1982, *17,* 199–222.

Jeste, D. V., Linnoila, M., Wagner, R. L., *et al.* Serum neuroleptic concentrations and tardive dyskinesia. *Psychopharmacology,* in press.

Jeste, D. V., Neckers, L. M., Wagner, R. L., *et al.* Lymphocyte monoamine oxidase and plasma prolactin and growth hormone in tardive dyskinesia. *Journal of Clinical Psychiatry,* 1981, *42,* 75–77.

Jeste, D. V., Olgiati, S. G., & Ghali, A. Y. Masking of tardive dyskinesia with four-times-a-day administration of chlorpromazine. *Diseases of the Nervous System,* 1977, *38,* 755–758.

Jeste, D. V., Phelps, B., Wagner, R. L., *et al.* Platelet monoamine oxidase and plasma dopamine-β-hydroxylase in tardive dyskinesia. *Lancet,* 1979, *2,* 850–851.

Jeste, D. V., Potkin, S. G., Sinha, S., *et al.* Tardive dyskinesia: Reversible and persistent. *Archives of General Psychiatry,* 1979, *36,* 585–590.

Jeste, D. V., Rosenblatt, J. E., Wagner, R. L., *et al.* High serum neuroleptic levels in tardive dyskinesia? *The New England Journal of Medicine,* 1979, *301,* 1184.

Jeste, D. V., Stoff, D. M., Potkin, S. G., *et al.* Amphetamine sensitivity and tardive dyskinesia—An animal model. *Indian Journal of Psychiatry,* 1979, *21,* 362–369.

Jeste, D. V., Wagner, R. L., Weinberger, D. R., *et al.* Evaluation of CT scans in tardive dyskinesia. *American Journal of Psychiatry,* 1980, *137,* 247–248.

Jeste, D. V., Weinberger, D. R., Zalcman, S. J., *et al.* Computed tomography in tardive dyskinesia. *British Journal of Psychiatry,* 1980, *136,* 606–607.

Jeste, D. V., & Wyatt, R. J. Changing epidemiology of tardive dyskinesia. *American Journal of Psychiatry,* 1981, *138,* 297–309.

Jeste, D. V., Zalcman, S., Weinberger, D. R., *et al. Apomorphine response and subtyping of schizophrenia.* Paper presented at the annual meeting of the American Psychiatric Association, New Orleans, May 1981.

Jick, I. I. The discovery of drug-induced illness. *The New England Journal of Medicine,* 1977, *296,* 481–485.

Jones, M., & Hunter, R. Abnormal movements in patients with chronic psychiatric illness. In G. E. Crane & R. Gardner, Jr. (Eds.), *Psychotropic drugs and dysfunctions of the basal ganglia* (U.S. Public Health Service Publication No. 1938)). Washington, D.C.: U.S. Government Printing Office, 1969.

Joyce, R. P., & Gunderson, C. H. Carbamazepine-induced orofacial dyskinesia. *Neurology,* 1980, *30,* 1333–1334.

Jus, A., Jus, K., & Fontaine, P., Long-term treatment of tardive dyskinesia. *Journal of Clinical Psychiatry,* 1979, *40,* 72–77.

Jus, A., Jus, K., Gautier, J., *et al.* Studies on the action of certain pharmacological agents on tardive dyskinesia and on the rabbit syndrome. *International Journal of Clinical Pharmacology,* 1974, *9,* 138–145.

Jus, A., Pineau, R., Lachance, R., *et al.* Epidemiology of tardive dyskinesia: Part I. *Diseases of the Nervous System,* 1976, *37,* 210–214.(a)

Jus, A., Pineau, R., Lachance, R., *et al.* Epidemiology of tardive dyskinesia: Part II. *Diseases of the Nervous System,* 1976, *37,* 257–261.(b)

Jus, A., Villeneuve, A., Gautier, J., *et al.* Deanol, lithium and placebo in the treatment of tardive dyskinesia. *Neuropsychobiology,* 1978, *4,* 140–149.

Kane, J., Struve, F., Woerner, M., *et al.* Preliminary findings with regard to risk factors in the development of tardive dyskinesia. *Psychopharmacology Bulletin,* 1981, *17,* 47–49.

Kane, J., Wegner, J., Stenzler, S., *et al.* The prevalence of presumed tardive dyskinesia in psychiatric inpatients and outpatients. *Psychopharmacology,* 1980, *69,* 247–251.

Kaplan, S. R., & Murkofsky, C. Oral–buccal dyskinesia symptoms associated with low-dose benzodiazepine treatment. *American Journal of Psychiatry,* 1978, *135,* 1558–1559.

Karasuyama, N., Fujii, K., & Takahashi, R. Tardive dyskinesia. *Clinical Neurology,* 1972, *12,* 687.

Karson, C. N. Oculomotor signs in a psychiatric population: A preliminary report. *American Journal of Psychiatry,* 1979, *136,* 1057–1060.

Kataria, M., Traub, M., & Marsden, C. D. Extrapyramidal side effects of metoclopramide. *Lancet,* 1978, *2,* 1254–1255.

Kaufman, M. A. Alternative diagnoses to tardive dyskinesia: Neuropathologic findings in three suspected cases. In L. Roizin, H. Shiraki, & N. Grcevic (Eds.), *Neurotoxicology.* New York: Raven Press, 1977.

Kazamatsuri, H. Differentiation of tardive dyskinesia and drug-induced parkinsonism. *The New England Journal of Medicine,* 1971, *284,* 1383.

Kazamatsuri, H. Treatment of tardive dyskinesia with oxypertine: Preliminary clinical experience and a brief review of the literature. *Comprehensive Psychiatry,* 1980, *21,* 352–357.

Kazamatsuri, H., Chien, C., & Cole, J. O. Treatment of tardive dyskinesia: I. Clinical efficacy of a dopamine-depleting agent, tetrabenazine. *Archives of General Psychiatry,* 1972, *27,* 95–99.(a)

Kazamatsuri, H., Chien, C., & Cole, J. O. Treatment of tardive dyskinesia: II. Short-term efficacy of dopamine-blocking agents, haloperidol and thiopropazate. *Archives of General Psychiatry,* 1972, *27,* 100–103.(b)

Kazamatsuri, H., Chien, C., & Cole, J. O. Treatment of tardive dyskinesia: III. Clinical efficacy of a dopamine competing agent, methyl-dopa. *Archives of General Psychiatry,* 1972, *27,* 824–827.(c)

Kazamatsuri, H., Chien, C., & Cole, J. O. Long-term treatment of tardive dyskinesia with haloperidol and tetrabenazine. *American Journal of Psychiatry,* 1973, *130,* 479–483.

Kebabian, J. W., & Calne, D. B. Multiple receptors for dopamine. *Nature,* 1979, *277,* 93–96.

Kennedy, P. F., Hershon, H. I., & McGuire, R. J. Extrapyramidal disorders after prolonged phenothiazine therapy. *British Journal of Psychiatry,* 1971, *118,* 509–518.

Kiloh, L. G., Smith, J. S., & Williams, S. E. Antiparkinson drugs as causal agents in tardive dyskinesia. *Medical Journal of Australia,* 1973, *2,* 591–593.

Kinoshita, J., Inose, T., & Sakai, H. Tardive dyskinesia—Studies on its clinical survey and postmortem examination of a case. *Annual Reports of the Pharmacopsychiatry Research Foundation,* 1972, *4,* 221–228.

Kirschberg, G. J., Dyskinesia—An unusual reaction to ethosuximide. *Archives of Neurology,* 1975, *32,* 137–138.

Klawans, H. L., Jr. The pharmacology of tardive dyskinesia. *American Journal of Psychiatry,* 1973, *130,* 82–86.

Klawans, H. L. Therapeutic approaches to neuroleptic-induced tardive dyskinesia. In M. D. Yahr (Ed.), *The basal ganglia.* New York: Raven Press, 1976.

Klawans, H. L., Bergen, D., Bruyn, G. W., *et al.* Neuroleptic-induced tardive dyskinesia in nonpsychotic patients. *Archives of Neurology,* 1974, *30,* 338–339.

Klawans, H. L., Falk, D. K., Nausieda, P. A., *et al.* Gilles de la Tourette syndrome after long-term chlorpromazine therapy. *Neurology,* 1978, *28,* 1064–1066.

Klawans, H. L., Hitri, A., Nausieda, A., *et al.* Animal models of dyskinesia. In I. Hanin & E. Usdin (Eds.), *Animal models in psychiatry and neurology.* New York: Pergamon Press, 1977.

Klawans, H. L., Jr., Ilahi, M. M., & Shenker, D. Theoretical implications of the use of L-dopa in parkinsonism. *Acta Neurologica Scandinavica,* 1970, *46,* 409–441.

Klawans, H. L., & Margolin, D. I. Amphetamine-induced dopaminergic hypersensitivity in guinea pigs. *Archives of General Psychiatry,* 1975, *32,* 725–732.

Klawans, H. L., & McKendall, R. R. Observations on the effect of levodopa on tardive lingual–facial–buccal dyskinesia. *Journal of the Neurological Sciences,* 1971, *14,* 189–192.

Klawans, H. L., & Rubovits, R. An experimental model of tardive dyskinesia. *Journal of Neural Transmission,* 1972, *33,* 235.

Klawans, H. L., & Rubovits, R. Effect of cholinergic and anticholinergic agents on tardive dyskinesia. *Journal of Neurology, Neurosurgery and Psychiatry,* 1974, *27,* 941–947.

Klawans, H. L., Shenker, D. M., & Weiner, M. J. Observations on the dopaminergic nature of hyperthyroid chorea. In A. Barbeau, T. N. Chase, & G. W. Paulson, (Eds.), *Advances in neurology* (Vol. 1). New York: Raven Press, 1973.

Klawans, H. L., Topel, J. L., & Bergen, D. Deanol in the treatment of levodopa-induced dyskinesias. *Neurology (Minneapolis),* 1975, *25,* 290–293.

Klawans, H. L., Weiner, W. J., & Nausieda, P. A. The effect of lithium on an animal model of tardive dyskinesia. *Progress in Neuro-psychopharmacology,* 1977, *1,* 53–60.

Kleinman, J. E., Bridge, T. P., Karoum, F., *et al.* Catecholamines and metabolites in the brains of psychotics and normals: Postmortem studies. In E. Usdin, I. J. Kopin, & J. D. Barchas (Eds.), *Catecholamines: Basic and clinical frontiers.* New York: Pergamon Press, 1979.

Kline, N. Discussion. In G. E. Crane (Ed.), Tardive dyskinesia in schizophrenic patients treated with psychotropic drugs. *Agressologie*, 1968, *9*, 217–218.(a)

Kline, N. S. On the rarity of "irreversible" oral dyskinesia following phenothiazines. *American Journal of Psychiatry*, 1968, *124*, 48–54.(b)

Kobayashi, R. M., Fields, J. Z., Kruska, R. E., *et al*. Brain neurotransmitter receptors and chronic antipsychotic drug treatment: A model for tardive dyskinesia. In I. Hanin & E. Usdin (Eds.), *Animal models in psychiatry and neurology*. New York: Pergamon Press, 1977.

Koch-Weser, J. Fatal reactions to drug therapy. *The New England Journal of Medicine*, 1974, *291*, 302–303.

Koestner, A. Animal models for dyskinetic disorders. In A. Barbeau, T. N. Chase, & G. W. Paulson (Eds.), *Advances in neurology* (Vol. 1). New York: Raven Press, 1973.

Koller, W. C., Weiner, W. J., Klawans, H. L., *et al*. Oral contraceptive-induced chorea: Clinical and experimental observations. *Neurology*, 1979, *29*, 604.

Korczyn, A. D. Pathophysiology of drug-induced dyskinesias. *Neuropharmacology*, 1972, *11*, 601–607.

Kornetsky, C. Animal models: Promises and problems. In I. Hanin & E. Usdin (Eds.), *Animal models in psychiatry and neurology*. New York: Pergamon Press, 1977.

Korsgaard, S. Baclofen (Lioresal) in the treatment of neuroleptic-induced tardive dyskinesia. *Acta Psychiatrica Scandinavica*, 1976. *54*, 17–24.

Kraepelin, E. [*Dementia praecox and paraphrenia*.] (R. M. Barclay & G. M. Robertson, trans.) New York: Robert E. Krieger, 1971. (Originally published, 1919.)

Kruse, W. Persistent muscular restlessness after phenothiazine treatment: Report of 3 cases. *American Journal of Psychiatry*, 1960, *117*, 152–153.

Kucharski, L. T., Smith, J. M., & Dunn, D. D. Mortality and tardive dyskinesia. *American Journal of Psychiatry*, 1979, *136*, 1228.

Kucharski, L. T., Smith, J. M., & Dunn, D. D. Tardive dyskinesia and hospital discharge. *Journal of Nervous and Mental Disease*, 1980, *168*, 215–218.

Kuhar, M. J., Pert, C. B., & Snyder, S. H. Regional distribution of opiate receptor binding in monkey and human brain. *Nature*, 1973, *245*, 447–450.

Kulik, F. A., & Wilbur, R. Propranolol for tardive dyskinesia and extrapyramidal side effects (pseudoparkinsonism) from neuroleptics. *Psychopharmacology Bulletin*, 1980, *16*(3), 18–19.

Kumar, B. B. Treatment of tardive dyskinesia with deanol. *American Journal of Psychiatry*, 1976, *133*, 978.

Kunin, R. A. Manganese in dyskinesias. *American Journal of Psychiatry*, 1976, *133*, 105. (a)

Kunin, R. A. Manganese and niacin in the treatment of drug-induced dyskinesias. *Orthomolecular Psychiatry*, 1976, *5*, 4–27.(b)

Lake, C. R., Sternberg, D. E., van Kammen, D. P., *et al*. Schizophrenia: Elevated cerebrospinal fluid norepinephrine. *Science*, 1979, *207*, 331–333.

Lal, S., & Ettigi, P. Comparison of thiopropazate and trifluoperazine in oral dyskinesia: A double blind study. *Current Therapeutic Research*, 1974, *16*, 990–997.

Lambert, P. A., Wolff, P., DeManimy, B., *et al*. Le dimethylaminoethanol dans le traitement des dyskinésies tardives induites par les neuroleptiques. *Annales Médico-Psycologiques*, 1978, *136*, 625–629.

Langer, S. Z. Denervation supersensitivity. In L. L. Iversen, S. D. Iversen, & S. H. Snyder (Eds.), *Handbook of psychopharmacology* (Vol. 2). New York: Plenum Press, 1975.

Laska, E., Varga, E., Wanderling, J., *et al*. Patterns of psychotropic drug use for schizophrenia. *Diseases of the Nervous System*, 1973, *34*, 294–305.

Laterre, E. C., & Fortemps, E. Deanol in spontaneous and induced dyskinesias. *Lancet*,

1975, *1,* 301.

Lauciello, F., & Appelbaum, M. Prosthodontic implications of tardive dyskinesia. *New York State Dental Journal,* 1977, *43,* 214–217.

Lavy, S., Melamed, E., & Penchas, S. Tardive dyskinesia associated with metoclopramide. *British Medical Journal,* 1978, *1,* 77–78.

Lehmann, H. E. Psychopharmacological treatment of schizophrenia. *Schizophrenia Bulletin,* 1975, *1,* 27–45.

Lehmann, H. E., Ban, T. A., & Saxena, B. M. A survey of extrapyramidal manifestations in the inpatient population of a psychiatric hospital. *Laval Medica,* 1970, *41,* 909–916.

Lennox, W. G. *Epilepsy and related disorders.* Boston: Little, Brown, 1960.

Levinson, P., Malen, R., Hogben, A., *et al.* Psychological factors in susceptibility to drug-induced extrapyramidal symptoms. *American Journal of Psychiatry,* 1978, *135,* 1375–1376.

Lieberman, A. N., Freedman, L. S., & Goldstein, M. Serum dopamine-β-hydroxylase activity in patients with Huntington's chorea and Parkinson's disease. *Lancet,* 1972, *1,* 153–154.

Lindeboom, S. F., & Lakke, J. P. W. F. Deanol and physostigmine in the treatment of L-dopa-induced dyskinesias. *Acta Neurologica Scandinavica,* 1978, *58,* 134–138.

Linnoila, M., & Viukari, M. Sodium valproate and tardive dyskinesia. *British Journal of Psychiatry,* 1979, *134,* 223.

Linnoila, M., Viukari, M., & Hietala, O. Effect of sodium valproate on tardive dyskinesia. *British Journal of Psychiatry,* 1976, *129,* 114–119.

Lipper, S. Impairment of optokinetic nystagmus in patients with tardive dyskinesia. *Archives of General Psychiatry,* 1973, *28,* 331–333.

Lipsius, L. H. Barbiturates and tardive dyskinesia. *American Journal of Psychiatry,* 1977, *134,* 1162–1163.

Living Webster encyclopedic dictionary of the English language. Chicago: The English Language Institute of America, 1975.

Lloyd, K. G., Worms, P., Zivkovic, B., *et al.* Interaction of GABA mimetics with nigro-striatal dopamine neurons. *Brain Research Bulletin,* 1980, *5*(Suppl. 2), 439–445.

Lomax, D. Discussion, following Klawans, Hitri, Nausieda, *et al.,* Animal models of dyskinesia. In I. Hanin & E. Usdin (Eds.), *Animal models in psychiatry and neurology.* Oxford: Pergamon Press, 1977.

Lonowski, D. J., Sterling, F. E., & King, H. A. Electromyographic assessment of dimethyl-aminoethanol (deanol) in treatment of tardive dyskinesia. *Psychological Reports,* 1979, *45,* 415–419.

Lutrand, J. C., & Duncamin, J. P. Les syndromes dyskinétiques en milieu psychiatrique. *Semaine des Hôpitaux de Paris,* 1978, *54,* 1465–1468.

MacCallum, W. A. G. Tetrabenazine for extrapyramidal movement disorders. *British Medical Journal,* 1970, *1,* 760.

Mackay, A. V. P., & Sheppard, G. P. Pharmacotherapeutic trials in tardive dyskinesia. *British Journal of Psychiatry,* 1979, *135,* 489–499.

Majumdar, S. K. Mechanism of chloroquine-induced involuntary movements. *British Medical Journal,* 1977, *1,* 1350.

Makman, M. H., Ahn, H. S., Thal, L. J., *et al.* Aging and monoamine receptors in brain. *Federation Proceedings,* 1979, *38,* 1922–1926.

Mallya, A., Jose, C., Baig, M., *et al.* Antiparkinsonics, neuroleptics and tardive dyskinesia. *Biological Psychiatry,* 1979, *14,* 645–649.

Mann, D. M. A., Yates, P. C., & Barton, C. M. Neuromelanin and RNA in cells of substantia nigra. *Journal of Neuropathology and Experimental Neurology,* 1977, *36,* 379–383.

Marsden, C. D., Tarsy, D., & Baldessarini, R. J. Spontaneous and drug-induced movement disorders in psychotic patients. In D. F. Benson & D. F. Blumer (Eds.), *Psychiatric aspects of neurological diseases*. New York: Grune & Stratton, 1975.

Marwaha, J., Hoffer, B. J., Geller, H. M., *et al*. Electrophysiologic interactions of antipsychotic drugs with central noradrenergic pathways. *Psychopharmacology*, 1981, *73*, 126–133.

Massengil, R., Jr., & Nashold, B. A swallowing disorder denoted in tardive dyskinesia patients. *Acta Oto-Laryngologica*, 1969, *68*, 457–458.

Matthysse, S. Central catecholamine metabolism in psychosis. In H. M. van Praag & J. Bruinvels (Eds.), *Neurotransmission and disturbed behavior*. New York: SP Medical & Scientific Books, 1978.

Matthysse, S., & Haber, S. Animal models of schizophrenia. In D. J. Ingle & H. M. Shein (Eds.), *Model systems in biological psychiatry*. Cambridge, Mass.: MIT Press, 1975.

Mattson, R. H., & Calverley, J. R. Dextroamphetamine-sulfate-induced dyskinesias. *Journal of the American Medical Association*, 1968, *204*, 108–110.

Matz, E., Rick, W., Oh, D., *et al*. Clozapine: A potential antipsychotic drug without extrapyramidal manifestations. *Current Therapeutic Research*, 1974, *16*, 687–695.

Maxwell, S., Massengil, R., & Nashold, B. Tardive dyskinesia. *Journal of Speech and Hearing Disorders*, 1970, *35*, 33–36.

McAndrew, J. B., Case, Q., & Treffert, D. A. Effects of prolonged phenothiazine intake on psychotic and other hospitalized children. *Journal of Autism and Childhood Schizophrenia*, 1972, *2*, 75–91.

McCreadie, R. G., Dingwall, J. M., Wiles, D. H., *et al*. Intermittent pimozide versus fluphenazine decanoate as maintenance therapy in chronic schizophrenia. *British Journal of Psychiatry*, 1980, *137*, 510–517.

McDowell, F. H. Dyskinetic movements. In A. Barbeau & F. H. McDowell (Eds.), *L-Dopa and parkinsonism*. Philadelphia: F. A. Davis, 1970.

McGeer, E. G., & McGeer, P. L. GABA-containing neurons in schizophrenia, Huntington's chorea and normal aging. In P. Korsgaard-Larsen, J. Scheel-Kruger, & H. Kofod (Eds.), *GABA-Neurotransmitters*. New York: Academic Press, 1979.

McLean, P., & Casey, D. E. Tardive dyskinesia in an adolescent. *American Journal of Psychiatry*, 1978, *135*, 969–971.

McLeod, J. G., & Walsh, J. C. H reflex studies in patients with Parkinson's disease. *Journal of Neurology, Neurosurgery and Psychiatry*, 1972, *35*, 77–80.

Mehta, D., & Itil, T. Tardive dyskinesia. *British Journal of Psychiatry*, 1973, *123*, 491–492.

Mehta, D., Mallya, A., & Volavka, J. Mortality of patients with tardive dyskinesia. *American Journal of Psychiatry*, 1978, *135*, 371–372.

Mehta, D., Mehta, S., & Mathew, P. Failure of deanol in treating tardive dyskinesia. *American Journal of Psychiatry*, 1976, *133*, 1467.

Mehta, D., Mehta, S., & Mathew, P. Tardive dyskinesia in psychogeriatric patients: A five-year follow-up. *Journal of the American Geriatric Society*, 1977, *25*, 545–547.

Melmed, S., & Bank, H. Metoclopramide and facial dyskinesia. *British Medical Journal*, 1975, *1*, 331.

Meltzer, H. Y. Biochemical studies in schizophrenia. In L. Bellak (Ed.), *Disorders of the schizophrenia syndrome*. New York: Basic Books, 1979.

Meltzer, H. Y., Goode, D. J., Fang, V. S., *et al*. Dopamine and schizophrenia. *Lancet*, 1976, *2*, 1142.

Merren, M. D. Amantadine in tardive dyskinesia (cont.). *The New England Journal of Medicine*, 1972, *286*, 268.

Messiha, F. S. Biochemical studies after chronic administration of neuroleptics to monkeys. In W. E. Fann, R. C. Smith, J. M. Davis, *et al*. (Eds.), *Tardive dyskinesia: Research and treatment.* New York: SP Medical & Scientific Books, 1980.

Mettler, F. A., & Crandell, A. Neurologic disorders in psychiatric institutions. *Journal of Nervous and Mental Disease,* 1959, *128,* 148–159.

Miller, E. M. Dimethylaminoethanol in the treatment of blepharospasm. *The New England Journal of Medicine,* 1973, *289,* 697.

Miller, E. M. Deanol in the treatment of levodopa-induced dyskinesias. *Neurology,* 1974, *24,* 116–119.(a)

Miller, E. M. Deanol: A solution for tardive dyskinesia? *The New England Journal of Medicine,* 1974, *291,* 796–797.(b)

Millington, W. R., McCall, A. L., & Wurtman, R. J. Deanol acetamidobenzoate inhibits the blood–brain transport of choline. *Annals of Neurology,* 1978, *4,* 302–306.

Mizrahi, E. M., Holtzman, D., & Tharp, B. Haloperidol-induced tardive dyskinesia in a child with Gilles de la Tourette's disease. *Archives of Neurology,* 1980, *37,* 780.

Moline, R. A. Atypical tardive dyskinesia. *American Journal of Psychiatry,* 1975, *132,* 534–535.

Mones, R. J. Experimental dyskinesias in normal rhesus monkey. In A. Barbeau, T. N. Chase, & G. W. Paulson (Eds.), *Advances in neurology* (Vol. 1). New York: Raven Press, 1973.

Moore, D. C., & Bowers, M. B., Jr. Identification of subgroup of tardive dyskinesia patients by pharmacologic probes. *American Journal of Psychiatry,* 1980, *137,* 1202–1205.

Moore, K. E., & Demarest, K. T. Effects of baclofen on different dopaminergic neuronal systems. *Brain Research Bulletin,* 1980, *5,* (Suppl. 2), 531–535.

Moreira, M. J. C., & Karnio, I. G. Improvement of tardive dyskinesia with high doses of propranolol: A case report. *Revista Paulista de Medicina,* 1979, *93,* 76–78.

Morris, J. N. *Uses of epidemiology* (3rd ed.). New York: Churchill Livingstone, 1975.

Murphy, D. L. Animal models for human psychopathology: Observations from the vintage point of clinical psychopharmacology. In G. Serban & A. Kling (Eds.), *Animal models in human psychobiology.* New York: Plenum Press, 1976.

Myrianthopoulos, N. C., Kurland, A. A., & Kurland, L. T. Hereditary predisposition in drug-induced parkinsonism. *Archives of Neurology,* 1962, *6,* 19–23.

Nagao, T., Ohshimo, T., Mitsunobu, K., *et al.* Cerebrospinal fluid monoamine metabolites and cyclic nucleotides in chronic schizophrenic patients with tardive dyskinesia or drug-induced tremor. *Biological Psychiatry,* 1979, *14,* 509–523.

Naik, S. R., Kelkar, M. R., & Sheth, U. K. Attenuation of stereotyped behavior by sex steroids. *Psychopharmacology,* 1978, *57,* 211–215.

Nair, N. P. V., Yassa, R., Ruiz-navarro, J., *et al.* Baclofen in the treatment of tardive dyskinesia. *American Journal of Psychiatry,* 1978, *135,* 1562–1563.

Nashold, B. S. The effects of central tegmental lesions on tardive dyskinesia. In G. E. Crane & R. Gardner (Eds.), *Psychotropic drugs and dysfunctions of the basal ganglia* (U.S. Public Health Service Publication 1938). Washington, D.C.: U.S. Government Printing Office, 1969.

Nasrallah, H. A., Pappas, N. J., & Crowe, R. R. Oculogyric dystonia in tardive dyskinesia. *American Journal of Psychiatry,* 1980, *137,* 850–851.

Nausieda, P. A., Koller, W. C., Weiner, W. J., *et al.* Modification of postsynaptic dopaminergic sensitivity by female sex hormones. *Life Sciences,* 1979, *25,* 521–526.

Nauta, W. J. H., & Domesick, V. B. Crossroads of limbic and striatal circuitry: Hypothalamo-nigral connections. In K. E. Livingston & O. Hornykiewicz (Eds.), *Limbic mechanisms.* New York: Plenum, 1978.

Nauta, W. J. H., & Mehler, W. R. Fiber connections of the basal ganglia. In G. E. Crane & R. Gardner (Eds.), *Psychotropic drugs and dysfunctions of the basal ganglia* (U.S.

Public Health Service Publication No. 1938). Washington, D.C.: U.S. Government Printing Office, 1969.

Nesse, R., & Carroll, B. J. Cholinergic side-effects associated with deanol. *Lancet*, 1976, *2*, 50–51.

Ng, L. K. Y., Gelhard, R. E., Chase, T. N., *et al.* Drug-induced dyskinesia in monkeys: A pharmacologic model employing 6-hydroxydopamine. In A. Barbeau, T. N. Chase, & G. W. Paulson, (Eds.), *Advances in neurology* (Vol. 1). New York: Raven Press, 1973.

Norris, J. P., & Sams, R. E. More on the use of manganese in dyskinesia. *American Journal of Psychiatry*, 1977, *134*, 1448.

O'Flanagan, P. M. Clonazepam in the treatment of drug-induced dyskinesia. *British Medical Journal*, 1975, *1*, 269–270.

Ogita, K., Yagi, G., & Itoh, H. Comparative analysis of persistent dyskinesia of long-term usage with neuroleptics in France and Japan. *Folia Psychiatrica et Neurologica Japonica*, 1975, *29*, 315–320.

Olsson, R., & Roos, B. E. Concentration of 5-hydroxyindoleacetic acid and homovanillic acid in the cerebrospinal fluid after treatment with probenecid in patients with Parkinson's disease. *Nature*, 1968, *219*, 502–503.

Pandurangi, A. K., Ananth, J., & Channabasavanna, S. M. Dyskinesia in an Indian mental hospital. *Indian Journal of Psychiatry*, 1978, *20*, 339–342.

Pandurangi, A. K., Devi, V., & Channabasavanna, S. M. Caudate atrophy in tardive dyskinesia (A pneumoencephalographic study). *Journal of Clinical Psychiatry*, 1980, *41*, 229–231.

Pandye, G. N., Garver, D. L., Tamminga, C., *et al.* Postsynaptic supersensitivity in schizophrenia. *American Journal of Psychiatry*, 1977, *134*, 518–522.

Patton, C. M. Rapid induction of acute dyskinesia by droperidol. *Anesthesiology*, 1975, *43*, 126–127.

Paulson, G. W. "Permanent" or complex dyskinesias in the aged. *Geriatrics*, 1968, *23*, 105–110.(a)

Paulson, G. W. An evaluation of the permanence of the " tardive dyskinesias." *Diseases of the Nervous System*, 1968, *29*, 692–694.(b)

Paulson, G. W. Dyskinesias in rhesus monkeys. *Transactions of the American Neurological Association*, 1972, *97*, 109–111.

Paulson, G. W. Dyskinesias in monkeys. In A. Barbeau, T. N. Chase, & G. W. Paulson (Eds.), *Advances in neurology* (Vol. 1). New York: Raven Press, 1973.

Paulson, G. W. Tardive dyskinesia. *Annual Review of Medicine*, 1975, *26*, 75–81.

Paulson, G. W. Tardive dyskinesia. *New York State Journal of Medicine*, 1979, *79*, 193–195.

Paulson, G. W., Rizvi, C. A., & Crane, G. E. Tardive dyskinesia as a possible sequel of long-term therapy with phenothiazine. *Clinical Pediatrics*, 1975, *14*, 953–955.

Pearce, J. Mechanism of action of amantadine. *British Medical Journal*, 1970, *3*, 529.

Peet, M., Middlemiss, D. N., & Yates, R. A. Propranolol in schizophrenia: II. Clinical and biochemical aspects of combining propranolol with chlorpromazine. *British Journal of Psychiatry*, 1981, *138*, 112–117.

Penovich, P., Morgan, J. P., Kerzner, B., *et al.* Double-blind evaluation of deanol in tardive dyskinesias. *Journal of the American Medical Association*, 1978, *239*, 1997–1998.

Perényi, A., & Aratō, M. Tardive dyskinesia on Hungarian psychiatric wards. *Psychosomatics*, 1980, *21*, 904–909.

Peroutka, S. J., & Snyder, S. H. Relationship of neuroleptic drug effects at brain dopamine, serotonin, α-adrenergic, and histamine receptors to clinical potency. *American Journal of Psychiatry*, 1980, *137*, 1518–1522.

Perris, C., Dimitrijevic, P., Jacobson, L., *et al.* Tardive dyskinesia in psychiatric patients treated with neuroleptics. *British Journal of Psychiatry,* 1979, *135,* 509–514.

Pert, A., Rosenblatt, J. E., Sivit, C., *et al.* Long-term treatment with lithium prevents the development of dopamine receptor supersensitivity. *Science,* 1978, *201,* 171–173.

Pert, C. B., & Snyder, S. H. Opiate receptor: Demonstration in nervous tissue. *Science,* 1973, *179,* 1011–1014.

Petit, H., & Milbled, G. Anomalies of conjugate ocular movements in Huntington's chorea: Application to early detection. In A. Barbeau, T. N. Chase, & G. W. Paulson (Eds.), *Advances in neurology* (Vol. 1). New York: Raven Press, 1973.

Petty, L. K., & Spar, C. J. Haloperidol-induced tardive dyskinesia in a 10-year-old girl. *American Journal of Psychiatry,* 1980, *137,* 745–746.

Pfeiffer, C. C., Groth, D. P., & Bain, J. A. Choline versus deanol as possible precursors of cerebral acetylcholine. *Biological Psychiatry,* 1959, *259,* 20.

Pfeiffer, C. C., Jenney, E. H., Gallagher, W., *et al.* Stimulant effects of 2-dimethylamino-ethanol, possible precursor of brain acetylcholine. *Science,* 1957, *126,* 610–6ll.

Physicians' desk reference (36th ed.). Oradell, N.J.: Medical Economics Co., 1982.

Pickar, D., & Davies, R. K. Tardive dyskinesia in younger patients. *American Journal of Psychiatry,* 1978, *135,* 385–386.

Pind, K., & Faurbye, A. Concentration of homovanillic acid and 5-hydroxyindoleacetic acid in the cerebrospinal fluid after treatment with probenecid in patients with drug-induced tardive dyskinesia. *Acta Psychiatrica Scandinavica,* 1970, *46,* 323–326.

Pletscher, A., & Kyburz, E. Neuroleptic drugs: Chemical versus biochemical classification. In D. Kemali, G. Bartholini, & D. Richter (Eds.), *Schizophrenia today.* New York: Pergamon Press, 1976.

Pöldinger, W. Therapy of extrapyramidal side effects, with particular reference to persistent dyskinesia and lithium tremor. *International Pharmacopsychiatry,* 1978, *13,* 230–233.

Polizos, P., Engelhardt, D. M., & Hoffman, S. P. CNS consequences of psychotropic drug withdrawal in schizophrenic children. *Psychopharmacology Bulletin,* 1973, *9,* 34–35.(a)

Polizos, P., Engelhardt, D. M., Hoffman, S. P., *et al.* Neurological consequences of psychotropic drug withdrawal in schizophrenic children. *Journal of Autism and Childhood Schizophrenia,* 1973, *3,* 247–253.(b)

Portnoy, R. A. Hyperkinetic dysarthria as an early indicator of impending tardive dyskinesia. *Journal of Speech and Hearing Disorders,* 1979, *44,* 214–219.

Post, R. M. Intermittent versus continuous stimulation: Effect of time interval on the development of sensitization or tolerance. *Life Sciences,* 1980, *26,* 1275–1282.

Post, R. M., & Kopanda, R. T. Cocaine, kindling and psychosis. *American Journal of Psychiatry,* 1976, *133,* 672–684.

Pradhan, S. N. Central neurotransmitters and aging. *Life Sciences,* 1980, *26,* 1643–1656.

Prange, A. J., Sisk, J. L., & Wilson, I. C. Balance, permission and discrimination among amines: A theoretical consideration of the actions of L-tryptophan in disorders of movement and affect. In J. D. Barchas & E. Usdin (Eds.), *Serotonin and behavior.* New York: Academic Press, 1973.

Prange, A. J., Wilson, I. C., Morris, C. E., *et al.* Preliminary experience with tryptophan and lithium in the treatment of tardive dyskinesia. *Psychopharmacology Bulletin,* 1973, *9,* 36–37.

Price, T. R. P., & Levin, R. The effects of electroconvulsive therapy on tardive dyskinesia. *American Journal of Psychiatry,* 1978, *135,* 991–993.

Pryce, I. G., & Edwards, H. Persistent oral dyskinesia in female mental hospital patients.

British Journal of Psychiatry, 1966, *112,* 983–987.

A psychiatric glossary (5th ed.). Boston: Little, Brown, 1980.

Quitkin, F., Rifkin, A., Gochfeld, L., *et al.* Tardive dyskinesia: Are first signs reversible? *American Journal of Psychiatry,* 1977, *134,* 84–87.

Ray, I. Tardive dyskinesia treated with deanol acetamidobenzoate. *The Canadian Medical Association Journal,* 1977, *117,* 129.

Re, O. N. Deanol in L-dopa and tardive dyskinesias: A review. *Current Therapeutic Research,* 1975, *18,* 872–875.

Reda, F. A., Escobar, J. I., & Scanlan, J. M. Lithium carbonate in the treatment of tardive dyskinesia. *American Journal of Psychiatry,* 1975, *132,* 560–562.

Reibling, A., Reyes, P., & Jameson, H. D. Dimethylaminoethanol ineffective in Huntington's disease. *The New England Journal of Medicine,* 1975, *293,* 724.

Ringel, S. P., & Klawans, H. L. Differentiation of tardive dyskinesias and drug-induced parkinsonism. *The New England Journal of Medicine,* 1971, *284,* 1382–1383.

Ringwald, E. Behandlung von neuroleptischen spathyperkinesien mit antiparkinsonika. *Pharmacopsychiatrica,* 1978, *11,* 294–298.

Rivera-Calimlim, L., Gift, T., Nasrallah, H. A., *et al.* Low plasma levels of CPZ in patients chronically treated with neuroleptics. *Communications in Psychopharmacology,* 1978, *2,* 113–121.

Robbins, N., & Fischbach, G. Effect of chronic disuse of rat soleus neuromuscular junctions on post synaptic function. *Journal of Neurophysiology,* 1971, *34,* 570.

Robin, M. M., Pelfreyman, M. G., & Schechter, P. J. Dyskinetic effects of intrastriatally injected GABA-transaminase inhibitors. *Life Sciences,* 1979, *25,* 1103–1110.

Robinson, S. E., Berney, S., Mishra, R., *et al.* The relative role of dopamine and norepinephrine receptor blockade in the action of antipsychotic drugs: Metoclopramide, thiethylperazine and molindone as pharmacological tools. *Psychopharmacology,* 1979, *64,* 141–147.

Roccatagliata, G., Albano, C., & Besio, G. Discinesie croniche tardive da neurolettici — Data farmacologici e liquorali. *Rivista di Patologia Nervosa e Mentale,* 1977, *98,* 228–232.

Roccatagliata, G., Albano, C., Cocito, L., *et al.* Interactions between central monoaminergic systems: Dopamine-serotonin. *Journal of Neurology, Neurosurgery and Psychiatry,* 1979, *42,* 1159–1162.

Roizin, L., True, C., & Knight, M. Structural effects of tranquilizers. *Research Publications of the Association of Nervous and Mental Disorders,* 1959, *37,* 285–324.

Rosenbaum, A. H., & De La Fuente, J. R. Benzodiazepines and tardive dyskinesia. *Lancet,* 1979, *2,* 900.

Rosenbaum, A. H., Maruta, T., Duane, D. D., *et al.* Tardive dyskinesia in depressed patients: Successful therapy with antidepressants and lithium. *Psychosomatics,* 1980, *21,* 715–719.

Rosenbaum, A. H., Maruta, T., Jiang, N., *et al.* Endocrine testing in tardive dyskinesia: Preliminary report. *American Journal of Psychiatry,* 1979, *136,* 102–103.

Rosenbaum, A. H., Niven, R. G., Hanson, N. P., *et al.* Tardive dyskinesia: Relationship with a primary affective disorder. *Diseases of the Nervous System,* 1977, *38,* 423–427.

Rosenbaum, A. H., O'Connor, M. K., & Duane, D. D. Treatment of tardive dyskinesia in an agitated, depressed patient. *Psychosomatics,* 1980, *21,* 765–766.

Rosenblatt, J. E., Pary, R. J., Bigelow, L. B., *et al.* Measurement of serum neuroleptic concentrations by radioreceptor assay: Concurrent assessment of clinical response and toxicity. *Psychopharmacology Bulletin,* 1980, *16*(3), 78–80.

Rosin, A. J. & Exton-Smith, A. N. Persistent oral dyskinesia in treatment with phenothiazine derivatives. *Lancet,* 1965, *1,* 650-651.

Roxburgh, P. A. Treatment of persistent phenothiazine-induced oral dyskinesia. *British Journal of Psychiatry,* 1970, *116,* 277-280.

Rubovits, R., & Klawans, H. L. Implications of amphetamine-induced stereotyped behavior as a model of tardive dyskinesia. *Archives of General Psychiatry,* 1972, *21,* 502-507.

Sassin, J. F., Taub, S., & Weitzman, E. D. Hyperkinesia and changes in behavior produced in normal monkeys by L-dopa. *Neurology,* 1972, *22,* 1122-1125.

Sato, S., Daly, R., & Peters, H. Reserpine therapy of phenothiazine induced dyskinesia. *Diseases of the Nervous System,* 1971, *32,* 680-685.

Sayers, A. C., Burki, H. R., Ruch, W., *et al.* Neuroleptic-induced hypersensitivity of striatal dopamine receptors in the rat as a model of tardive dyskinesias. Effects of clozapine, haloperidol, loxapine and chlorpromazine. *Psychopharmacologia (Berlin),* 1975, *41,* 97-104.

Sax, D. S., Butters, N., Tomlinson, E. B., *et al.* Effects of serial caudate lesions and L-dopa administration upon the cognitive and motor behavior of monkeys. In A. Barbeau, T. N. Chase, & G. W. Paulson (Eds.), *Advances in neurology* (Vol. 1). New York: Raven Press, 1973.

Scatton, B., Garret, C., & Julou, L. Acute and subacute effects of neuroleptics on dopamine synthesis and release in the rat striatum. *Archives of Pharmacology,* 1975, *289,* 419.

Scheel Krüger, J., & Randrup, A. Pharmacological evidence for a cholinergic mechanism in brain involved in a special stereotyped behavior of reserpinized rats. *British Journal of Pharmacology,* 1968, *34,* 217p-218p.

Schelkunov, E. L. Adrenergic effect of chronic administration of neuroleptics. *Nature,* 1967, *214,* 1210-1212.

Schiele, B. C., Gallant, D., Simpson, G., *et al.* A persistent neurological syndrome associated with antipsychotic drug use. *Annals of Internal Medicine,* 1973, *79,* 99-100.

Schmidt, W. R., & Jarcho, L. W. Persistent dyskinesia following phenothiazine therapy. *Archives of Neurology,* 1966, *14,* 369-377.

Schöcken, D. D., & Roth, G. S. Reduced β-adrenergic receptor concentrations in aging man. *Nature,* 1977, *27,* 856-858.

Schönecker, M. Ein eigentumliches Syndrom im oralen Bereich bei Megaphen Applikation. *Nervenarzt,* 1957, *28,* 35.

Sedivec, V., Valenova, Z., & Paceltova, L. Persistent extrapyramidal oral dyskinesias following treatment with thymoleptics. *Activitas Nervosa Superior,* 1970, *12,* 67-68.

Sedman, G. Clonazepam in the treatment of tardive oral dyskinesia. *British Medical Journal,* 1976, *2,* 583.

Seeman, M. V., Patel, J., & Pyke, J. Tardive dyskinesia with Tourette-like syndrome. *Journal of Clinical Psychiatry,* 1981, *42,* 357-358.

Seeman, P., & Lee, T. Antipsychotic drugs: Direct correlation between clinical potency and presynaptic action on dopamine neurons. *Science,* 1975, *188,* 1217-1219.

Shapiro, A. K., Shapiro, E., Bruun, R. D., *et al. Gilles de la Tourette's syndrome.* New York: Raven Press, 1978.

Shapiro, M. B., Post, F., Lofring, B., *et al.* Memory function in psychiatric patients over sixty: some methodological and diagnostic implications. *Journal of the Mental Sciences,* 1956, *102,* 233-246.

Sharman, D. F. Brain dopamine metabolism and behavioral problems of farm animals. In P. J. Roberts, G. N. Woodruff, & L. L. Iversen (Eds.), *Advances in biochemical psychopharmacology* (Vol. 19). New York: Raven Press, 1978.

Sharpless, S. K. Isolated and deafferented neurons: Disuse supersensitivity. In H. H. Japser,

A. A. Ward, & A. Pope (Eds.), *Basic mechanisms of the epilepsies*. Boston: Little, Brown, 1969.

Sharpless, S. K. Supersensitivity-like phenomena in the central nervous system. *Federation Proceedings*, 1975, *34*, 1990–1997.

Sheppard, C., Collins, L., Fiorentino, D., *et al.* Polypharmacy in psychiatric treatment: Incidence at a state hospital. *Current Therapeutic Research*, 1969, *11*, 765–774.

Sherman, R. A. Successful treatment of one case of tardive dyskinesia with electromyographic feedback from the masseter muscle. *Biofeedback and Self-Regulation*, 1979, *4*, 367–370.

Shoulson, I., & Chase, T. N. Fenfluramine and dyskinesias. *The New England Journal of Medicine*, 1974, *291*, 850–851.

Siede, H., & Muller, H. F. Choreiform movements as side effects of phenothiazine medication in geriatric patients. *Journal of American Geriatric Society*, 1967, *15*, 517–522.

Sigwald, J., Bouttier, D., Raymondeaud, C., *et al.* Quatre cas de dyskinésie facio-bucco-lingui-masticatrice à évolution prolongée secondaire à un traitment par les neuroleptiques. *Revue Neurologique*, 1959, *100*, 751–755.

Simpson, G. M. Tardive dyskinesia. *British Journal of Psychiatry*, 1973, *122*, 618.

Simpson, G. M. The current status of tardive dyskinesia. *International Drug Therapy Newsletter*, 1980, *15*, 22–24.

Simpson, G. M., Branchey, M. H., Lee, J. H., *et al.* Lithium in tardive dyskinesia. *Pharmakopsychiatrie*, 1976, *9*, 76–80.

Simpson, G. M., Cooper, T. B., Bark, N., *et al.* Effect of antiparkinsonian medication on plasma levels of chlorpromazine. *Archives of General Psychiatry*, 1980, *37*, 205–208.

Simpson, G. M., & Kline, N. S. Tardive dyskinesia: Manifestations, incidence, etiology and treatment. In M. D. Yahr (Ed.), *The basal ganglia*. New York: Raven Press, 1976.

Simpson, G. M., Lee, J. H., & Shrivastava, R. K. Clozapine in tardive dyskinesia. *Psychopharmacology*, 1978, *56*, 75–80.

Simpson, G. M., Lee, J. H., Shrivastava, R. K., *et al.* Baclofen in the treatment of tardive dyskinesia and schizophrenia. *Psychopharmacology Bulletin*, 1978, *14*, 16–18.

Simpson, G. M., Lee, J. H., Zoubok, B., *et al.* A rating scale for tardive dyskinesia. *Psychopharmacology*, 1979, *64*, 171–179.

Simpson, G. M., & Shrivastava, R. K. Abnormal gaits in tardive dyskinesia. *American Journal of Psychiatry*, 1978, *135*, 865.

Simpson, G. M., & Varga, E. Clozapine: A new antipsychotic agent. *Current Therapeutic Research*, 1974, *16*, 679–686.

Simpson, G. M., Varga, E., Lee, J. H., *et al.* Tardive dyskinesia and psychotropic drug history. *Psychopharmacology*, 1978, *58*, 117–124.

Simpson, G. M., Voitaschevsky, A., Young, M. A., *et al.* Deanol in the treatment of tardive dyskinesia. *Psychopharmacology*, 1977, *52*, 257–261.

Singer, K., & Cheng, N. M. Thiopropazate hydrochloride in persistent dyskinesia. *British Medical Journal*, 1971, *4*, 22–25.

Singh, M. M. Diazepam in the treatment of tardive dyskinesia. *International Pharmacopsychiatry*, 1976, *11*, 232–234.

Singh, M. M., Nasrallah, H. A., Lal, H., *et al.* Treatment of tardive dyskinesia with diazepam: Indirect evidence for the involvement of limbic, possibly GABAergic mechanisms. *Brain Research Bulletin*, 1980, *5*(Suppl. 2), 673–680.

Skinner, T., Gochnauer, R., & Linnoila, M. Liquid chromatographic method to measure thioridazine and its active metabolites in biological samples. *Acta Pharmacologica et Toxicologica*, 1981, *48*, 223–226.

Smith, J. M., & Baldessarini, R. J. Changes in prevalence, severity and recovery in tardive dyskinesia with age. *Archives of General Psychiatry*, 1980, *37*, 1368–1373.

Smith, J. M., Dunn, D. D., & Burke, M. P. Tardive dyskinesia and body weight. *American Journal of Psychiatry*, 1980, *137*, 1272–1274.

Smith, J. M., Kucharski, L. T., Eblen, C., *et al.* An assessment of tardive dyskinesia in schizophrenic outpatients. *Psychopharmacology*, 1979, *64*, 99–104.

Smith, J. M., Kucharski, L. T., Oswald, W. T., *et al.* A systematic investigation of tardive dyskinesia in inpatients. *American Journal of Psychiatry*, 1979, *136*, 918–922.

Smith, J. M., Oswald, W. T., Kucharski, L. T., *et al.* Tardive dyskinesia: Age and sex differences in hospitalized schizophrenics. *Psychopharmacology*, 1978, *58*, 207–211.

Smith, J. S., & Kiloh, L. G. Six month evaluation of thiopropazate hydrochloride in tardive dyskinesia. *Journal of Neurology, Neurosurgery and Psychiatry*, 1979, *42*, 576–579.

Smith, R. C., & Davis, J. M. Behavioral supersensitivity to apomorphine and amphetamine after chronic high dose haloperidol treatment. *Psychopharmacology Communications*, 1975, *1*, 285–293.

Smith, R. C., & Davis, J. M. Behavioral evidence for supersensitivity after chronic administration of haloperidol, clozapine or thioridazine. *Life Sciences*, 1976, *19*, 725–732.

Smith, R. C., & Leelavathi, D. E. Behavioral and biochemical effects of chronic neuroleptic drugs: Interaction with age. In W. E. Fann, R. C. Smith, J. M. Davis, *et al.* (Eds.), *Tardive dyskinesia: Research and treatment*. New York: SP Medical & Scientific Books, 1980.

Smith, R. C., Tamminga, C., & Davis, J. M. Behavioral effects of apomorphine and amphetamine in tardive dyskinesia patients. In W. E. Fann, R. C. Smith, J. M. Davis, *et al.* (Eds.), *Tardive dyskinesia: Research and treatment*. New York: SP Medical & Scientific Books, 1980.

Snyder, S. H. The dopamine hypothesis of schizophrenia: Focus on the dopamine receptor. *American Journal of Psychiatry*, 1976, *133*, 197–202.

Sovner, R., & Loadman, A. More on barbiturates and tardive dyskinesia. *American Journal of Psychiatry*, 1978, *135*, 382.

Sovner, R., & DiMascio, A. The effect of benztropine mesylate in the rabbit syndrome and tardive dyskinesia. *American Journal of Psychiatry*, 1977, *134*, 1301–1302.

Sovner, R., DiMascio, A., Berkovitz, D., *et al.* Tardive dyskinesia and informed consent. *Psychosomatics*, 1978, *19*, 172–177.

Stadler, H., Lloyd, K. G., Gadea-Ciria, M., *et al.* Enhanced striatal acetylcholine release by chlorpromazine and its reversal by apomorphine. *Brain Research*, 1973, *55*, 476–480.

Stafford, J. R., & Fann, W. E. Deanol acetamidobenzoate (Deaner) in tardive dyskinesia. *Disorders of the Nervous System*, 1977, *38*(Suppl.), 3–6.

Stahl, S. M. Tardive Tourette syndrome in an autistic patient after long-term neuroleptic administration. *American Journal of Psychiatry*, 1980, *137*, 1267–1269.

Stancer, H. C. Tardive dyskinesia not associated with neuroleptics. *American Journal of Psychiatry*, 1979, *136*, 727.

Standefer, M. J., & Dill, R. E. The role of GABA in dyskinesias induced by chemical stimulation of the striatum. *Life Sciences*, 1977, *21*, 1515–1520.

Stanley, M., Lautin, A., Rotrosen, J., *et al.* Metoclopramide: Antipsychotic efficacy of a drug lacking potency in receptor models. *Psychopharmacology*, 1980, *71*, 219–225.

Stavraky, G. W. *Supersensitivity following lesions of the nervous system*. Toronto: University of Toronto Press, 1961.

Stevens, J. R. Eye blink and schizophrenia: Psychosis or tardive dyskinesia? *American Journal of Psychiatry*, 1978, *135*, 223–225.

Stevens, J. R., Wilson, K., & Foote, W. GABA blockage, dopamine and schizophrenia: Experimental studies in the cat. *Psychopharmacologia,* 1977, *39,* 105–119.

Stimmel, G. L. Tardive dyskinesia with low-dose short-term neuroleptic therapy. *American Journal of Hospital Pharmacy,* 1976, *33,* 961–963.

Stoff, D. M., Gillin, J. C., & Wyatt, R. J. Animal models of drug-induced hallucinations. In R. C. Stillman & R. E. Willette (Eds.), *The psychopharmacology of hallucinations.* New York: Pergamon Press, 1978.

Stone, A. A. Informed consent: Special problems for psychiatry. *Hospital and Community Psychiatry,* 1979, *30,* 321–327.

Stone, A. A. The right to refuse treatment. *Archives of General Psychiatry,* 1981, *38,* 358–362.

Struve, F. A., & Klein, D. F. Diagnostic implications of the B-mitten EEG pattern: Relationship to primary and secondary affective dysregulation. *Biological Psychiatry,* 1976, *11,* 599–611.

Sutcher, H. D., Underwood, R. B., Beatly, R. A., *et al.* Orofacial dyskinesia: A dental dimension. *Journal of the American Medical Association,* 1971, *216,* 1459–1463.

Sweet, R. D., Bruun, R. D., Shapiro, A., *et al.* The pharmacology of Gilles de la Tourette's syndrome (chronic multiple tics). In H. L. Klawans (Ed.), *Clinical neuropharmacology* (Vol. 1). New York: Raven Press, 1976.

Taber's cyclopedic medical dictionary (12th ed.). Philadelphia: F. A. Davis, 1973.

Tamminga, C. A., & Chase, T. N. Bromocriptine and CF 25-397 in the treatment of tardive dyskinesia. *Archives of Neurology,* 1980, *37,* 204–205.

Tamminga, C. A., Crayton, J. W., Chase, T. N. Improvement in tardive dyskinesia after muscimol therapy. *Archives of General Psychiatry,* 1979, *36,* 595–598.

Tamminga, C. A., Smith, R. C., & Davis, J. M. The effects of cholinergic drugs on the involuntary movements of tardive dyskinesia. In W. E. Fann, R. C. Smith, J. M. Davis, *et al.* (Eds.), *Tardive dyskinesia: Research and treatment.* New York: SP Medical & Scientific Books, 1980.

Tamminga, C. A., Smith, R. C., Ericksen, S. E., *et al.* Cholinergic influences in tardive dyskinesia. *American Journal of Psychiatry,* 1977, *134,* 769–774.

Tamminga, C. A., Smith, R. C., Pandye, G., *et al.* A neuroendocrine study of supersensitivity in tardive dyskinesia. *Archives of General Psychiatry,* 1977, *34,* 1199–1203.

Tanner, R. H., & Domino, E. F. Exaggerated response to (+) amphetamine in geriatric gerbils. *Gerontology,* 1977, *23,* 165–173.

Tarsy, D. Dopamine–acetylcholine interaction in the basal ganglia. In W. S. Fields (Ed.), *Neurotransmitter function.* New York: Stratton, 1977.

Tarsy, D. Personal communication, 1981.

Tarsy, D., & Baldessarini, R. J. Pharmacologically induced behavioral supersensitivity to apomorphine. *Nature (New Biology),* 1973, *245,* 262.

Tarsy, D., & Baldessarini, R. J. Behavioral supersensitivity to apomorphine following chronic treatment with drugs which interfere with the synaptic function of catecholamines. *Neuropharmacology,* 1974, *13,* 927–940.

Tarsy, D., & Baldessarini, R. J. The pathophysiologic basis of tardive dyskinesia. *Biological Psychiatry,* 1977, *12,* 431–450.

Tarsy, D., & Bralower, M. Deanol acetamidobenzoate treatment in choreiform movement disorders. *Archives of Neurology,* 1977, *34,* 756–758.

Tarsy, D., Granacher, R., & Bralower, M. Tardive dyskinesia in young adults. *American Journal of Psychiatry,* 1977, *134,* 1032–1034.

Tarsy, D., Leopold, N., & Sax, D. Physostigmine in choreiform movement disorders. *Neurology (Minneapolis),* 1973, *23,* 392.

Tarsy, D., Leopold, N., & Sax, D. S. Physostigmine in choreiform movement disorders. *Neurology*, 1974, *24*, 28–33.

Thach, B. T., Chase, T. N., & Bosma, J. F. Oral facial dyskinesia associated with prolonged use of antihistaminic decongestants. *The New England Journal of Medicine*, 1975, *293*, 486–487.

Tolosa, E. S. Modification of tardive dyskinesia and spasmodic torticollis by apomorphine. *Archives of Neurology*, 1978, *35*, 459–462.(a)

Tolosa, E. S. *Reversal by levodopa of dopamine "hypersensitivity" in tardive dyskinesia.* Paper presented at the second World Congress of Biological Psychiatry, Barcelona, October 1978.(b)

Tolosa, E. S. Clinical features of Meige's disease (idiopathic orofacial dystonia) — A report of 17 cases. *Archives of Neurology*, 1981, *38*, 147–151.

Trendelenburg, U. Supersensitivity and subsensitivity to sympathomimetic amines. *Pharmacological Reviews*, 1963, *15*, 225–276.

Turek, I. S. Drug-induced dyskinesia: Reality or myth? *Diseases of the Nervous System*, 1975, *36*, 397–399.

Turek, I. S., Kurland, A. A., Hanlon, T. E., *et al.* Tardive dyskinesia: Its relation to neuroleptic and antiparkinson drugs. *British Journal of Psychiatry*, 1972, *121*, 605–612.

Turunen, S., & Achte, K. A. Buccolingual masticatory syndrome as a side effect of neuroleptic therapy. *Psychiatric Quarterly*, 1967, *41*, 268–279.

Uhrbrand, L., & Faurbye, A. Reversible and irreversible dyskinesia after treatment with perphenazine, chlorpromazine, reserpine, and electroconvulsive therapy. *Psychopharmacologia*, 1960, *1*, 408–418.

Umez-Eronini, E. M., & Eronini, E. A. Chloroquine-induced involuntary movements. *British Medical Journal*, 1977, *1*, 945–946.

Ule, G., & Struwe, O. Hirnveranderungen bei dyskinesie nach neuroleptica-medikation. *Nervenarzt*, 1978, *49*, 268–270.

Ungerstedt, U. Postsynaptic supersensitivity after 6-hydroxydopamine-induced degeneration of the nigro-striatal dopamine system. *Acta Physiologica Scandinavica*, 1971, *367*(Suppl.), 69–93.

Ungerstedt, U., Avemo, A., Avemo, E., *et al.* Animal models of parkinsonism. *Advances in Neurology*, 1973, *3*, 257–271.

Ungerstedt, U., Butcher, L., Butcher, S. G., *et al.* Direct chemical stimulation of dopaminergic mechanisms in the nigrostriatum of the rat. *Brain Research*, 1969, *14*, 461–471.

Vale, S., & Espejel, M. A. Amantadine for dyskinesia tarda. *The New England Journal of Medicine*, 1971, *284*, 673.

Van Woert, M. H., Jutkowitz, R., Rosenbaum, B., *et al.* Gilles de la Tourette's syndrome: Biochemical approaches. In M. D. Yahr (Ed.), *The basal ganglia.* New York: Raven Press, 1976.

Verwoert, A. *Clinical geropsychiatry.* Baltimore: Williams & Wilkins, 1976.

Vick, N. A. *Grinker's neurology* (7th ed.). Springfield, Ill.: Charles C Thomas, 1976.

Villeneuve, A. The rabbit syndrome: A peculiar extrapyramidal reaction. *Canadian Psychiatric Association Journal*, 1972, *12*, 69–72.

Villeneuve, A., & Boszormenyi, Z. Treatment of drug-induced dyskinesias. *Lancet*, 1970, *1*, 353–354.

Villeneuve, A., Cazejust, T., & Cote, M. Estrogens in tardive dyskinesias in male psychiatric patients. *Neuropsychobiology*, 1980, *6*, 145–151.

Villeneuve, A., Langelier, P., & Bedard, P. Estrogens, dopamine and dyskinesias. *Canadian Psychiatric Association Journal*, 1978, *23*, 68–70.

Viukari, M., & Linnoila, M. Effect of methyldopa on tardive dyskinesia in psychogeriatric patients. *Current Therapeutic Research,* 1975, *18,* 417–424.

Viukari, M., & Linnoila, M. Effect of fusaric acid on tardive dyskinesia and mental state in psychogeriatric patients. *Acta Psychiatrica Scandinavica,* 1977, *56,* 57–61.

Voogd, R. N. J., & Huijzen, C. V. *The human central nervous system: A synopsis and atlas.* New York: Springer-Verlag, 1979.

Walker, J. E., Hoehn, M., Sears, E., *et al.* Dimethylaminoethanol in Huntington's chorea. *Lancet,* 1973, *1,* 1512–1513.

Walsh, C. H. Involuntary facial movements. *British Medical Journal,* 1975, *1,* 737.

Walton, D., White, J. G., & Black, D. A. A modified word-learning test: A cross-validation study. *British Journal of Medical Psychology,* 1959, *32,* 213–220.

Warne, R. W., & Gubbay, S. S. Choreiform movements induced by anticholinergic therapy. *Medical Journal of Australia,* 1979, *1,* 465.

Wegner, J. T., Struve, F. A., Kantor, J. S., *et al.* Relationship between the B-mitten EEG pattern and tardive dyskinesia. *Archives of General Psychiatry,* 1979, *36,* 599–603.

Weinberger, D. R., Torrey, E. F., Neophytides, A. N., *et al.* Lateral cerebral ventricular enlargement in chronic schizophrenia. *Archives of General Psychiatry,* 1979, *36,* 735–739.

Weiner, W. J., & Bergen, D. Prevention and management of the side effects of levodopa. In H. L. Klawans (Ed.), *Clinical neuropharmacology* (Vol. 2). New York: Raven Press, 1977.

Weiner, W. J., Carvey, P., Nausieda, P. A., *et al.* The effect of chronic levodopa on haloperidol induced behavioral supersensitivity in the guinea pig. *Life Sciences,* 1981, *28,* 2173–2178.

Weiner, W. J., Goetz, C. G., Nausieda, P. A., *et al.* Respiratory dyskinesias — Extrapyramidal dysfunction and dyspnea. *Annals of Internal Medicine,* 1978, *88,* 327–331.

Weiner, W. J., Nausieda, P. A., & Klawans, H. L. Regional brain manganese levels in an animal model of tardive dyskinesia. In W. E. Fann, R. C. Smith, J. M. Davis, *et al.* (Eds.), *Tardive dyskinesia: Research and treatment.* New York: SP Medical & Scientific Books, 1980.

Weinhold, P., Wegner, J. T., & Kane, J. M. Familial occurrence of tardive dyskinesia. *Journal of Clinical Psychiatry,* 1981, *42,* 165–166.

Weiss, B., Greenberg, L., & Cantor, E. Age-related alterations in the development of adrenergic denervation supersensitivity. *Federation Proceedings,* 1979, *38,* 1915–1921.

Weiss, B., & Santelli, S. Dyskinesia evoked in monkeys by weekly administration of haloperidol. *Science,* 1978, *200,* 799–801.

Weiss, B., Santelli, S., & Lusink, G. Movement disorders induced in monkeys by chronic haloperidol treatment. *Psychopharmacology,* 1977, *53,* 289–293.

Weiss, K. J., Ciraulo, D. A., & Shader, R. I. Physostigmine test in rabbit syndrome and tardive dyskinesia. *American Journal of Psychiatry,* 1980, *137,* 627–628.

Widrowe, H. J., & Heisler, S. Treatment of tardive dyskinesia. *Diseases of the Nervous System,* 1976, *37,* 162–164.

Williams, R. J. *Biochemical individuality.* New York: Wiley, 1956.

Winsberg, B. G., Hurwic, M. J., & Perel, J. Neurochemistry of withdrawal emergent symptoms in children. *Psychopharmacology Bulletin,* 1977, *13,* 38–40.

Woogen, S., Graham, J., & Angrist, B. A tardive dyskinesia-like syndrome after amitriptyline treatment. *Journal of Clinical Psychopharmacology,* 1981, *1,* 34–36.

Wurtman, R. J., Hirsch, M. J., & Growdon, J. H. Lecithin consumption raises serum free choline levels. *Lancet,* 1977, *2,* 68–69.

Wyatt, R. J. Biochemistry of schizophrenia (Pt. 4). *Schizophrenia Bulletin,* 1976, *12,* 5–50.

Wyatt, R. J., Gillin, J. C., Stoff, D. M., *et al.* β-Phenylethylamine (PEA) and the neuropsychiatric disturbances. In E. Usdin, J. Barchas, & D. Hamburg (Eds.), *Neuroregulators and psychiatric disorders.* New York: Oxford University Press, 1977.

Wyatt, R. J., & Torgow, J. S. A comparison of equivalent clinical potencies of neuroleptics as used to treat schizophrenia and affective disorders. *Journal of Psychiatric Research,* 1976, *13,* 91–98.

Yagi, G. *Irreversible extrapyramidal disturbance induced by psychotropic drugs.* Paper presented at the meeting of the Kanagowaken Seishin Igakukai, 1970 (cited in Yagi *et al.,* 1976).

Yagi, G., Ogita, K., Ohtsuka, N., *et al.* Persistent dyskinesia after long-term treatment with neuroleptics in Japan. *Keio Journal of Medicine,* 1976, *25,* 27–35.

Yahr, M. D. Abnormal involuntary movements induced by dopa: Clinical aspects. In A. Barbeau & F. H. McDowell (Eds.), *L-Dopa and parkinsonism.* Philadelphia: F. A. Davis, 1970.

Yahr, M. D., & Duvoisin, R. C. *The treatment of parkinsonism with L-dopa.* Paper presented at the Ninth International Congress of Neurology, New York, October 1969.

Yamadori, A., & Albert, M. L. Involuntary movement disorder caused by methyldopa. *The New England Journal of Medicine,* 1972, *286,* 610.

Yarden, P. E., & Discipio, W. J. Abnormal movements and prognosis in schizophrenia. *American Journal of Psychiatry,* 1971, *128,* 317–323.

Yesavage, J. A., Becker, J., Werner, P. D., *et al.* Serum level monitoring of thiothixene in schizophrenia: Acute single-dose levels at fixed doses. *American Journal of Psychiatry,* 1982, *139,* 174–178.

Zahniser, N. R., Chou, D., & Hanin, I. Is 2-dimethylaminoethanol (deanol) indeed a precursor of brain acetylcholine? A gas chromatographic evaluation. *Journal of Pharmacology and Experimental Therapeutics,* 1977, *200,* 545–559.

Zimmer, R., Teelken, A. W., Meier, K. D., *et al.* Preliminary studies of CSF gamma-aminobutyric acid levels in psychiatric patients before and during treatment with different psychotropic drugs. *Progress in Neuro-psychopharmacology,* 1981, *4,* 613–620.

Author Index

Italicized page numbers indicate material in tables and figures.

337

Subject Index

Italicized page numbers indicate material in tables and figures.

353